Anthropology of Violent Death

Published and forthcoming titles in the Forensic Science in Focus series

Published

The Global Practice of Forensic Science
Douglas H. Ubelaker (Editor)

Forensic Chemistry: Fundamentals and Applications
Jay A. Siegel (Editor)

Forensic Microbiology
David O. Carter, Jeffrey K. Tomberlin, M. Eric Benbow and Jessica L. Metcalf (Editors)

Forensic Anthropology: Theoretical Framework and Scientific Basis
Clifford Boyd and Donna Boyd (Editors)

The Future of Forensic Science
Daniel A. Martell (Editor)

Forensic Anthropology and the U.S. Judicial System
Laura C. Fulginiti, Alison Galloway, and Kristen Hartnett-McCann (Editors)

Forensic Science and Humanitarian Action: Interacting with the Dead and the Living
Roberto C. Parra, Sara C. Zapico, and Douglas H. Ubelaker (Editors)

Disaster Victim Identification in the 21st Century: A US Perspective
John Williams and Victor Weedn (Editors)

The Forensic Evaluation of Burnt Human Remains
Sarah Ellingham, Joe Adserias Garriga, Sara C. Zapico, and Douglas H. Ubelaker (Editors)

Anthropology of Violent Death: Theoretical Foundations for Forensic Humanitarian Action
Roberto C. Parra and Douglas H. Ubelaker (Editors)

Forthcoming

AI In Forensic Science
Zeno Geradts and Karin Franke (Editors)

An Illustrated Guide to Forensic Skeletal Trauma Analysis
Donna Boyd

Anthropology of Violent Death

Theoretical Foundations for Forensic Humanitarian Action

EDITED BY

Roberto C. Parra

Technical Assistance Team, United Nations Joint Human Rights Office (UNJHRO), MONUSCO, Democratic Republic of Congo
Unité mixte de recherche d'Anthropologie bio-culturelle, Droit, Éthique & Santé (UMR 7268 - ÁDES), Aix Marseille University, Marseille, France

Douglas H. Ubelaker

Smithsonian Institution, National Museum of Natural History, Washington, DC, USA

AAFS AMERICAN ACADEMY OF FORENSIC SCIENCES

WILEY

This edition first published 2023

Registered Offices
John Wiley & Sons, Inc., 111 River Street, Hoboken, NJ 07030, USA
John Wiley & Sons Ltd, The Atrium, Southern Gate, Chichester, West Sussex, PO19 8SQ, UK

Editorial Office
The Atrium, Southern Gate, Chichester, West Sussex, PO19 8SQ, UK

For details of our global editorial offices, customer services, and more information about Wiley products visit us at www.wiley.com.

Wiley also publishes its books in a variety of electronic formats and by print-on-demand. Some content that appears in standard print versions of this book may not be available in other formats.

Library of Congress Cataloging-in-Publication Data

Names: Parra, Roberto C., 1979– editor. | Ubelaker, Douglas H., editor.
Title: Anthropology of violent death : theoretical foundations for forensic humanitarian action / edited by Roberto C. Parra, Douglas H. Ubelaker.
Other titles: Forensic science in focus
Description: Hoboken, NJ : Wiley, 2023. | Series: Forensic science in focus | Includes index.
Identifiers: LCCN 2022052849 (print) | LCCN 2022052850 (ebook) | ISBN 9781119806363 (hardback) | ISBN 9781119806370 (adobe pdf) | ISBN 9781119806387 (epub)
Subjects: MESH: Forensic Anthropology | Violence | Homicide | Body Remains | Sociological Factors
Classification: LCC RA1059 (print) | LCC RA1059 (ebook) | NLM W 750 | DDC 614/.17—dc23/eng/20230103
LC record available at https://lccn.loc.gov/2022052849
LC ebook record available at https://lccn.loc.gov/2022052850

Cover Design: Wiley
Cover Image: Courtesy of Roberto C. Parra

Set in 10.5/13.5pt Meridien LT Std by Straive, Chennai, India

Contents

About the editors

Roberto C. Parra, MA, DLAF 005, is a Peruvian anthropologist who graduated from the School of Anthropology of the Universidad Nacional del Altiplano in Puno, Peru. He did an internship during his undergraduate studies at the Centro Mallqui, the Bio-anthropology foundation of Peru, under the direction of Dr. Sonia Guillen and Dr. Marvin Allison. As a product of this experience, Roberto earned his graduation with a thesis linked to the field of bioanthropology. To complement his professional perspective, he reached the level of physiologist in the master's program in physiology at the graduate school of the Faculty of Medicine of the Universidad Nacional Mayor de San Marcos, Lima, Peru. Currently, Roberto is a career forensic anthropologist and received his master's degree in forensic anthropology at the graduate School of Pontificia Universidad Catolica del Peru, as well as a specialization diploma in forensic anthropology at the same university. Furthermore, he was certified as Forensic Anthropologist by the Latino American Board of Forensic Anthropology (DLAF in Spanish) of the Latino American Association of Forensic Anthropology (ALAF), of which he is an active member and was a former President for two years. He is a specialist in ISO 9001 Quality Management Issues and ISO 17025 Laboratory Quality Management and has focused on issues related to forensic sciences and quality management.

Roberto has 20 years of experience in the field of forensic sciences, humanitarian action, and human rights investigations, mainly in the management of the dead in armed conflicts, catastrophes, and migration crises. He has served as an expert witness, reporting on more than 1500 cases including air crash and shipwreck victims, human rights violations, and domestic criminal cases. He has testified in several legal proceedings in Peru.

In 2002, he began his forensic career in the Peruvian context as part of the forensic staff of the Institute of Legal Medicine and Forensic Sciences of Peru. In this institution, Roberto has been an assistant in the forensic anthropology department of the Central Morgue of Lima, later was the national coordinator of the Specialized Forensic Team, and was also the National Coordinator of the Peruvian Forensic Response System for Disasters, which includes the Peruvian DVI team. For several years, he was forensic analyst at the Laboratory of Molecular Biology and Forensic Genetics. Finally, Roberto reached the position of advisor to the Head of the Institute of Legal Medicine and Forensic Sciences of Peru for the Quality Management in Forensic Science. As part of his scientific advice, he was one of the founders of the Ibero-American network of Institutions of Legal Medicine and Forensic Sciences.

Since 2012, Roberto has developed several international missions in Latin America, Africa, and the Middle East as part of the Staff of the Forensic Unit of the International Committee of the Red Cross and as part of the staff of forensic scientists of the Human Rights Office of the High Commissioner (OHCHR) of the United Nations where currently he is a staff of United Nations Joint Human Rights Office (UNJHRO), like forensic specialist for the Democratic Republic of Congo. Roberto has also been a Research Collaborator and Affiliate, Bioarchaeology and Stable Isotope Research Lab (BSIRL), at Vanderbilt University, Nashville, Tennessee. Roberto is currently academically linked to the Faculty of Medicine – Timone Sector, Biological Anthropology Service of the University of Aix-Marseille where he is a PhD candidate.

Douglas H. Ubelaker, PhD, is a curator and senior scientist at the Smithsonian Institution's National Museum of Natural History in Washington, DC, where he has been employed for nearly four decades. Since 1978, he has served as a consultant in forensic anthropology. In this capacity he has served as an expert witness, reporting on more than 900 cases, and has testified in numerous legal proceedings. He was for many years a Professorial Lecturer with the Departments of Anatomy and Anthropology at the George Washington University, Washington, DC, and is an Adjunct Professor with the Department of Anthropology, Michigan State University, East Lansing, Michigan. Dr. Ubelaker has published extensively in the general field of human skeletal biology with an emphasis on forensic applications. He has served on the editorial boards of numerous leading scientific publications, including the *Journal of Forensic Sciences*, *Forensic Sciences Research* and *Science and Justice*, the *Open Forensic Science Journal*, *International Journal of Legal Medicine*, *Human Evolution*, *Homo*, *Journal of Comparative Human Biology*, *Anthropologie*, *International Journal of the Science of Man*, *Forensic Science Communications*, *Human Evolution*, and the *International Journal of Anthropology and Global Bioethics*. Dr. Ubelaker received a Bachelor of Arts degree and a Doctor of Philosophy from the University of Kansas. He has been a Member of the American Academy of Forensic Sciences since 1974 and achieved the status of Fellow in 1987 in the Physical Anthropology Section. He served as the 2011–2012 President of the AAFS. He is a Fellow of the Washington Academy of Sciences and a Diplomate of the American Board of Forensic Anthropology. He is a member of the American Association of Physical Anthropology and the Paleopathology Association.

Dr. Ubelaker has received numerous honors, including the Memorial Medal of Dr. Aleš Hrdlička, Humpolec, Czech Republic; the Anthropology Award of the Washington Academy of Sciences; the T. Dale Stewart Award by the Physical Anthropology Section of the American Academy of Forensic Sciences; the FBI Director's Award for Exceptional Public Service; the Federal Highway Administration Pennsylvania Division Historic Preservation Excellence Award; a special recognition award from the FBI; and was elected Miembro Honorario of the Sociedad de Odontoestomatologos Forenses IberoAmericanos and of the Asociación Latinoamericana de Antropología Forense (ALAF).

List of contributors

Ahmed Al-Dawoody
Legal Advisory Service on IHL
International Committee of the Red Cross (ICRC)
Geneva
Switzerland

Élisabeth Anstett
UMR 7268 ADES anthropologie bio-culturelle
droit, éthique et santé, Faculté des sciences médicales et paramédicales
Aix-Marseille Université
Marseille
France

Valérie Robin-Azevedo
University of Paris, Migrations and Society Research Unit (URMIS)
Paris
France
Co-director of the research project "Transfunerary: Mass violence and funerary practices in Europe and Latin America."

Antoon De Baets
Faculty of Arts
University of Groningen
Groningen
The Netherlands

Stephen Cordner
Department of Forensic Medicine
Monash University
Australia

Francisco Ferrándiz
Institute for Language, Literature and Anthropology (ILLA)
Center for Human and Social Sciences (CCHS)
Spanish National Research Council (CSIC)

Ryan Harrod
Academic Affairs
Garrett College
McHenry, MD
USA

Tricia Redeker Hepner
MA Program in Social Justice and Human Rights
School of Social and Behavioral Sciences
Arizona State University
USA

Jaymelee J. Kim
Forensic Sciences Program
Department of Justice Sciences
University of Findlay
Findlay, OH
USA

Melanie Klinkner
Department of Humanities and Law
Bournemouth University
UK

Krista E. Latham
Department of Biological and Anthropology
University of Indianapolis
USA
and
Human Identification Center
University of Indianapolis
USA

Avril Maddrell
Department of Geography and Environmental Science
University of Reading
UK

Debra Martin
Department of Anthropology
University of Nevada
Las Vegas, NV
USA

Alyson J. O'Daniel
Department of Anthropology
University of Indianapolis
USA

Anna Osterholtz
Department of Anthropology and Middle Eastern Cultures
Mississippi State University
Mississippi, MS
USA

Roberto C. Parra
United Nations Joint Human Rights Office (UNJHRO)
Specialized Forensic Team, MONUSCO
Democratic Republic of Congo
and
Unité mixte de recherche d'Anthropologie bio-culturelle
Droit, Éthique & Santé (UMR 7268 -ÁDES)
Aix Marseille University
Marseille
France

Pierre Perich
Forensic Department, Hôpital de la Timone
Aix Marseille University
Marseille
France

Tanya Ramos
Department of Biology
University of Indianapolis
USA

Antonius C. G. M. Robben
Department of Anthropology
Utrecht University
Utrecht
The Netherlands

Adam Rosenblatt
International Comparative Studies
Duke University
Durham, NC
USA

Alfredo González-Ruibal
Instituto de Ciencias de Patrimonio (INCIPIT)
Consejo Superior de Investigaciones Cientificas (CSIC)
Madrid
Spain

Alexandra Ortiz Signoret
Legal Advisory Service on IHL
International Committee of the Red Cross (ICRC)
Geneva
Switzerland

Dawnie W. Steadman
Department of Anthropology
University of Tennessee
USA

Morris Tidball-Binz
UN Special Rapporteur on Extra-judicial
Summary or Arbitrary Executions
OHCHR-UNOG
Geneve, Switzerland

Douglas H. Ubelaker
Smithsonian Institution
National Museum of Natural History
Washington, DC
USA

Digna M. Vigo-Corea
Unité mixte de recherche d'Anthropologie bio-culturelle, Droit
Éthique & Santé (UMR 7268 -ÁDES)
Unidad Medico Legal II Ancash
Instituto de Medicina Legal y Ciencias Forenses
Ministerio Publico del Perú

Laura Wittman
Department of French and Italian
Stanford University
Stanford, CA
USA

Foreword

The loss of human life as a result of violence anywhere is a matter of central concern for my mandate as United Nations special Rapporteur of extrajudicial, summary, or arbitrary executions. I therefore welcome this publication which stands as a testimony and a landmark of the remarkable evolution of knowledge and experience gained over the past 40 years in forensic anthropology applied to human rights and humanitarian action, for the investigation, documentation, analysis, and understanding of lethal violence.

During the first systematic use in the early 1980s of forensic anthropology and related forensic disciplines to investigate human rights violations in Argentina, few at that time could have foreseen the remarkable contribution which those investigations would make to the development of forensic science, human rights standards, and humanitarian action.

Also, when we carried out those pioneering forensic investigations into human rights violations in Argentina using forensic anthropology, there was no reference made to forensic science in existing international human rights standards and documents. Similarly, there was no reference made to human rights or humanitarian investigations in the forensic science literature of the time. This would change dramatically in the years, which followed and led to the growing intertwining of forensic science with human rights and humanitarian action.

The remarkable synergy which followed those first steps, between evolving forensic sciences and international human rights and humanitarian law, made these developments possible. This was triggered and is still guided by the plight of victims of violence, in particular the relatives of those killed or "disappeared." Above all, they are the result of the extraordinary and innovative contribution from a growing community of activists, including families of victims, on one hand; and academics on the other, including jurists, social scientists, and, principally, forensic scientists from the world over.

Today, it would be inconceivable to carry out any large-scale investigation into violent death resulting from violations of human rights, of international humanitarian law, or from natural causes, without the central concourse of forensic science, principally forensic anthropology; and the use of multiple human rights and humanitarian standards which have been developed since to guide such investigations. As a result, atrocities which in the past would have remained undocumented and often contested, with resulting impunity for perpetrators and the risk of recurrence, can today be reliably documented to help ensure the necessary reparatory and preventive measures.

Forensic science understandably plays a growingly important role in supporting the United Nations (U.N.) efforts to protect and promote human rights worldwide.

In particular, the Geneva-based United Nations human rights bodies, including the Human Rights Commission and its successor the Human Rights Council, as well as the Office of the High Commissioner for Human Rights and many U.N. human rights Special Procedures have made growing use, since the early 1990s, of forensic expertise in support of many of their activities, from the investigation and documentation of human rights violations to technical cooperation and advice for governments to help enhance their forensic capacity and improving compliance with human rights obligations.

At the same time, the United Nations has been instrumental in developing, promoting, and helping implement important standards of forensic best practices applied to human rights investigations. Some of these, such as the *Minnesota Protocol on the Investigation of Potentially Unlawful Death,* published by the United Nations in 2017,[1] are today considered as universal standards and are positively impacting forensic practice, research, and training worldwide.

It is also fair to say that the forensic profession has been enriched by its incorporation of human rights standards to a range of fields of forensic research and practice. An example of this is humanitarian forensic action, a novel discipline of forensic sciences applied to humanitarian activities, the development of which is rooted in the experience gained from forensic human rights investigations. Humanitarian forensic action is today recognized as essential for ensuring the proper and dignified management of the dead from armed conflicts and disasters and their reliable identification. For example, the *Guiding Principles for Dignified Management of the Dead in Humanitarian Emergencies and to Prevent them Becoming Missing Persons,* published in 2021 by the International Committee of the Red Cross,[2] reaffirms the central role of forensic science, in particular forensic anthropology, for the proper management, documentation, and identification of those who died a violent death.

In summary, against the background of the relatively recent upsurge of forensic knowledge, standards, and investigative capacity to document violent death, normative standards of justice included in national and international instruments also came progressively to the forefront, to help ensure truth, justice, accountability, and non-repetition. Forensic anthropology's contribution to these developments has been paramount.

Reminding us all about the millions of children, women, and men who have been victims over the last century of unimaginable atrocities that deeply shock the conscience of humanity, the Preamble of the Rome Statute of the International Criminal Court underlines the shared determination to put an end to impunity for the perpetrators of these crimes and to contribute to their prevention.[3]

Combating impunity and preventing atrocities worldwide requires, first and foremost, effective and reliable investigations, made possible today by forensic science applied to human rights investigations and humanitarian action.

Forensic anthropology, with its practical understanding of violent death, plays an essential role in this noble endeavor, for which this important and welcome publication will undoubtedly stand as an important milestone.

Morris Tidball-Binz[4]
UN Special Rapporteur on Extra-judicial,
Summary or Arbitrary Executions

Notes

1. Available at: https://www.ohchr.org/Documents/Publications/MinnesotaProtocol.pdf Last visited on March 1, 2022.
2. Available at: https://shop.icrc.org/guiding-principles-for-dignified-management-of-the-dead-in-humanitarian-emergencies-and-to-prevent-them-becoming-missing-persons-pdf-en.html Last visited on March 1, 2022.
3. Preamble of the Rome Statute of the International Criminal Court. Available at: https://legal.un.org/icc/statute/99_corr/preamble.htm Last visited on March 1, 2022.
4. United Nations Special Rapporteur on extrajudicial, summary or arbitrary executions; adjunct clinical professor in Forensic Medicine, School of Public Health and Preventive Medicine, Faculty of Medicine Nursing and Health Sciences, Monash University, Australia visiting professor, Department of Forensic Medicine, Ethics and Medical Law, University of Coimbra; visiting professor, Department of Biomedical Health Sciences, Faculty of Medicine, University of Milano, Italy; directorate member of the University of Coimbra Centre for Humanitarian and Human Rights Forensic Research and Training.

Preface

"As damning as a signed confession left in the grave": When the dead open the eyes of the living

Whenever we witness violent death brought about by contexts which fall outside the bounds of everyday experience – international crimes, extreme political violence, epidemics and natural disasters, the migration crisis – we find ourselves radically confronted with the realities of mass death and the complexity of the phenomena that give rise to it. These phenomena have been the subject of interdisciplinary research for some time now. It is only recently, however – in the last decade or so – that the social sciences have begun getting to grips in a thorough and systematic manner with the remains of the victims. For a long time, then, the complex issues surrounding dead bodies and their treatment were under-explored, and all the more so when it came to dealing with corpses on a mass scale. For is it not the case that, in the west at any rate, death, accursed and repressed, has long been the "central taboo" of the modern world, following centuries of what Philippe Ariès described as "tamed death"?[1]

Following the end of the Cold War, the 1990s saw a proliferation of practices of transitional justice, the enshrining of the right to truth, the expansion of international criminal justice, the implementation of memory policies in the name of the "duty to remember," the outlawing of genocide denial in most European states, to name a few. These developments went hand-in-hand with the theorization of the doctrine of the "fight against impunity" for massive violations of human rights, based on the famous Louis Joinet report of 1997.[2] It was also in the mid-1990s that what is now referred to as the "forensic turn," to use the term employed by the historian Robert Jan van Pelt and reprised by Elisabeth Anstett and Jean-Marc Dreyfus, came about.[3] This "turn," made possible by the emergence of new technologies (specifically DNA testing) to facilitate the identification of dead bodies, normalizes exhumations as a method of dealing with human remains *en masse*. It mobilizes interdisciplinary knowledge, brings together a wide variety of actors (experts, survivors and victims' families, civil society, NGOs, and national and international entities), and has unquestionably contributed to the expansion of human rights investigations and forensic humanitarian action across the globe. This should not surprise us given that, as the American forensic anthropologist Clyde Snow, a crucial figure who helped found the Argentinian Forensic Anthropology Team (EAAF) in 1984, so aptly put it at the dawn of the forensic turn: "The bones don't lie and they don't forget."[4] Indeed, bones defy time, denial, and forgetting.

This turning point, marked in particular by the increasing prosecution of human rights violations in the name of the fight against impunity, has favored the adoption of normative texts (at both domestic and international levels) setting out the need to document violent deaths, provide a framework for the handling of human remains, and preserve the traces of disasters. This need is constantly reactivated by the reality of ongoing situations that force us to pursue new approaches not only *in situ* but also on the paths of exile and in the lands of refuge. On every continent, human remains are being searched for, exhumed, gathered, stored, (re)buried, and where possible identified, whether this is carried out in the context of judicial or extra-judicial processes, by professionals or families, within or outside the scope of the law. First and foremost, the work carried out on and around these remains gives the families of the disappeared the opportunity to mourn their loved ones. Importantly, however, it also allows light to be shed on the causes of death, on the modus operandi of the perpetrators where applicable, and on a whole array of indicators that can tell us more about the specific and diverse character of the phenomena, whether criminal or natural, behind their presence.

This work takes on a unique dimension when carried out as part of investigations, such as those opened on March 2, 2022 by the office of the Prosecutor of the International Criminal Court (ICC) and, in parallel, by the UN Commission of Inquiry on the situation in Ukraine stemming from the Russian aggression, with a view to launching future prosecutions. All perpetrators, as Clyde Snow put it, drop "a trail of clues which, when properly collected, preserved and analyzed, are as damning as a signed confession left in the grave."[5] In this respect, the Ukrainian situation will perhaps bring about a paradigm shift in the international (criminal) system. For here we are seeing the beginnings of a model that sets out explicitly to achieve "effective coordination and communication" at the international level in support of "forensic and investigative actions on the ground," through close collaboration with national authorities in order to "strengthen the impact of [the] collective work in establishing the truth."[6]

Violent death, and the transversal challenges created by dead bodies and their treatment in these extra-ordinary contexts, is now at the center of multiple political, professional, and societal practices, sometimes working in synergy, sometimes at odds with one another, involving various instruments of hard and soft law, and a rapidly growing volume of scientific studies. Whether treated as a person, as a physical trace, or as a piece of evidence, the corpse – the legal status of which continues to raise many uncertainties – is the focus of much attention, of many demands, and of important strategic considerations. Whether present or absent, identified or anonymous, whole or fragmented, recognized or denied, exhibited or concealed, honored or desecrated, protected or instrumentalized, preserved or destroyed, it bears witness. At once an object and a means of investigation, it provides eloquent testimony of the inevitable, indissoluble link between the living and the dead. It is this link, the fundamental questions it poses, the manifold practices to which it gives rise, and the different ways in which these are regulated, that form the central thread running through the present volume. A volume that is not only timely but also crucial to a better understanding of how and why the dead are asked to open the eyes of the living.[7]

Sévane Garibian
May 2022
Faculty of Law
Département de droit pénal
University of Geneva
Right to Truth, Truth(s) through Rights:
Mass Crimes Impunity and Transitional Justice

Notes

1. Philippe Ariès, *The hour of our death* (transl. Helen Weaver), New York, Alfred A. Knopf, 1981.
2. Named after the French magistrate Louis Joinet, who produced the report for the UN High Commission on Human Rights: *Question of the impunity of perpetrators of human rights violations (civil and political)*, Final report prepared by Louis Joinet pursuant to Sub-Commission decision 1996/119, E/CN.4/Sub.2/1997/20, June 26, 1997.
3. Elisabeth Anstett and Jean-Marc Dreyfus ed., *Human remains and identification: mass violence, genocide, and the 'forensic turn'*, Manchester, Manchester University Press, 2015.
4. Interviewed by Jeff Guntzel, a *National Catholic Reporter* journalist (July 30, 2004, available online).
5. *Idem.*
6. Statement of the ICC Prosecutor, Karim Khan, announcing the deployment of a forensics and investigative team to Ukraine (42 investigators, forensic experts, and support personnel), which "represents the largest ever single field deployment by [his] Office since its establishment" (May 17, 2022, available online).
7. To quote the Bulgarian proverb: "The living close the eyes of the dead, the dead open the eyes of the living" ("Живите затварят очите на мъртвите, мъртвите отварят очите на живите", transliterated "Zhivite zatvaryat ochite na mŭrtvite, mŭrtvite otvaryat ochite na zhivite").

Series Preface

The forensic sciences represent diverse, dynamic fields that seek to utilize the very best techniques available to address legal issues. Fueled by advances in technology, research, and methodology, as well as new case applications, the forensic sciences continue to evolve. Forensic scientists strive to improve their analyses and interpretations of evidence and to remain cognizant of the latest advancements. This series results from a collaborative effort between the American Academy of Forensic Sciences (AAFS) and Wiley to publish a select number of books that relate closely to the activities and objectives of the AAFS. The book series reflects the goals of the AAFS to encourage quality scholarship and publication in the forensic sciences. Proposals for publication in the series are reviewed by a committee established for that purpose by the AAFS and also reviewed by Wiley. The AAFS was founded in 1948 and represents a multidisciplinary professional organization that provides leadership to advance science and its application to the legal system. The 11 sections of the AAFS consist of Criminalistics, Digital and Multimedia Sciences, Engineering Sciences, General, Pathology/Biology, Questioned Documents, Jurisprudence, Anthropology, Toxicology, Odontology, and Psychiatry and Behavioral Science. There are over 7000 members of the AAFS, originating from all 50 States of the United States and many countries beyond. This series reflects global AAFS membership interest in new research, scholarship, and publication in the forensic sciences.

Zeno Geradts
Senior forensic scientist at the Netherlands Forensic
Institute of the Ministry of Justice. Netherlands
Series Editor

Douglas H. Ubelaker
Senior Scientist, Smithsonian Institution, National Museum
of Natural History, Washington, DC, USA
Series Editor

Acknowledgments

The editors wish to thank the chapter contributors and the American Academy of Forensic Science for supporting this volume. The editors would also like to thank the anonymous reviewers who contributed greatly to the reading of the documents. All our thanks to Morris Tidball-Binz and Sévane Garibian for their kind words for this volume.

CHAPTER 1

The anthropology of violent death and the treatment of the bodies: an introduction

Roberto C. Parra[1,2*] and Douglas H. Ubelaker[3]

[1]*Technical Assistance Team. United Nations Joint Human Rights Office (UNJHRO), MONUSCO, Democratic Republic of Congo*
[2]*Unité mixte de recherche d'Anthropologie bio-culturelle, Droit, Éthique & Santé (UMR 7268 - ÁDES), Aix Marseille University, Marseille, France*
[3]*Smithsonian Institution, National Museum of Natural History, Washington, DC, USA*
**The views expressed herein are those of the author and do not necessarily reflect the views of the United Nations.*

Anthropological approaches to death abound in the classical literature (Bloch and Parry 1982; Dreyfus and Anstett 2017; Ferguson 2006; Hertz 1960; Laqueur 2002, 2015; Martin et al. 2012; Metcalf and Huntington 1991; Carr 1995; Parker Pearson 2016; Robben 2018a, 2018b; Ucko 1969; Van Gennep 1960; Verdery 1999; Whitehead 2002, 2004a, 2005, 2007; among others). On the one hand, the anthropology of death has focused on elucidating how the dead continue to live in the collective imagination through a wide variety of mortuary and funerary rites. These rituals reinforce the meaning of death as an alternative way of living, prolonging their bonds, facing loss, and turning that death into a "good death." On the other hand, the representation of the body carries a symbolic load of meanings, such as the "brute stuff of death itself",[1] and it sets up a wide range of traditions and customs for an appropriate commemoration. Hertz (1960) contributions have constituted the starting point to address both issues, and they have strongly driven the advancement of knowledge in the field of the anthropology of death. According to Engelke (2019, p. 31), "what we can take from Hertz is that the anthropology of death always begins and ends with the stuff of death, above all the materiality of the corpse, but more generally speaking the things that matter to making death good." Additionally, Hertz's

Anthropology of Violent Death: Theoretical Foundations for Forensic Humanitarian Action, First Edition.
Edited by Roberto C. Parra and Douglas H. Ubelaker.

approach does not focus only on how people remember their dead but also on how the dead prompt the living to remember them (Robben 2018a). These memories can be good to think about, but they can also be damaging, disturbing, and intrusive, and they can even be politically used to dominate or destroy others (Anstett and Dreyfus 2014; Dreyfus and Anstett 2017; Stepputat 2014; Verdery 1999).

Throughout its history, humanity has been closely – and somewhat ironically – linked to violent episodes that have resulted in the death of millions of people (Fry 2013). In the twentieth century alone, between 170 and 230 million people have died violently as a result of human actions (Hobsbawm 1994; Leitenberg 2006; Robinson 1998; Rummel 1996). Between 1990 and 2017, lethal violence in the form of criminal activity in particular and armed conflicts in general have produced nearly 14 million victims as well as countless social, humanitarian, economic, and cultural consequences. Paradoxically, all this has happened during an era distinguished by the positioning of science and technology, as well as the solid defense of human rights, but at the same time, it is clear that profound issues of disrespect for life, death, and human dignity still persist. This reality does not concur with those arguments stating that we have become less violent as we have become more civilized, as proposed, for example, by Pinker (2011). Rather, as Whitehead (2004c) and Sorel (1999) have highlighted, there is no straightforward correlation between violence and progress; violence always takes different forms and emerges in diverse contexts, and anthropologists have been exploring these expressions for quite a long time (Domínguez 2018).[2]

Pinker's arguments gathered support from popular sources, such as the recommendations made by Bill Gates and Mark Zuckerberg in 2018,[3] but they also sparked opposing reactions, including the criticisms expressed in John Gray's (2011) *Delusions of Peace*[4] and later (2015) in "Steven Pinker is wrong about violence and war".[5] In both pieces, Gray offers a series of solid reasons to doubt that violence is declining. Ferguson (2013) also contradicted Pinker's thesis, arguing that what Pinker points out might be actually true but in the complete opposite direction. Other critiques point out Pinker's inappropriate use of statistical information to build his case (Cirillo and Taleb 2016; Falk and Hildebolt 2017) as well as the limitations and exaggerations in his use of data regarding violence in the prehistoric past (Ferguson 2013; Martin and Harrod 2015; Martin and Tegtmeyer 2017; Martin et al. 2012).

Historical documentation has played an important role in establishing and understanding the magnitude of violent episodes as part of armed conflicts (Hobsbawm 1994, 2002, 2008; Keegan 1976, 2012; Leitenberg 2006), and archaeology has contributed to the interpretive analysis of these events of prehistoric violence through the collection of data from the various bodies and contexts observed (Arkush and Allen 2008; Anderson and Martin 2018; Arkush and

Allen 2006; Ferguson 2008; Martin and Anderson 2014; Ralph 2013; Redfern 2017; Nielsen and Walker 2009; Smith and Knusel 2014). Likewise, forensic anthropology[6] has dealt with the analysis of violent events in recent history (Baraybar 2015; Doretti and Fondebrider 2001; Ferllini 2003, 2007; Fondebrider 2002, 2016; Kimmerle and Baraybar 2008; Komar and Lathrop 2012; Márquez-Grant and Errickson 2021; Rosenblatt 2010; Schmitt 2002; Snow 1984; Snow et al. 1989; Ubelaker 1996, 2017; Ubelaker et al. 2019; among others). Other anthropological approaches have also formulated explanations regarding the meaning of violence dynamics (Domínguez 2018; Ferguson 1984; Ferguson and Whitehead 1999; Fry 2013; Riches 1986, 1991; Schmidt and Schroder 2001; Whitehead 2004a, 2005, 2007; among others). However, the dissemination of anthropological knowledge regarding death and endemic violence is still a pending challenge and highly relevant in order to inform the opinion of the non-specialized public community (Buikstra 2019).

Evidence shows that the causes and processes behind violent deaths extend far beyond warfare; currently, intentional homicide due to criminal activities, interpersonal relationships, and a myriad of sociopolitical and cultural factors are the leading causes of death worldwide (UNODC 2019).[7] Violent death, played out in all these different scenarios, has catapulted societies across the world into a humanitarian crisis, with tens of thousands of clandestine dump sites.[8] In most situations, these places present a devastating image that is difficult to grasp due to the harshness of its cruelty and misery. Humans are experiencing a period of history that has accelerated to a "dizzying pace" and advancing at a speed that endangers our species (Hobsbawm 2008). All evidence indicates that political, ideological, racial, and religious motivations have been exacerbating our own destruction (Anstett and Dreyfus 2014). According to Parra and colleagues (2020, p. 79), "all these bloody episodes require new thoughts for humanitarian action to be conducted in an appropriate way. In many ways, social sciences and forensic sciences need to unite to face such humanitarian challenges". Within this context, the anthropology of violent death aims to become a framework for understanding what we should avoid as humanity and what we should embrace in terms of humanitarian action looking forward. During the first decades of the last century, Boas (1928, p. 11) argued "that a clear understanding of the principles of anthropology illuminates the social processes of our own times and may show us, if we are ready to listen to its teachings, what to do and what to avoid". Certainly, anthropology must keep contributing to this task by drawing attention to and explaining various events that have involved violent deaths, as well as their multiple forms of expression, the reasons behind them, and the meanings that these deaths hold within the affected communities (Anstett and Dreyfus 2014; Ferrándiz and Robben 2015; Fontein 2014; Kwon 2006, 2008; Robben 2018a, 2018b; Rojas-Pérez 2017; Uribe 1990).

Cruel or extreme violence has been a predominant behavior in many different times and contexts, and it has caused a strong impact on the living, the dead, and their symbolic environment (Sémelin 2007; Sofsky 2006; Whitehead 2002, 2004 a, 2005, 2007). Apparently, when people exert extreme violence, the biological death of their victims is not the end of their aggression, much less the types of behaviors expressing surrender and submission that in other species – even including chimpanzees, which have shown a high rate of intragroup lethal aggression (Wilson et al. 2014) – would stop the attack (Baumeister 1997; Smith 2020). Rather, among humans, it seems that the behaviors signaling submission and defeat become a strong force that empowers and drives the aggressor to initiate the destruction of his victim (Baumeister 1997; Sémelin 2007; Sofsky 2006; Whitehead 2004b). Why humans have the urge to destroy one another? Why is death not enough? Why should the body of the deceased also be attacked? There is certainly no single or simple answer to these questions.

Whitehead (2007) argues that violence should be understood as an important information exchange system modulated by cultural content, where there is a "recognition that violence is as much a part of meaningful and constructive human living as it is an imagination of the absence and destruction of all cultural and social order" (Whitehead 2007, p. 41). Cruelty – or extreme humiliation – continues to be the mechanism that contributes to the information exchange between the actors involved (victim and perpetrators, including witnesses), and its specific expressions depend on the characteristics of the local culture (White head 2004a, 2004b, 2004c). Baumeister (1997) argued that the origin of these violent actions and limitless violent impulses could be explored within our own behavioral roots and the way we relate to each other. According to Baumeister, among the main triggers of these impulses and actions are, first, the yearn for material security, which includes access to money and the way to obtain it, in addition to the desire for power, in different social and cultural spheres. Second, if egotism is threatened, then resentment is activated and violence begins, and it can escalate to a higher level of aggressiveness when the "favorable image of the person is questioned or contested by someone else" (Baumeister 1997), through humiliation, lack of respect, or a direct attack upon one's honor and dignity. The response to these aggressions can turn into revenge, with extreme and limitless consequences depending on the injuries caused. Third is idealism: when people firmly believe that they are on the right side and are working to make this world a better place, they see the use of extreme force as justified to ensure that those interests are cared for. Fourth is the pursuit of sadistic pleasure, which encompasses the pathological pleasure derived from killing and seeing their victims suffer, something closely linked to pleasure, arousal, and sexual desire. Various documented examples, such as several forms of mutilation – both of living people and of corpses – as well as other expressions less common in modern times – such as cannibalism, framed as a sign of power – show us that the diverse combinations of factors that originate violence, such as cultural differences, damaged social relationships, and the intensity of the exchange of information have contributed to create a message that leads to extreme and violent deaths.

Some scholars argue that cruel actions are caused by a dehumanizing process, by which the minimization of the victims' existence gradually escalates in intensity until the victims reach non-human levels, making them comparable to cockroaches, rats, or chickens and therefore justifying – in the perpetrator's mind – their extermination (Smith 2020; Taylor 2004; Uribe 2018). All these specific forms of violence are not produced by a feverish excess of savage, dehumanized, or pathological minds but are rather cultural representations of meaning derived from the history and the sociocultural relationships endemic to a particular place, just as these signs are used performatively through time (Hinton 2002, 2005; Taylor 1999; Whitehead 2004b). Whitehead (2004b) has highlighted that violence is always a matter of intensity, degree, and cultural notions that drive the development of actions from vehement to violent. This approach:

> "Is therefore intended to call attention to the way in which the meaning of a violent death cannot be entirely understood by reference to biological origins, sociological functions, or material and ecological necessities but has to be appreciated for the way in which it is also a cultural expression of the most fundamental and complex kind. Such cultural expression itself, if it is to be understood, must necessarily involve competence in the manipulation of signs and symbols" (Whitehead 2004b, p. 68).

The manipulation of signs and symbols referred to by Whitehead has led to an enormous capacity for the production of bodies and inert body parts, which are the result of a growing variety of sophisticated ways to destroy human lives (Anderson and Martin 2018; Anstett 2018; Dreyfus and Anstett 2017; Parra et al. 2020; Sofsky 2006; Uribe 1990) as well as the very essence of their human condition (Kristeva 1982; Sémelin 2007; Sofsky 2006). Anthropology has not only made substantial progress in understanding how the destruction of bodies has been integrated into the social and symbolic space of societies affected by violence but has also devoted abundant attention to contextualize the meaning and role of corpses, their parts, and their bodily fluids in those spaces of violence (Anstett and Dreyfus 2014). The body has been used as a mechanism for the transmission of cruelty that has a significant power to annihilate social structures and the social order (Uribe 1990); while the body can be an object of worship, loaded with symbolic charge and rituality, and could contribute to the construction of complex cultural processes, it can also be a powerful weapon of destruction (Sémelin 2007; Uribe 1990); the cruelty of these actions has extermination – understood as a way of kill, kill again, and over-kill[9] – as its main and final purpose. Aware of the profound significance that the manipulation of the victims' bodies carries, the perpetrators get encouraged by these cruel actions and facilitate their exposure according to their own interests, including the creation of sophisticated forms of representation. The body then becomes a means for the transmission and representation of messages that include, but are not limited to, spectacle, humiliation, power, terror, domination, and misery.

Cruelty is the common component underlying such violent expressions that do not cease until the destruction of all physical traces of their victim is complete – that is, until annihilation is achieved. Violent death threatens and damages the social order of the living and the dead, including violence against the "brute stuff of death itself", and rearranges our worldview to transform these events into a bad death; in this new and negative context, the body and its own identity can be devalued or destroyed to the extreme point of social death (Engelke 2019; Parra et al. 2020), and therefore, it becomes an impure and dangerous entity that pollutes space (Kwon 2006, 2008; Korman 2014; Rojas-Pérez 2017).

Social death goes beyond the biological realm, creating a situation where the social and cultural memory of the individual is consciously vanishing, where the dead lose their identity and their constructive social connection with the living, and where all traces of the existence of the individual are finally destroyed. Social death deals with the loss of all bonds of affection and commemoration, status, and moral positions, and taken to the extreme, it refers to the non-recognition of the human condition (Králová and Walter 2017; Parra et al. 2020). Social death embodies entirely the opposite of what is defended by the principles of the anthropology of death, which, as we have already highlighted, imply the persistence and positive continuity of the social life of the deceased, "in one form or another, to the peace of human association" (Hertz 1960, p. 78), making death a good death and preserving the bonds between individuals and communities (Engelke 2019).

Douglas (1966), Turner (1969), and Kristeva (1982) agree on the need to resolve liminal perceptions of the body when death comes. Kristeva (1982) refers to this condition of the body as an "abject state", Turner (1969) calls it "unclassified matter", and Douglas (1966) relates this matter to something "dirty" and culturally "out of place". In her pioneering work "Purity and Danger: An Analysis of the Concept of Pollution and Taboo", Douglas introduced the concept of "matter out of place" to highlight everything that does not fit into a specific cultural category. Douglas argues that each culture perceives the world through a system of categories and that these categories define the natural order of their worldview. In a world in which everything has an assigned place, the notion of purity is reduced to a state where things are in their proper place within the scheme. However, things that do not fit in that order represent a system anomaly or a "matter out of place", and as such, they are considered dirty, impure, and threatening. This is precisely what happens with a bad death and the deathscapes: when there is no mortuary ritual, the corpse and its body parts become abject (Kristeva 1982).

When the dead are not attended adequately, they do not resolve their liminal status; those who are socially dead become social specters that are culturally encoded and classified. All of them reflect negative qualities due to their seedy condition, so they are considered repulsive and dirty as well as powerful, threatening, and highly dangerous; they are bad phenomena to think about. The persistence of the bad death sets up negative deathscapes or impure places where these powerful specters haunt; these spaces remain in liminality with a strong polluting load if they are not addressed and culturally resolved. Impure and contaminated deathscapes cause the dead to threaten the social order of communities in various regions of the world. The ways in which corpses are disposed, hidden, manipulated, discussed, and exhibited are proportional to the perception of how deaths are understood and internalized by communities (Anstett and Dreyfus 2014; Martin et al. 2012). In addition to the tragedy that violent death represents, the social order is altered as well. In this regard, Crossland and Joyce (2015, p. 17) have highlighted the following:

> "A means to transfer the dead body from its liminal location in a temporary grave to a final resting place, where the dead can be reincorporated into society. If the work is successful, the human remains uncovered in forensic excavations will ultimately be reunited with their relatives and undergo the proper funerary rites, once again located in their proper place".

Forensic science has been contributing both to justice and to social order not only by restoring the ties of connection between the deceased and their loved ones but also by liberating communities from deathscapes tainted with seedy death. In this sense, after a forensic intervention, communities may have the opportunity to reincorporate the dead into social life within their own social realm. The processes of recovery of corpses and human body parts require symbolic sensitivity when confronted to numerous factors: turbulent political contexts, diverse interests in dispute that must be evaluated, and varied cultural rituals of death, among others. It also requires a careful analysis of the ways in which bodies and body parts are manipulated, considering a broad regional approach to the cultural context, and the question of how the manipulation of the corpse would affect local perception and stories in the process of memory creation and commemoration (Martin et al. 2012; Verdery 1999). In this regard, Moon (2012) has argued that human remains transform into what Star and Griesemer (1989) have called "boundary objects", that is, "an object that lives in multiple social worlds and which has different identities in each" (Star and Griesemer (1989, p. 409). Moon (2012) considers that boundary objects remain, although they are linked to different interests, and they can be used and interpreted differently; they can offer the opportunity to establish points of mediation and negotiation because they are very flexible to adapt to local needs and different identities, but they are also extremely solid to sustain a common identity in all those convergent spaces. As stated by Parra et al. (2020) forensic sciences need to generate new models and strategies in humanitarian action and human rights, where the needs of the various parties in litigation can be met throughout the rescue of the boundary objects.

Notes

1. As stated by Engelke (2019, p. 30).
2. https://anthrosource.onlinelibrary.wiley.com/hub/journal/15481433/violence
3. https://www.theguardian.com/books/2018/jan/12/davos-bill-gates-mark-zuckerberg-what-to-read
4. https://www.prospectmagazine.co.uk/magazine/john-gray-steven-pinker-violence-review
5. https://www.theguardian.com/books/2015/mar/13/john-gray-steven-pinker-wrong-violence-war-declining
6. Forensic anthropology as a discipline takes multiple dimensions from anthropology, which has a recognized history of development and which is nurtured by a diversity of conceptual perspectives, theoretical foundations, and methods (Boyd Jr and Boyd 2018; Christensen et al. 2014; Dirkmaat et al. 2008; Dirkmaat 2012; Komar and Buikstra 2008; Steadman 2013; Ubelaker 1996, 2017, among others). This discipline has played a fundamental role for the study of skeletal biology in forensic contexts, which has contributed to the documentation of the deceased's profile, including variables such as sex, age, phenotypic characteristics, health, and disease conditions as well as the circumstances of death through the study of traumatic injury to bone (Wedel and Galloway 2014; Komar and Buikstra 2008; Symes et al. 2012; Kimmerle and Baraybar 2008, among others). The archaeological approach to forensic anthropology has also contributed to the identification and uncovering of contexts where bodies were deposited as well as the treatment of the body and the effects of post-depositional processes (Dirkmaat et al. 2008; Ubelaker 1996; Groen et al. 2015, among others). Forensic anthropology has also used sociocultural approaches to collect information from witnesses and survivors from communities affected by violence (Baraybar 2008; Parra et al. 2020; Webster 1998), with the purpose of gathering as much legal evidence as possible and contrasting it with data from the sites where the bodies were deposited and the bodies themselves (Ta'ala et al. 2006). In addition to the legal and humanitarian issues, forensic anthropology has also played a very important social role in the processes of memory reconstruction (Baraybar and Blackwell 2014; Ferrándiz 2006; Renshaw 2007; Sant Cassia 2006, among others).Other new approaches to forensic anthropology have begun to emerge from the cultural perspective (Rodríguez 2021).

7. See UNODC 2019: *Various circumstances, motivations, and relationships can act as driving forces of homicide, and they are often overlapping and multifaceted. Although it can sometimes be difficult to distinguish between the different elements that drive homicide, the Global Study on Homicide uses a classification of homicide into three main typologies: homicide related to interpersonal conflict, homicide related to criminal activities, and homicide related to sociopolitical agendas.*
8. See the Report of the Special Rapporteur of the Human Rights Council on extrajudicial, summary, or arbitrary executions. A/75/384.
9. We are using the phrase "to kill, kill again, and over-kill" (originally in Spanish, "matar, rematar y contramatar") in the sense proposed by Uribe (1990) and Sémelin (2007).

References

Anderson, C.P. and Martin, D.L. (2018). *Massacres: Bioarchaeology and Forensic Anthropology Approaches*. Gainesville: University Press of Florida.

Anstett, É. (2018). What is a mass grave? Toward an anthropology of human remains treatment in contemporary context of mass violence. In: *A Companion to the Anthropology of Death* (ed. A.C.G.M. Robben), 177–188. Chichester: John Wiley and Sons.

Anstett, É. and Dreyfus, J.M. (eds.) (2014). *Destruction and Human Remains: Disposal and Concealment in Genocide and Mass Violence*. Manchester: Manchester University Press.

Arkush, E.N. and Allen, M.W. (2008). *The Archaeology of Warfare: Prehistories of Raiding and Conquest*. Gainesville: University Press of Florida.

Baraybar, J.P. (2008). When DNA is not available, can we still identify people? Recommendations for best practice. *Journal of Forensic Sciences* **53**: 533–540.

Baraybar, J.P. (2015). Variation of gunshot injury patterns in mortality associated with human rights abuses and armed conflict: an exploratory study. *Science and Justice* **55**: 355–362.

Baraybar, J.P. and Blackwell, R. (2014). Where are they? Missing, forensics, and memory. *Annals of Anthropological Practice* **38**(1): 22–42.

Baumeister, R.F. (1997). *Evil: Inside Human Violence and Cruelty*. New York: W.H. Freeman.

Bloch, M. and Parry, J. (eds.) (1982). *Death and the Regeneration of Life*. Cambridge: Cambridge University Press.

Boas, F. (1928). *Anthropology and Modern Life*. New York: W.W. Norton and Company.

Boyd, C.C. Jr. and Boyd, D.C. (eds.) (2018). *Forensic Anthropology: Theoretical Framework and Scientific Basis*. Hoboken: John Wiley and Sons.

Buikstra, J.E. (2019). Knowing your audience: reactions to the human Body, Dead and Undead. In: *Bioarchaeologists Speak Out: Deep Time Perspectives on Contemporary Issues* (ed. J.E. Buikstra), 19–58. Cham: Springer.

Carr, C. (1995). Mortuary practices: their social, philosophical-religious, circunstancial, and physical determinants. *Journal of Archaeological Method and Theory* **2**(2): 105–200.

Christensen, A., Passalacqua, N., and Bartelink, E. (2014). *Forensic Anthropology: Current Methods and Practice*, 1 e. San Diego: Academic Press.

Cirillo, P. and Taleb, N.N. (2016). On the statistical properties and tail risk of violent conflicts. *Physica A: Statistical Mechanics and its Applications* **452**: 29–45.

Crossland, Z. and Joyce, R.A. (eds.) (2015). *Disturbing Bodies: Perspectives on Forensic Anthropology*. Santa Fe: School for Advanced Research Press.

Dirkmaat, D.C. (eds.) (2012). *A Companion to Forensic Anthropology*. Chichester: Wiley-Blackwell.

Dirkmaat, D.C., Cabo, L.L., Ousley, S.D., and Symes, S.A. (2008). New perspectives in forensic anthropology. *Yearbook of Physical Anthropology* **51**: 33–52.

Domínguez, V.R. (2018). Violence: anthropologists engaging violence, 1980–2012. *American Anthropologist*. Virtual Issue. Retrieved from https://anthrosource.onlinelibrary.wiley.com/hub/journal/15481433/violence.

Doretti, M. and Fondebrider, L. (2001). Science and human rights: truth, justice, reparation, and reconciliation: a long way in Third World countries. In: *Archaeologies of the Contemporary Past* (eds. V. Buchli and L. Gavin), 138–144. London: Routledge.

Douglas, M. (1966). *Purity and Danger: An Analysis of Concepts of Pollution and Taboo*. London and New York: Routledge.2002.

Dreyfus, J.M. and Anstett, É. (2017). *Human Remains in Society. Curation and Exhibition in the Aftermath of Genocide and Mass Violence*. Manchester: Manchester University Press.

Engelke, M. (2019). The anthropology of death revisited. *Annual Review of Anthropology* **48**(1): 29–44.

Falk, D. and Hildebolt, C. (2017). Annual war deaths in small-scale versus state societies scale with population size rather than violence. *Current Anthropology* **58**: 805–813.

Ferguson, R.B. (eds.) (1984). *Warfare, Culture, and Environment*. Orlando: Academic Press.

Ferguson, R.B. (2006). Archaeology, cultural anthropology, and the origins and intensification of war. In: *The Archaeology of Warfare: Prehistories of Raiding and Conquest* (eds. E.N. Arkush and M.W. Allen), 469–523. Gainesville: University Press of Florida.

Ferguson, R.B. (2008). War before history. In: *The Ancient World at War* (ed. P. De Souza). London: Thames and Hudson.

Ferguson, R.B. (2013). Pinker's list: exaggerating prehistoric war mortality. In: *War, Peace, and Human Nature: The Convergence of Evolutionary and Cultural Views* (ed. D.P. Fly), 112–131. Cambridge: Oxford University Press.

Ferguson, R.B. and Whitehead, N.L. (1999). *War in the Tribal Zone: Expanding States and Indigenous Warfare*. Santa Fe: School of American Research Press.

Ferllini, R. (2003). The development of human rights investigations since 1945. *Science and Justice* **43**(4): 219–224.

Ferllini, R. (eds.) (2007). *Forensic Archaeology and Violation of Human Rights*. Springfield: Charles C. Thomas.

Ferrándiz, F. (2006). The return of Civil War ghosts: the ethnography of exhumations in contemporary Spain. *Anthropology Today* **22**: 7–12.

Ferrándiz, F. and Robben, A.C.G.M. (eds.) (2015). *Necropolitics: Mass Graves and Exhumations in the Age of Human Rights*. Philadelphia: University of Pennsylvania Press.

Fondebrider, L. (2002). Reflections on the scientific documentation of human rights violations. *International Review of the Red Cross* **84**(848): 885–891.

Fondebrider, L. (2016). The application of forensic anthropology to the investigation of cases of political violence: perspectives from South America. In: *Handbook of Forensic Anthropology and Archaeology* (eds. S. Blau and D.H. Ubelaker), 2 e, 65–74. New York: Routledge.

Fontein, J. (2014). Remaking the dead, uncertainty and the torque of human materials in Northern Zimbabwe. In: *Governing the Dead* (ed. F. Stepputat), 114–140. Manchester: Manchester University Press.

Fry, D.P. (eds.) (2013). *War, Peace, and Human Nature: The Convergence of Evolutionary and Cultural Views*. Oxford: Oxford University Press.

Gray, J. (2011). Delusions of peace. Prospect Magazine. Retrieved from https://www.prospectmagazine.co.uk/magazine/john-gray-steven-pinker-violence-review.

Gray, J. (2015). Steven Pinker is wrong about violence and war. The Guardian. Retrieved from https://www.theguardian.com/books/2015/mar/13/john-gray-steven-pinker-wrong-violence-war-declining.

Groen, M.W.J., Márquez-Grant, N., and Janaway, R.C. (2015). *Forensic Archaeology: A Global Perspective*. Chichester: Wiley-Blackwell.

Hertz, R. (1960). *A Contribution to the Study of the Collective Representation of Death and Right Hand*. London: Cohen and West.

Hinton, A.L. (2002). *Annihilating Difference: The Anthropology of Genocide*. Berkeley: University of California Press.

Hinton, A.L. (2005). *Why Did they Kill: Cambodia in the Shadow of Genocide*. Berkeley: University of California Press.

Hobsbawm, E. (1994). *The Age of Extremes: A History of the World, 1914–1991*. London: Michael Joseph.

Hobsbawm, E. (2002). War and peace in the 20th Century. In: *War and Peace in the 20th Century and Beyond* (eds. G. Lundestad and O. Njølstad), 25–40. River Edge: World Scientific Publishing Co.

Hobsbawm, E. (2008). War, peace and hegemony at the beginning of the twenty-first century. In: *War, Peace and Hegemony in a Globalized World: The changing balance of power in the twenty-first century* (ed. C. Chari), 15–24. Oxon: Routledge.

Keegan, J. (1976). *The Face of Battle*. London: Penguin Books.

Keegan, J. (2012). *A History of Warfare*. New York: Vintage Books.

Kimmerle, E.H. and Baraybar, J.P. (2008). *Skeletal Trauma: Identification of Injuries Resulting from Human Rights Abuse and Armed Conflict*. Boca Ratón: CRC Press.

Komar, D.A. and Buikstra, J.E. (2008). *Forensic Anthropology: Contemporary Theory and Practice*. New York: Oxford University Press.

Komar, D.A. and Lathrop, S.L. (2012). Patterns of trauma in conflict victims from Timor Leste. *Journal of Forensic Sciences* **57**(1): 3–5.

Korman, R. (2014). The Tutsi body in the 1994 genocide: ideology, physical, destruction and memory. In: *Destruction and Human Remains: Disposal and Concealment in Genocide and Mass Violence* (eds. É. Anstett and J.M. Dreyfus), 226–242. Manchester: Manchester University Press.

Králová, J. and Walter, T. (eds.) (2017). *Social Death: Questioning the Life-death Boundary*. London: Routledge.

Kristeva, J. (1982). *Powers of Horror: An Essay on Abjection*. New York: Colombia University Press.

Kwon, H. (2006). *After the Massacre: Commemoration and Consolation in Ha My and My Lai*. Berkeley: University of California Press.

Kwon, H. (2008). *Ghosts of War in Vietnam*. Cambridge: Cambridge University Press.

Laqueur, T. (2002). The dead body and human rights. In: *The Body* (eds. S.T. Sweeney and I. Hodder), 75–93. Cambridge/New York: Cambridge University Press.

Laqueur, T. (2015). *The Work of the Dead: A Cultural History of the Mortal Remains*. Princeton: Princeton University Press.

Leitenberg, M. (2006). Death in Wars and Conflict in the 20th Century 3 Cornell University Peace Studies Program Occasional Paper 29.

Márquez-Grant, N. and Errickson, D. (2021). The legislation, search, recovery, identification and repatriation of conflict casualties worldwide: Introducing the WWI and WWII Special Issue. *Forensic Science International* ***320***: 110716.

Martin, D.L. and Anderson, C.P. (eds.) (2014). *Bioarchaeological and Forensic Perspectives on Violence: How Violent Death is Interpreted from Skeletal Remains.* Cambridge: Cambridge University Press.

Martin, D.L. and Harrod, R.P. (2015). Bioarchaeological contributions to the study of violence. *American Journal of Physical Anthropology* **156**: 116–145.

Martin, D.L. and Tegtmeyer, C. (eds.) (2017). *Bioarchaeology of Women and Children in Times of War: Case Studies from the Americas.* New York: Springer.

Martin, D.L., Harrod, R.P., and Pérez, V.R. (2012). *The Bioarchaeology of Violence.* Gainesville: University Press of Florida.

Metcalf, P. and Huntington, R. (1991). *Celebrations of Death: The Anthropology of Mortuary Ritual,* 2 e. Cambridge: Cambridge University Press.

Moon, C. (2012). Interpreters of the dead: forensic knowledge, human remains and the politics of the past. *Social and Legal Studies* **22**(2): 149–169.

Nielsen, A. and Walker, W. (eds.) (2009). *Warfare in Cultural Context: Practice Agency, and the Archaeology of Conflict.* Tucson: University of Arizona Press.

Parker Pearson, M. (2016). From corpse to skeleton: dealing with the dead in prehistory. *Bulletins et Mémoires de la Société d'Anthropologie de Paris* **28**(1–2): 4–16.

Parra, R.C., Anstett, É., Perich, P., and Buikstra, J.E. (2020). Unidentified deceased persons: social life, social death and humanitarian action. In: *Forensic Science and Humanitarian Action: Interacting with the Dead and the Living* (eds. R.C. Parra, S.C. Zapico, and D.H. Ubelaker), 1 e. Hoboken, NJ: John Wiley and Sons.

Pinker, S. (2011). *The Better Angels of our Nature: Why Violence has Declined.* New York: Viking.

Ralph, S. (eds.) (2013). *The Archaeology of Violence: Interdisciplinary Approaches.* Albany: State University of New York Press.

Redfern, R.C. (2017). *Injury and trauma in bioarchaeology.* In: *Interpreting Violence in Past Lives.* Cambridge: Cambridge University Press.

Renshaw, L. (2007). The iconography of exhumation: representations of mass graves from the Spanish Civil War. In: *Archaeology and the Media* (eds. T. Clack and M. Brittain), 237–251. Walnut Creek, CA: Left Coast Press.

Riches, D. (eds.) (1986). *The Anthropology of Violence.* New York: Basil Blackwell.

Riches, D. (1991). Aggression, war, violence: Space/time and paradigm. *Man* **26**: 281–297.

Robben, A.C.G.M. (eds.) (2018a). *A Companion to the Anthropology of Death.* Chichester: John Wiley and Sons.

Robben, A.C.G.M. (2018b). *Death, Mourning, and Burial: A Cross-Cultural Reader,* 2 e. Chichester: John Wiley and Sons.

Robinson, M. (1998). Opening address. Paper presented at the Conference on Genocide and Crimes Against Humanity: Prevention and Early Warning, United States Holocaust Memorial Museum, Washington, DC

Rodríguez, L. (eds.) (2021). *Culture as Judicial Evidence.* Cincinnati: University of Cincinnati Press.

Rojas-Pérez, I. (2017). *Mourning Remains: State Atrocity, Exhumations, and Governing the Disappeared in Peru's Postwar Andes.* Palo Alto: Stanford University Press.

Rosenblatt, A. (2010). International forensic investigations and the human rights of the dead. *Human Rights Quarterly* **32**(4): 922–951.

Rummel, R. (1996). *Death by Government.* New Brunswick: Transaction.

Sant Cassia, P. (2006). Recognition and emotion: exhumations of missing persons in Cyprus. In: *Divided Cyprus: Modernity, History, and an Island in Conflict* (eds. Y. Papadakis, N. Peristianis, and G. Welz), 194–214. Bloomington: Indiana University Press.

Schmidt, B.E. and Schroder, I.W. (eds.) (2001). *Anthropology of Violence and Conflict.* New York: Routledge.

Schmitt, S. (2002). Mass graves and the collection of forensic evidence: genocide, war crimes and crimes against humanity. In: *Advances in Forensic Taphonomy; Method, Theory and Archaeological Perspectives* (eds. W.D. Haglund and M.H. Sorg), 277–292: CRC Press Boca Raton.

Sémelin, J. (2007). *Purify and Destroy: The Political Uses of Massacre and Genocide.* New York: Columbia University Press.

Smith, D.L. (2020). *On Inhumanity: Dehumanization and How to Resist It.* New York: Oxford University Press.

Smith, M. and Knusel, C. (eds.) (2014). *The Routledge Handbook of the Bioarchaeology of Human Conflict.* London: Routledge.

Snow, C. (1984). The investigation of human remains of the "disappeared" in Argentina. *American Journal of Medicine and Pathology* **5**: 297–299.

Snow, C., Stover, E., and Hannibal, K. (1989). Scientists as detectives. *Investigating Human Rights: Technology Review* **92**(2): 43–51.

Sofsky, W. (2006). *Tratadosobre la violencia.* Madrid: AbadaEditores.

Sorel, G. (1999). In: *Reflections on Violence* (ed. J. Jennings). Cambridge: Cambridge University Press.

Star, S.L. and Griesemer, J.R. (1989). Institutional ecology, 'translations' and boundary objects: Amateurs and professionals in Berkeley's Museum of Vertebrate Zoology 1907–1939. *Social Studies of Science* **19**(3): 387–420.

Steadman, D.W. (2013). The places we will go: paths forward in forensic anthropology. In: *Forensic Science: Current Issues, Future Directions* (ed. D.H. Ubelaker), 131–151. West Sussex: Wiley-Blackwell.

Stepputat, F. (2014). *Governing the Dead: Sovereignty and the Politics of Dead Bodies.* Manchester: Manchester University Press.

Symes, S.A., Lábbé, E.N., Chapman, E.N., Wolff, I., et al. (2012). Interpreting traumatic injury to bone in medicolegal investigation. In: *A Companion to Forensic Anthropology* (ed. D.C. Dirkmaat), 340–389. West Sussex: Wiley-Blackwell.

Ta'ala, S.C., Berg, G.E., and Haden, K. (2006). Blunt force cranial trauma in the Cambodian killing fields. *Journal of Forensic Sciences* **51**: 996–1001.

Taylor, C.C. (1999). *Sacrifice as terror: the Rwandan Genocide of 1994.* New York: Routledge.

Taylor, C.C. (2004). Deadly images: king sacrifice, president habyarimana, and the iconography of pregrnocidal rwandan political literature. In: Violence (ed. N.L. Whitehead): School of Americal Research Press.

Turner, V. (1969). *The ritual process: structure and anti structure.* Chicago: Aldine.

Ubelaker, D.H. (1996). Skeletons Testify: Anthropology in Forensic Science. Presented at the AAPA Luncheon Address: April 12, 1996. *Yearbook of Physical Anthropology* **39**: 229–244.

Ubelaker, D.H. (2017). A history of forensic anthropology. *American Journal of Physical Anthropology* **165**(4): 915–923. doi: 10.1002/ajpa.23306.

Ubelaker, D.H., Shamlou, A., and Kunkle, A.E. (2019). Forensic anthropology in the global investigation of humanitarian and human rights abuse: perspective from the published record. *Science and Justice* **59**(2): 203–209.

Ucko, P.J. (1969). Ethnography and archaeological intepretation of funerary remains. *World Archaeology* **1**(2): 262–280.

UNODC (2019). Global Study on Homicide. Executive Summary. Vienna: United Nations Office on Drugs and Crime.

Uribe, M.V. (1990). Matar, rematar y contramatar. Las masacresenel Tolima 1948–1964. Bogotá: CINEP.

Uribe, M.V. (2018). *Antropología de la Inhumanidad: un ensayointerpretativosobreel terror en Colombia*, 2 e. Bogotá: Universidad de los Andes.

Van Gennep, A. (1960 [1908]). *The Rites of Passage*. Chicago: University of Chicago Press.

Verdery, K. (1999). *The Political Lives of Dead Bodies: Reburial and Postsocialist Change*. New York: Columbia University Press.

Webster, A.D. (1998). Excavation of a Vietnam-era aircraft crash site: use of cross-cultural understanding and dual forensic recovery methods. *Journal of Forensic Sciences* **43**(2): 277–283.

Wedel, V.I. and Galloway, A. (2014). *Broken Bones: Anthropological Analysis of Blunt Force Trauma*, 2 e. Springfield: Charles C. Thomas.

Whitehead, N.L. (2002). *Dark Shamans: Kanaimà and the Poetics of Violent Death*. Durham: Duke University Press.

Whitehead, N.L. (eds.) (2004a). *Violence*. Santa Fe: School of American Research Press.

Whitehead, N.L. (2004b). Introduction: cultures, conflicts, and the poetics of violent practice. In: *Violence* (ed. N.L. Whitehead), 3–24. Santa Fe: School of American Research Press.

Whitehead, N.L. (2004c). On the poetics of violence. In: *Violence* (ed. N.L. Whitehead), 57–78. Santa Fe: School of American Research Press.

Whitehead, N.L. (2005). War and violence as cultural expression. *Anthropology News* **46**: 23–26.

Whitehead, N.L. (2007). Violence and the cultural order. *Daedalus* **136**(1): 40–50. doi: 10.2307/20028088.

Wilson, M.L., Boesch, C., Fruth, B., Furuichi, T., et al. (2014). Lethal aggression in Pan is better explained by adaptative strategies than human impacts. *Nature* **513**: 414–417.

CHAPTER 2
The posthumous dignity of dead persons

Antoon De Baets
Faculty of Arts, University of Groningen, Groningen, The Netherlands

2.1 Introduction: generations and posthumous dignity

Observing humanity from a long-term perspective, we can easily see that the chain of succeeding generations forms a single *historical community*. And since these generations have passed and will pass their heritage on to each other, we can add that they also form a single *moral community*: if all the living together constitute "humanity," then the living, the dead, and the unborn together constitute "humanity at large." But there are notable differences among these three groups.

In 2020, demographers Carl Haub and Toshiko Kaneda calculated the number of people that have ever lived on earth. They guesstimated that the total number of individuals who have been born since the dawn of humanity is 108 billion. Of these, nearly 8 billion are alive and about 100 billion dead (Toshiko and Haub 2020). Others have recently calculated the number of future people on earth. If we look at the next 50 000 years only, and assume a birth rate over that period that equals the rate in this century, the unborn would count around 6.75 trillion people (Krznaric 2020, pp. 82–83, 264).

On top of these vast demographic differences between the dead, the living, and the unborn, there are three striking asymmetries between them. The dead and the unborn do not exist in the same sense as the living as the former are no more alive and the latter not yet alive. Moral principles cover not only the living, that is, people who can reciprocate or can harm and benefit each other, but also the dead and the unborn (Parfit 1984, p. 357; White 1984, pp. 60–62, 86–89; Meyer 2021, § 1). The latter, however, are vulnerable in that they are unable to

---

Anthropology of Violent Death: Theoretical Foundations for Forensic Humanitarian Action, First Edition. Edited by Roberto C. Parra and Douglas H. Ubelaker.

represent and defend themselves. Therefore, we need to speak about the living in terms of rights and duties and about the dead and the unborn in terms of respect and protection. This first asymmetry is already reflected in the fact that while there is a *Universal Declaration of Human Rights* for the living, no such thing exists for the dead or the unborn.

UNESCO drafted a declaration of duties of the living to the unborn in 1997 (UNESCO 1997), and this author, inspired by it, drew up a declaration of duties of the living to the dead in 2004 (De Baets 2004).[1] These declarations of duties to the unborn and the dead, respectively, show a second asymmetry because they do not mirror each other; there is even hardly any overlap between them. Why? The dead have existed and were once living individuals with own personalities; therefore, they are, in principle, individually identifiable. The unborn lack this trait. The declaration about past persons is cast in individual terms, whereas the declaration about future persons is written in collective and abstract terms (Prior 1978, p. 171). And there is even a third asymmetry. In contrast to the future that is unknown but open ended and for which we can make plans, the past is irreversible and unalterable (see also Parfit 1984, pp. 149–186).[2] While we can harm or benefit future people, albeit indirectly, our capacity to harm or benefit the dead is, strictly speaking, nonexistent. Moral questions regarding the dead may therefore look less urgent.

In the following, I will study the community of the 100 billion dead and build a theory on how to approach them best. My thesis is the posthumous dignity thesis: the dead should be viewed as *past* human beings who have posthumous dignity.[3] My argument provides evidence for posthumous dignity and identifies its constituent elements. It shows that the posthumous dignity of the dead is the reason why the living have duties of respect and protection toward the dead. It operationalizes these two duties into more specific ones. I also discuss some disputes to which posthumous dignity gives rise, the breaches it can suffer, and the ways to repair them.

I must add from the outset that in defending the thesis, my approach is scientific. Unlike many others, I do not assume that the dead have agency,[4] and I avoid agential concepts (such as afterlife, immortality, spirits, or souls). The burden of proof for the agency thesis is on those who claim it, not on those who, as I do, find it unconvincing. Nevertheless, I do think that the dead are influential in two ways. First, they *influence* the living not only substantially (as remains) but also genetically (as offspring), materially (as legacy), and biographically (as memories and life stories). Second, the fact that many *believe* that the dead have agency is in itself a major form by which the dead are influential. I hold that the posthumous dignity thesis, even with its flaws and unresolved puzzles, is more consistent than other theories about the dead.[5]

2.2 The dead and posthumous dignity

The term "the dead" is not self-explanatory. The dead are not well described as merely dead bodies. A dead body is not an ordinary object, neither from a medical nor from a legal perspective. One of the guiding medical principles is: "Purchasing . . . cells, tissues or organs for transplantation, or their sale by living persons or by the next of kin for deceased persons, should be banned."[6] And legally, relatives of the dead do not *own* the latter's body – which is considered a *res nullius* (a thing of nobody) or a *nullius in bonis* (among nobody's property) – but they have a right to custody over it between death and burial.[7] It follows that "*who* are the dead" is a better question than "*what* are the dead."

The proper perspective is to compare and contrast the dead not to objects but to human beings. Human beings are not only bodies but also persons, not only biology but also psychology. The bodily and the personal are dual aspects of the dead also. However, in contrast to what many philosophers following John Locke have done, I will not make hard distinctions between the concept of human beings and the concept of persons because in the dominion of the dead, such distinctions are merely important in a heuristic and epistemological sense, not in an ontological sense.[8] Therefore, I will use "persons" as a synonym for "human beings" here. Hence, when we compare human beings – or persons – to the dead, the crucial difference is that human beings have interests, needs, rights, and duties and make claims and choices, while the dead are incapable of having or making these, either now or in the future. The crucial similarity is that without exception all the dead *have been* human beings (and persons). The dead are no longer human beings (or persons) but are still *reminiscent* of them, marking them with powerful symbolism (Feinberg 1985, pp. 53–57, 70–71, 94–95, 116–117). It follows that there is only one possible definition for the dead: *the dead are past human beings or past persons.*

My definition of the dead has one important consequence: since the dead are not human beings, they have neither full nor residual human rights (and even no rights at all).[9] That is the reason why no *Universal Declaration of Human Rights of the Dead* exists: it is impossible by definition. Equally important, if the dead do not have human rights, they are not covered by the core concept uniting these rights, namely, human dignity.[10]

We need another moral language to talk about the dead. This language is one of duties on the part of living based on the "fact" that the dead have posthumous dignity. The fact that the living have these duties toward the dead does not mean that the dead are entitled to corresponding rights. This position does not imply, however, that the rights that individuals exercise while alive do not have legal consequences after they die nor that there are no claims related to the dead; quite the contrary.

With its dual claim that the dead do not have rights and the living have duties toward the dead, the posthumous dignity thesis is situated halfway between the legal maxim of *actio personalis moritur cum persona* ("personal action dies with the person") in common law and the dignitarian approach in civil law. The thesis rejects two extreme and mutually exclusive positions: one that sees the dead as mere bodies without any influence and one that allocates full agency to the dead with own lives separate from the living. My thesis is neither a strategy to delay the inevitable conclusion that death equals destruction nor a door to full-scale metaphysical realities. Rather, it occupies a middle ground, which is compatible with both science and minimalist but quasi-universally held conceptions of dignity and respect.

2.3 Evidence for posthumous dignity

It is impossible to prove conclusively the existence of posthumous dignity as a dimension of the dead. The required evidence is not empirical in the usual, experiential sense because it is out of the question to ask the dead whether they experience such a thing as posthumous dignity. Rather, it is *phenomenological*: one can observe posthumous dignity only indirectly through the prism of its consequence (respect) or its opposite (indignity). Evaluating attitudes of respect and indignity toward the dead yields the following set of facts.

In anthropology, we see that quasi-universally the living *do* respect the dead and believe that the latter have dignity. For many, respect for the dead is a core value of life. In archaeology, traces of funerary rites are seen as proof of the presence of human activity. In biology, we notice that although grief is a feature of several animals, only human beings develop a sustained and deeply ritual relationship with their dead. In the legal domain, all countries have elaborated burial and cemetery regulations. In international humanitarian law, the universally ratified Geneva Conventions prescribe that human remains of the war dead should be respected. Infringements of posthumous dignity serve as powerful proof *a contrario* for its existence. If the reasonable person is the standard, then we can safely say that the disrespectful treatment of dead bodies and the desecration of burial sites meet with quasi-universal indignation, that is, are generally recognized as outrages. The International Criminal Court has stipulated that, when occurring in war, such "outrages upon the dignity of dead persons" are war crimes.[11]

The evidence thus shows that the dead are quasi-universally approached and treated with respect – with the important caveat that the evidence is far more compelling for recent than for remote times. I shall discuss this aspect later, but for now suffice it to say that this caveat cannot avoid the further conclusion from this brief phenomenological analysis that the best way to understand the quasi-universal respect for the dead is to *postulate* the posthumous dignity of the dead.[12]

2.4 Duties flowing from posthumous dignity

From our quest for evidence, we concluded that the dead have posthumous dignity, and therefore deserve respect and protection. Since the dead *deserve* respect and protection, we can say that respect and protection are duties.[13] But who exactly are those who hold the duties and those who benefit from them? Here, we should sharply distinguish respect from protection. While all the living without exception hold the duty to respect the dead, this is not the case with the duty to protect: given practical limits (see, e.g. Barker 2020), only specific groups hold the latter duty.[14] Indeed, in discussing the protection of posthumous dignity, we should differentiate between thick and thin relations. The dead with whom we have thick relations – the few we admire and love – can summon our protection; the others can command our respect. In thick relations, duties of protection are individual; in thin relations, they are collective – as embodied in archives, museums, public commemorations, and the like. This essential distinction is the reason why I avoid speaking about a "duty of care for the dead" as many authors do: "care" conflates "respect" and "protection."

Specific groups act or are entitled to act as representatives of the dead and to perform duties of protection. To begin with, there are the dead themselves when they were alive: some designed a strategy for their afterlife preferences and posthumous legacy (including their posthumous digital legacy) (see, e.g. Zhao 2016). Their family members, friends, and wider solidarity networks usually take over that role when they die. This is the inner circle of concerned individuals. In the next circle, we find various community caretakers. Depending on the tasks at hand, it includes executors of wills, estate administrators, religious counselors, forensic scientists, and the medical, legal, or historical professions.[15] In a third circle, we reach the classical trias of state duties: a state duty to respect (the state should show respect for the dead itself); a state duty to protect (the state should prevent third parties from infringing the duties to the dead); and a state duty to fulfill (the state should facilitate the discharge of duties by its citizens by means of legislative, political, cultural, and other measures). At the official level, a panoply of guardians is available: governments and parliaments promulgating laws and regulations for cemeteries or archives, in the first place, but also the judiciary and enquiry commissions. At the international level, courts guided by custom and treaty are in charge. Guardianship to protect the dead is never straightforward: the wishes of the dead are often misinterpreted, intentionally or not.[16]

Now that the duty-bearers are identified, who is benefiting from these duties? The dead are not the beneficiaries of the duties of respect and protection in any real sense as they are unaware of any such duties performed on their behalf: they are beneficiaries *in the perception* of the living. To the extent that the duties to the dead are fulfilled, they comfort the latter's surviving near and dear and of society at large; to the extent that they are breached, the relatives suffer, others are outraged, and the overall trust in a decent posthumous treatment is diminished. So much so that we can say that society in its entirety is the main beneficiary of the duties to the dead.

The general duties of respect and protection can be broken down in more specific duties. A "universal declaration of duties of the living to the dead" would look as follows:

UNIVERSAL DECLARATION OF THE DUTIES OF THE LIVING TO THE DEAD

Considering that the dead have posthumous dignity, they deserve respect and protection as specified in the following duties to be discharged in a culture-sensitive manner:

Identity-related duties to the dead

Art. 1 IDENTITY: The duty to search for and identify the dead.

Body-related duties to the dead

Art. 2 BODY: The duty to protect the physical integrity of the dead.

Art. 3 FUNERAL: The duty to honor the dead with last rites.

Art. 4 DISPOSAL: The duty to bury or cremate the dead decently and not to disturb their resting places.

Personality-related duties to the dead

Art. 5 IMAGE: The duty to show the dead only after balancing their posthumous privacy and reputation against the public interest.

Art. 6 SPEECH: The duty to comment on the dead only after balancing their posthumous privacy and reputation against the public interest.

Legacy-related duties to the dead

Art. 7 WILL: The duty to respect the will of the dead regarding their reasonable body-related wishes and their property.

Art. 8 HERITAGE: The duty to safeguard the heritage of the dead.

Rights needed by the living when performing duties to the dead

Art. 9 HISTORY: The right to know the truth about past human rights violations.

Art. 10 MEMORY: The right to mourn and commemorate.

The duties to the dead in the Declaration are multifaceted as they cover biological, cultural, religious, economic, and psychological aspects, among others. They are structured according to a chronological logic though there are many overlaps.

The first group contains a single *identity-related duty*. Article 1 encompasses the search, localization, rescue, and identification of the dead – and in their wake, the legal recognition of death. Identifying the dead and the causes and circumstances of their deaths is demanded as an elementary form of truth by surviving relatives. There is a generalized, quasi-universal aversion against anonymous death. Proper identification prevents the dead from becoming missing persons.

Body-related duties (Articles 2–4) evoke quasi-timeless posthumous dignity (even skeletons from prehistory are treated with respect)[17] in contrast to personality- and legacy-related duties (Articles 5–8) that gradually fade away. The violation of the dead body and the resting place is usually punished more severely than the violation of personality aspects. Although universal,[18] body-related duties should take into account cultural and religious traditions with their variations in funeral and disposal practices. Herodotus already observed that the death rituals of one people were abhorred by another. The usual pattern has three distinct moments: death, the last rite, and disposal below, on, or above the earth. But there are many deviations from this pattern: a funeral can be held without a body or a burial without a rite. One can think of the "tomb of the unknown soldier." The concept of a resting place should be taken to encompass burial grounds, funeral architecture, and grave goods, including objects that function as doubles of the dead. When ashes are ritually dispersed, no final resting place exists. Accepted practices such as organ and tissue donation; using bodies for scientific, educational, or therapeutic purposes; exhumation and autopsy for forensic purposes; emergency burials; and cemetery clearance require a fair balance of all interests involved, including the consent of relatives.

Body-related duties have a strong privacy dimension. As an empirically retrievable expression of posthumous dignity, posthumous privacy is a characteristic of the dead, *not* a right, and the evidence for it is considerable. Physicians have professional obligations of confidentiality after the deaths of their patients.[19] Families have the right to take the dead body of their relative in custody; unwanted public intrusion into funerals and other expressions of mourning is seen as an outrage. Funerals have unique characteristics: they are semi-public meetings of great intimacy and privacy, yet have the power, in the presence of the dead body as their focal point, to strengthen the bonds among families and wider social networks for the future. In the case of political personalities, they can even transform into rallying points for political resistance.

Personality–related duties (Articles 5–6) also satisfy deeply felt needs to honor the dead.[20] Funerals (Article 3) often reflect the personality of the deceased. Articles 5–6 propose duties regarding posthumous privacy and reputation.[21] The saying "you cannot defame the dead" is correct only in the sense that the dead themselves do not feel the defamation anymore. Evidence for posthumous privacy and reputation is considerable here also. Criminal or civil codes in many countries, data protection and archival legislation, and medical codes of ethics have provisions for the responsible handling of information about the dead, including embargo terms. In showing images or footage of the dead, privacy and reputation concerns may be overridden by the public interest if the images are shown in historical works, artistic endeavors, and reports about war or human rights violations.[22] "Commenting on" the dead refers to many genres, from tape recordings of funerals over obituaries, epitaphs, funerary orations, and genealogies to biographies. The balancing problem revolves around the problem of how to respect posthumous privacy and reputation without blocking access to sensitive archives or paralyzing critical research and writing (Schauer 1992, pp. 179, 185–186). If posthumous dignity is sacralized in overbroad legal provisions about "the memory of the dead" and "defamation of the dead," the expression of ideas about the dead can be seriously hampered, if not censored (De Baets 2021). The exercise of free expression about the past should not become too burdensome: the default presumption should be in favor of disclosure of information about the dead.[23] The passage of time should be taken into account: the longer after death the disclosure occurs, the stronger this default presumption. Even so, there may be circumstances in which authors prefer to exercise a right to silence regarding some sensitive posthumous aspects of their subjects.

Legacy-related duties (Articles 7–8) bifurcate into (personal) will and (collective) heritage. At the individual level, wills regarding funeral and burial belong to the privacy aspects and, if unambiguously expressed and reasonable, count heavily in any balancing with other interests.[24] Wills also regulate the estate (the tangible, including pecuniary, and intangible property of the dead). While many individuals do not wish to be forgotten, some, by stipulating that their personal papers be destroyed and digital records erased, do not wish to be remembered. At the collective level, the preservation and transmission of tangible and intangible cultural heritage is regulated in UNESCO conventions and international humanitarian law.[25] Legacy-related duties may raise complicated issues of posthumous mecenate, publicity, copyright, and intellectual property.[26]

The *rights to memory and history* (Articles 9–10), finally, help the living to properly fulfil their duties. These two rights are strong manifestations of the human rights to thought, opinion, expression, assembly, and association. They enable survivors to be informed about past breaches of posthumous dignity and to mourn and commemorate their dead decently so as to give painful past events a proper context, interpretation, and meaning.[27] It should be noted, however, that the right to memory is different from a duty to remember. A duty of remembrance imposed by oneself is acceptable, but when it is imposed by the state or by others, it should be rejected for several reasons. It confuses respect and protection. It forces us to commemorate the dead for all eternity, granting them an immortality that human beings do not possess. It is vulnerable to abuse if those who impose the duty make biased selections of whom to remember and whom to forget. Above all, human rights clearly stipulate that the right to hold opinions, including memories, without interference and express them also includes the right not to hold such opinions and memories and not to express them.[28] Sacralizing the dead is a dangerous game.

2.5 The nature of posthumous dignity

Posthumous dignity has some salient characteristics. I tentatively suggest that it is:

- A dimension, not a right,
- Non-discriminatory,
- Fading over time,
- Relative, not absolute,
- Attributed, not intrinsic.

Posthumous dignity is *not a right*. The dead do not have rights and therefore no right to either posthumous dignity or posthumous respect. Rather, posthumous dignity is *a dimension* of the dead, consisting of the aspects of identity, body, personality, and legacy and concretely expressed as posthumous privacy and posthumous reputation.

A second feature of posthumous dignity is its non-discriminatory character, meaning that it is applicable to all the dead without distinction. We can identify concentric layers of relations: those loved in small circles (the near and dear), those loved in large circles (the wise ancestors, the heroes of humanity, the benefactors), those to whom we remain indifferent (the overwhelming majority), and the few considered morally repugnant (tyrants and mass murderers in particular) – with the understanding that those to whom we are indifferent or inimical are somebody else's near and dear. Such a *moral typology* is important to identify to which dead we have duties of respect and protection but does not exclude posthumous dignity for anyone. Being an ancestor or leaving a heritage to posterity is not a condition for granting posthumous dignity; being a dead tyrant or instigator of mass murder is not a condition for not granting it (Parfit 2011: Volume 1, pp. 184, 240, 244, 374).[29] Moral merit is no criterion. The non-discriminatory character of posthumous dignity is the only real sense in which it is universal. This does not mean, however, that we cannot intervene in the administration of the *protection* to dead tyrants and mass murderers: they deserve posthumous dignity in private, but in the interests of society, it is legitimate to prevent any public or institutionalized commemoration. A democratic state has a right to prevent graves of mass murderers from becoming places of pilgrimage.

The third feature is that posthumous dignity *endures but fades over time*. Although much evidence for posthumous dignity is found in the past, it is far from historically universal: for centuries, many have assumed that posthumous dignity was solely applicable to the own cultural group. Archaeologists have often treated the human remains of indigenous peoples with disrespect. In other words, the ascription of posthumous dignity varied according to time, place, and perspective. Philippe Ariès, the leading historian of Western attitudes toward death, wrote: "The lavish expression of grief about the loss of a loved one and the need to commemorate that life . . . came to the fore in Western culture only in the nineteenth century . . . The individual tombstone . . . was a modern invention."[30] The problem is how we deal with our incomplete knowledge of the remote dead. We can construct an *epistemological typology* consisting of those who left traces from which to extract knowledge (the recently dead, the powerful, the famous, and the rich) and those about whom we are ignorant (the millions of anonymous dead in history). Although in principle, posthumous dignity has no time bar, this fading effect erodes any duties of protection in practice.

The fourth feature has already been noted earlier, namely, that posthumous dignity is *relative, not absolute*. Most duties to the dead are regulated by law and tradition, and all have to be balanced against the interests of the living, including public health, public order, and free expression.

The final characteristic is fundamental. Some may argue that the evidence for posthumous dignity is, in fact, evidence for posthumous respect and that it would therefore be better to build the thesis around posthumous respect alone, skipping the allegedly underlying posthumous dignity altogether. But these critics do not offer an explanation for posthumous respect, whereas my thesis does. The deeper problem, then, is why posthumous dignity exists. There are three views: posthumous dignity is an intrinsic property of the dead *recognized* by the living; a potential property of the dead *becoming manifest* each time the living approach them; or a property *attributed* by the living to the dead. The first two positions reintroduce by the backdoor what we waved goodbye near the front door: that, like the living, the dead are assigned agency entitling them to dignity claims. Consistent with my overall position, I take the last view: posthumous dignity is attributed. This is the reason why I hesitate to call posthumous dignity *inalienable*: in principle, it cannot be lost or removed entirely; in practice, it is sometimes breached. Attribution is not completely universal.

The living attribute posthumous dignity to the dead because it is a *social practice*. Society as a whole has an interest in attributing dignity to its dead and cultivating respect for them because doing so provides its citizens with reasonable expectations of being treated decently after their deaths themselves. Attribution thus contributes to norms of civility and to peace. Funerals and wills would make no sense if everyone saw that they were poorly respected. If that were so, the living would lose trust in these practices, and if enough people would lose that trust, they would eventually disappear. But these practices *have not* disappeared; on the contrary, they have increased over time.[31]

2.6 Semantic debates about posthumous dignity

Meanwhile, it should have become clear that talking about the dead is a semantic minefield packed with metaphors and euphemisms and with the pathetic fallacy (the tendency to ascribe human traits to inanimate phenomena). This minefield is a result of the ambiguous ontological status of the dead. Language plays tricks upon us each time we try to catch the essence of the dead. A few examples will show this. I defined the dead as past human beings and still called the historical community formed by the dead, the living, and the unborn "humanity at large." Furthermore, my definition of the dead as "past human beings" is negative, whereas the rules of logic prescribe that definitions should state the *essential* attributes of a species and not be negative where they can be affirmative. The definition of the dead is the rare case where the negative form – derived from and contrasted with the living – appropriately expresses the essential characteristic. Some avoid the term "the dead" (presumably for its blunt impact), and replace it with "the deceased," but the latter term encompasses the recent dead alone, whereas "the dead" emphasizes duration and covers the state of being dead completely.

Furthermore, the International Committee of the Red Cross, the United Nations Human Rights Commission, and the International Criminal Court, among others, do not speak of "past persons" (or "past human beings") but rather of "dead persons"[32] to indicate the dead, but this is less correct. The term "dead persons" suggests that there are two classes of persons – those with the property to live and those with the property to be dead – which is absurd because, by definition, personhood is a property of the living alone.[33] Despite its problematic meaning, I have adopted the term "dead persons" because it has two considerable *practical* advantages. First, as a "subcategory" of persons, "dead persons" fall – at least symbolically – within the legal provisions for persons generally, which increases their protection. Second, legal instruments that use the "dead persons" concept also tend to describe the dignity of the dead not as "posthumous dignity" as would be the proper logic, but as "the personal dignity of the dead," bringing human rights and humanitarian provisions such as the prohibition of "outrages upon personal dignity" within their purview.

The pressure to follow the international tradition to speak about "dead persons" is visible in this essay's very title. To make things worse, the title – "The Posthumous Dignity of Dead Persons – is tautological: "posthumous" and "dead" express the same thought. This is done on purpose because shorter titles are not clearer: "Posthumous dignity" presupposes readers already acquainted with the problems involved; "The dignity of dead persons" does not acknowledge the crucial distinction between human and posthumous dignity.

I avoided the frequently used phrase "respect for the memory of the dead" throughout because "memory of the dead" is not correct: the dead do not have a memory. Rather, "memory of the dead" is a certain set of ideas *about* the life of a dead person lingering on in the minds of the living. In the same vein, I talk about duties *to* the dead, but since the dead are not human beings and do not reciprocate, it would be better to speak about duties *regarding* the dead. And should we label breaches of posthumous dignity "harms," "wrongs," "offenses," "abuses," or "violations" when we know that, strictly speaking, the dead cannot be harmed, wronged, offended, abused, or violated?[34]

There are more perplexing semantic puzzles, though. Time and again, I have repeated in my writings and lectures that my thesis is that the dead do not have human rights and that this fact does not exclude that the living have duties toward them. At least half of those who responded to my thesis summarize it as if I defend the thesis that the dead . . . have human rights! (e.g. Cotkin 2008, p. 312). This is due partly to sloppy interpretation, partly to the semantic traps that time and again confuse us. Some of the writings of those authors who argue, either on purpose, unthinkingly, or by mistake, that the dead have human rights are confusing, but – to my surprise, I must admit – most were inspiring. It is impossible to escape the semantic minefield in which the dead are buried.

2.7 Breaches of posthumous dignity

In practice, the dignity of the dead can be attacked, breached, or denied to the point of virtual destruction, thus shocking and offending humanity. An attempt to inventory all breaches of posthumous dignity and of the duties it entails yielded a list of sixty legal and moral wrongs to the dead (De Baets 2009a, pp. 133–137).[35] They included such widely varying wrongs as the disruption of funerals, the refusal to return dead bodies to relatives, the unwillingness to execute last wills, the tampering with identities of the dead, the cleansing of archives, the denial of atrocities, and the censorship of biographers, among others. Many are punishable by law, and if not, they are still moral wrongs to the dead. The inventory is incomplete and brings to mind a telling commentary by the International Committee of the Red Cross. Common Article 3 of the Geneva Conventions prohibits "acts which world public opinion finds particularly revolting" such as "violence to life and person" and "outrages upon personal dignity." In this context, the Committee wrote:

> One may ask if the list [of such revolting acts, *adb*] is a complete one. At one stage of the discussions, additions were considered . . . The idea was rightly abandoned . . . [I]t is always dangerous to try to go into too much detail – especially in this domain. However much care were taken in establishing a list of all the various forms of infliction, one would never be able to catch up with the imagination of future torturers who wished to satisfy their bestial instincts; and the more specific and complete a list tries to be, the more restrictive it becomes . . .[36]

The same is true for outrages upon the dignity of the dead: the variation is endless. I will briefly review here only three types of breaches that are recognized as war crimes or crimes against humanity. First, the crime of "outrages upon personal dignity" is a war crime under the Geneva Conventions and before the International Criminal Court. Its scope includes outrages upon the dignity of the dead, such as the mutilation of dead bodies and the refusal of a decent burial (Dörmann 2003, pp. 314–315, 323; Genocide Network 2018).[37] The material element of this crime must have a subjective and an objective component (Dörmann 2003, pp. 314–324). Crimes against the dead, however, do not possess a subjective component because the dead cannot be "personally" aware of the existence of any ill-treatment or humiliation.[38] At the same time, the objective component – the fact that the reasonable person must be outraged by the treatment[39] – is overwhelming. Second, the enforced disappearances of persons, when committed as part of a widespread or systematic attack against the civilian population, are crimes against humanity.[40] Insofar as they lead to executions and to concealment or non-identification of dead bodies, they are also breaches of posthumous dignity.[41] Finally, intentional attacks against buildings dedicated to "education, . . . [or] science . . . [or] historic monuments" are also war crimes.[42] These historical monuments are part of the heritage of the dead.

Who then are the victims of posthumous dignity breaches? Because the dead cannot be harmed by these breaches, the victims are surviving families and friends, indeed humanity as a whole. Outrages upon the dignity of the dead, disappearances leading to death, and the intentional destruction of historical heritage breach duties of respect and protection and the right to memory. However, the fact that some perpetrators *believe* that they can intentionally harm the dead by "dehumanizing" (disfiguring and de-identifying) them is an important fact in itself (De Baets 2009a, pp. 137–139). History has seen many cases of posthumous trial, including posthumous execution and denial of burial.

Two main motives for such breaches can be distinguished. One possibility is that the perpetrators aim at punishing the dead for their acts when they were still alive or at preventing the latter from returning as wandering spirits to take revenge. Another option is that they punish the dead in order to deter or humiliate the living. Deterrence occurs when graves are destroyed to prevent them from becoming the focus of a pilgrimage; humiliation when genocide deniers, by lying about the atrocities, target genocide survivors. If these indignities are inflicted with impunity, historical injustice is perpetuated. The question arises, therefore, whether these breaches can be redressed.

2.8 Restoration of posthumous dignity

The restoration of posthumous dignity has been a powerful motive behind the establishment of the International Criminal Court as we are reminded in the preamble of its statute: "*Mindful* that during this century millions of children, women and men have been victims of unimaginable atrocities that deeply shock the conscience of humanity."[43] When the judges of the court first met in 2003, United Nations Secretary-General Kofi Annan declared: "For those who have been slaughtered, all we can do is seek to accord them in death the dignity and respect they were so cruelly denied in life."[44]

I will therefore examine successively whether conceptions of victims, theories of historical injustice, and principles for reparation pay sufficient attention to the restoration of posthumous dignity. The first problem we meet is that most conceptions of victims do not include the dead. The earliest attempt to calculate damages in cases of wrongful death – in the *Lusitania* case of 1923 – avoided the language of victims: the beneficiaries of financial compensation in such cases were the heirs claiming that they had suffered losses. The calculation was executed according to a famous formula still in use today:

> Estimate the amounts (i) which the decedent, had he not been killed, would probably have contributed to the claimant; add thereto (ii) the pecuniary value to such claimant of the deceased's personal services in claimant's care, education, or supervision; and also add (iii) reasonable compensation for such mental suffering or shock, if any, caused by the violent severing of family ties, as claimant may actually have sustained by reason of such death. The sum of these estimates reduced to its present cash value will generally represent the loss sustained by claimant.[45]

The focus is on the survivors here. Likewise, the *United Nations Declaration of Basic Principles of Justice for Victims of Crime and Abuse of Power* (1985) does not talk about the dead. It distinguishes direct victims, who are those suffering harm through crime or abuse of power, and indirect victims, meaning the immediate family or dependents of the direct victims and those persons who suffer harm while trying to help direct victims. But it does not specify whether "those suffering harm through crime" include the dead.[46]

Recently, however, a judge of the International Criminal Court has entertained the view that dead persons *are* victims:

> The Single Judge finds it self-evident that a victim does not cease to be a victim because of his or her death . . . It is deemed appropriate, that the successors of a deceased person exercise the rights of deceased persons in proceedings in order to safeguard claims for any future reparations.[47]

We must conclude that the judge's opinion, including his phrase "rights of deceased persons," is not widely shared.

Theories of historical injustice, if they are to include the dead, should define the term "historical injustice" as the sum of all atrocity crimes committed in the past – crimes similar to genocide, crimes against humanity, and war crimes today. Historical injustice can be split into *remote* historical injustice, in which all perpetrators and victims are dead, and *recent* historical injustice, in which at least some perpetrators or victims are still alive.[48] Remote historical injustice is the most problematic form. Restoration of remote historical injustice has been defended *and* rejected vigorously. Opponents of the idea say that it is too long ago, that the injustice has been superseded by more recent events, that younger generations gradually become less aware of the injustice, that the evidence for it is lost or incomplete, that it revives old pain and old conflicts, that the prosecution of perpetrators and the reparation of victims are forever impossible, that the past cannot be altered, and that it is out of the question to reevaluate all of the past all of the time. Supporters of the idea argue that even atrocity crimes of longer ago still shock the conscience of humanity, that they are imprescriptible, and that the right to know the truth about these atrocities continues to exist after the death of the last perpetrators and last victims. This debate is undecided, and few agree on the right course.

Recent historical injustice can be tackled with the measures described in the *United Nations Reparation Principles*.[49] These principles distinguish five types of reparation: restitution (the complete reparation of the situation before the crime), compensation (the partial reparation of the situation before the crime), rehabilitation (medical and psychological), prevention (ensuring that the crimes do not happen again), and finally, symbolic reparation or satisfaction. The first four forms come too late for the dead, but they may help victims who survived. Only the last form is partly applicable to the dead.[50] Reiterating that any satisfaction is achieved solely *in the eyes* of the survivors and does not affect the dead, some measures of symbolic reparation mentioned in the *Reparation Principles* are applicable in situations of recent as well as remote historical injustice. In the following, I quote and comment upon these measures:

Scientific reparation: "Verification of the facts and full and public disclosure of the truth to the extent that such disclosure does not cause further harm or threaten the safety and interests of the victim." This corresponds to duties 1, 5–6, and 8 of our Declaration. The search for facts is the first stage in the search for causes and for historical truth: if corroborated, these facts fix the boundaries of any sound historical narrative and explanation of past atrocities. Such searches are protected by the right to the truth,[51] which must be complemented with a state duty to investigate atrocities, including by maintaining accessible archives.[52] Neither regime change nor amnesty laws nor the passage of time can affect this state duty. Because atrocity crimes are imprescriptible, the right to the truth forms the bridge between the realms of justice and history. In applying the right to the truth to temporally distant cases, two risks persist, however: the risk of anachronism in evaluating crimes of longer ago and the uncertainties in determining indirect victimhood over longer periods. Finally, the disclosure of the truth is conditional on its effect upon the victims – but if the dead are victims at all, the effects upon them are nonexistent and therefore cannot be negative.

Forensic reparation: "The search for the whereabouts of the disappeared, for the identities of the children abducted, and for the bodies of those killed, and assistance in the recovery, identification and reburial of the bodies in accordance with the expressed or presumed wish of the victims, or the cultural practices of the families and communities." This corresponds to duties 1–4 and 7 of our Declaration. Like scientific reparation, forensic reparation fosters "the search for clues, which may assist in the historical reconstruction of events."[53]

Legal reparation: "An official declaration or a judicial decision restoring the dignity, the reputation and the rights of the victim and of persons closely connected with the victim." This corresponds to duties 1 and 6–7 of our Declaration. Legal reparation restores property rights, reviews or annuls previous biased court judgments, and issues posthumous pardons. It dovetails with a strongly felt need among relatives to set the record straight and to clear names and reputations. It is also activated when courts declare that genocide denial is a form of hate speech.

Political reparation: "Public apology, including acknowledgement of the facts and acceptance of responsibility." Political measures such as apologies touch duties 1 and 6 of our Declaration. Political reparation is usually directed at groups of victims rather than individuals. It provides official acknowledgment of breaches committed by predecessor regimes and endorses other types of reparations made by successor regimes.

Memorial reparation: "Commemorations and tributes to the victims." This corresponds to duties 3 and 5–6 of our Declaration. Memorial reparation may be the sole reparation measure in cases of mass deaths, including in the remote past.

Educational reparation: "Inclusion of an accurate account of the violations that occurred in . . . law training and in educational material at all levels."

This corresponds to duties 1, 6, and 8 of our Declaration. It includes the rewriting of falsified history textbooks and the teaching of historical taboos. Educational reparation is a natural extension of scientific reparation. Both aim at preventing future falsification and denial of historical injustices and also encompass such measures as the rescue of manuscripts, the republication of works of dead authors previously censored, and the novel publication of biographies of those formerly fallen in disgrace.

All these forms of symbolic reparation have *immediate* effects on the restoration of the posthumous dignity of dead persons.

2.9 Conclusion: the impact of posthumous dignity

However, symbolic reparation of the posthumous dignity of the dead has ramifications beyond its immediate effects. *Substantially,* it brings comfort to the surviving relatives and to wider communities. *Morally,* it helps discontinue historical injustice, thus decreasing the risk of its repetition. *Socially,* it raises the awareness of historical injustice, adding to its preventive role. *Politically,* it strengthens the rights to memory and history, as robust forms of the right to freedom of expression, and directly supports democracy.

Posthumous dignity is a thesis providing a consistent perspective on the dead. Compliance with the duties it entails assists individual survivors in their years of grief and societies in their decades of building the rule of law, human rights, and democracy. Its restoration reminds the community of past atrocities and helps prevent their re-occurrence. Attributing posthumous dignity to the dead profoundly enhances the human dignity of the living. In doing so, the Golden Rule for the Dead is our guide: *do unto the dead as you would have others do unto you after you die.*

Notes

1. Also reproduced in De Baets (2009a, p. 123). An updated version is included in this chapter.
2. The comparison between the dead and fetuses is also ill-suited because the former's situation is definitive, the latter's open ended.
3. After a gestation process starting in 2000, I have introduced the posthumous dignity thesis in the 2004 essay, the 2009 book, and several articles. Others have defended comparable concepts. *The Minnesota Protocol on the Investigation of Potentially Unlawful Death* (2017), §§ 42, 90, 154, speaks about "respect for the dignity of the dead." Its 1991 predecessor did not mention this concept. In their preamble, the *Guiding Principles for the Dignified Management of the Dead in Humanitarian Emergencies and to Prevent Them Becoming Missing Persons* (Geneva: ICRC Missing Persons Project, 2021) state: "Respect

due to a human being does not cease with death." In the literature, various authors use the posthumous dignity concept, including, for example, Sian Cook, "Posthumous Dignity and the Importance in Returning Remains of the Deceased," and Roberto Parra, Elisabeth Anstett, Pierre Perich, and Jane Buikstra, "Unidentified Deceased Persons: Social Life, Social Death and Humanitarian Action," both in Roberto Parra, Sara Zapico, and Douglas Ubelaker, eds., *Forensic Science and Humanitarian Action: Interacting with the Dead and the Living* (Hoboken, NJ: Wiley, 2020), 67–99.

4. I do not go as far as Parra et al., "Unidentified Deceased Persons," 79–84, who speak of the (symbolic) agency of corpses. Using an expanded notion of "agency," they include what I call "influence" in it. For a discussion about dead-related agency issues, see Rosenblatt (2010) pp. 929–936.
5. This chapter is about being dead, not about dying or mourning. Dying is an experience (except, perhaps, in cases of sudden death), mourning is an experience, but being dead is not an experience.
6. World Health Organization, *Guiding Principles on Human Cell, Tissue and Organ Transplantation* (2010), Principle 5.
7. United Nations (UN) Commission on Human Rights, *Updated Set of Principles for the Protection and Promotion of Human Rights through Action to Combat Impunity* (UN Doc. E/CN.4/2005/102/Add.1) (2005) (hereafter *Impunity Principles*), Principle 34. The worldwide repatriation trend since the 1990s should also be noted here: in the case of remains of indigenous persons, custody belongs to the indigenous people who can prove cultural affiliation to the deceased, and the latter's remains should return to them. See also *UN Declaration on the Rights of Indigenous Peoples* (2007), Article 12. Since 1989, the World Archaeological Congress and some national archaeological societies have approved codes of ethics to deal with human remains.
8. I do not make the Lockean distinction between human beings and persons here, e.g., by arguing that persons are human beings with certain characteristics (conscious, rational, free, moral, etc.). The implication of that distinction (namely, that certain classes of human beings are not, not yet, no longer, or not fully persons, such as young children, the mentally ill, or the irreversibly comatose), while important for the living, disappears after death because young children, the mentally ill, and the irreversibly comatose, when deceased, do not differ in essence from other dead persons.
9. From my review of around a hundred philosophical essays about the dead for this chapter, I estimate that the thesis that the dead have rights is defended by about 10% of the authors: it is a minority position. The large majority departs from the premise that the living owe duties to the dead. As recently as 2018, the *Declaration for the Dignified Treatment of All Missing and Deceased Persons and Their Families as a Consequence of Migrant Journeys (The Mytilini Declaration)* has a part entitled "The rights of the missing and of the deceased and their bereaved families," but it identifies only the families as right-holders.
10. For an analysis of the human dignity concept, see De Baets (2007).
11. "List of Customary Rules of International Humanitarian Law," *International Review of the Red Cross*, 87, no. 857 (March 2005), Rules 90 and 113.
12. Additional reasons for broadly shared posthumous respect may be found in the quasi-universal feeling of perplexity about the borders of humanity, in fear of death, and in a widely shared urge for transcendental continuity of life. Following Martin Heidegger, Roger Scruton writes: "Our existence has no ultimate foundation: it is a

brute fact for which we can find no reason, since all our reasons are generated within life" (Scruton 1994, p. 315).

13. I prefer "duties" over "obligations" (which most often have a relational character) and "responsibilities" (duties is shorter and simpler).

14. It has been argued, unconvincingly I find, that dead victims of atrocity crimes form an exceptional category, deserving not only respect but also protection from *all* of us. Meyer, "Intergenerational Justice," § 5.4, calls this "surviving duties."

15. Legal standing with representation by guardians has been granted to corporations (everywhere), future generations (climate change cases in several countries), deities (India), nature (Bolivia, Ecuador, Uganda, India, Bangladesh), a river, a mountain, and a parc (New Zealand), rivers (Canada, Colombia), a lake (Spain), trees (Belgium), and an orangutan (Argentina).

16. Another problem is which legal norms should be followed when disputes arise about exhuming human remains, removing war cemeteries, or transferring war memorials: those in vigor at the time of the victim's death, the cemetery's establishment, the memorial's creation, or those at the time of the disputes. According to the principle of intertemporal law, the law as evolved at the time of the dispute should be applicable. See Petrig (2009) and De Baets (2022, pp. 1600–1601).

17. Posthumous dignity never expires completely as we can observe when archaeologists discover ancient remains, to which names ("Lucy", "Ötzi") are given.

18. Brown (1991) includes death rituals in his list of human universals.

19. "I will respect the secrets that are confided in me, even after the patient has died." World Medical Association, Declaration of Geneva (Geneva 1948, last revised 2017), sixth vow. This declaration is often called the "physician's oath."

20. See Zhao (2011, 2014).

21. Reputation and honor are closely related: reputation is the esteem given to a person by others; honor is a person's self-esteem. It follows that posthumous honor is impossible because the dead do not have self-esteem, whereas posthumous reputation exists because it is attributed by the living to the dead.

22. For legal cases, see United States Supreme Court, *National Archives and Records Administration v. Favish, et al.*, 124 S.Ct. 1570 (2004); European Court of Human Rights, *Case of Hachette Filipacchi Associés v. France* (Application no. 71111/01), Judgment (2007).

23. The 2016 General Data Protection Regulation of the European Union (EU Regulation 2016/679) is not applicable to personal data of "deceased persons," implying that the margins to use such data are broad: see its Considerations 27, 158, 160.1.

24. Conventions such as those drafted by the Hague Conference on Private International Law (1961) and Unidroit (1973) regulate the status of testamentary dispositions and last wills.

25. For a definition of cultural property, see *Convention for the Protection of Cultural Property in the Event of Armed Conflict* (1954), Article 1.

26. Regarding posthumous intellectual property, see Barkan and Bush (2002, pp. 201–223); regarding posthumous copyright, see *Berne Convention for the Protection of Literary and Artistic Works* (1886, 1979), Articles 6bis–7bis. Regarding posthumous publicity, see Gross et al. (1988) and Madoff (2010).

27. For best practices for commemorations and collective funerals, see International Committee of the Red Cross (ICRC), *Operational Best Practices Regarding the Management of Human Remains and Information on the Dead by Non-Specialists* (Geneva: ICRC, 2004),

18–19, and ICRC, *Mourning Process and Commemoration* (Geneva: ICRC, 2002), 27–28 (an overview of death conceptions in major religions).

28. See International Covenant on Civil and Political Rights (ICCPR) (1966), Articles 18–22 (Article 18.2 in particular); UN Human Rights Committee, *General Comment 34* (Freedoms of Opinion and Expression) (2011) (UN Doc. CCPR/C/GC/34), § 10. See also De Baets (2009a), 147–157, for an extensive discussion. For a discussion of the duty to grieve as a duty to oneself, not to the dead, see Cholbi (2021), pp. 149–165.

29. This view is the opposite of Smilansky (2018), a crazy plea to punish dead dictators.

30. As paraphrased in Hutton (1993, p. 104).

31. For the clearest formulation of the argument, see Partridge (1981). See also Winter (2010).

32. The term "dead person[s]" is used in the *Geneva Conventions* (1949) and their Additional Protocols (1977) and in the *Elements of Crimes* of the International Criminal Court (ICC). The term "the dead" is used in the *Hague Convention X* of 1907, the *Geneva Conventions* of 1906, 1929, and 1949; the *Additional Protocols* of 1977; and "List of Customary Rules", Rules 112–116. Other uses in, for example, UN Commission on Human Rights, "Human Rights and Forensic Science" (resolutions 1998/36; 2000/32; 2003/33; 2005/26).

33. A human being/person who is alive exists; a human being/person who dies goes out of existence; a human being/person who is dead does not exist (although the latter's remains may continue to exist for some time). As Immanuel Kant argued, the property of existence (or of being alive) is not a personal property as any other (such as being rational); it is a condition for these properties. See also Soll (1998, pp. 33–36, 182 note 26), Luper (2019, § 1.5) and Eser (2002, volume 1, 923, note 156).

34. Note that in his four-volume work *The Moral Limits of the Criminal Law*, Joel Feinberg discussed "the mistreatment of dead bodies" not under *Harm to Others*, *Harm to Self*, or *Harmless Wrongdoing*, but under *Offense to Others*, 72–77.

35. See De Baets (2009a, 133–137).

36. Jean Pictet, and others, *Commentary on Geneva Convention I* (Geneva: ICRC, 1952), 54.

37. See also the report of the UN Special Rapporteur on Extrajudicial, Summary or Arbitrary Executions on Mass Graves (UN Doc. A/75/384) (2020). For examples of trials involving charges of mutilation of dead bodies, cannibalism, and refusal of honorable burial, see UN War Crimes Commission, ed., *Law Reports of Trials of War Criminals*, volume 13 (London: UN War Crimes Commission, 1949), 151–152. See also European Court of Human Rights, Case of *Akpinar and Altun v. Turkey* (Application no. 56760/00): Judgment (2007), which was a case of corpse mutilation, at § 82: "[T]he Court has never applied Article 3 of the Convention [prohibition of torture, *adb*] in the context of disrespect for a dead body. The present Chamber concurs with this approach, finding that the human quality is extinguished on death, and therefore, the prohibition on ill-treatment is no longer applicable to corpses . . . despite the cruelty of the acts concerned." See also the partly dissenting opinion of Judge Fura-Sandström.

38. Recognized in ICC, *Elements of Crimes* (2002), Articles 8 (2) (b) (xxi), and 8 (2) (c) (iv), Element 1 (notes 49 and 57 respectively).

39. Recognized in ICC, *Elements of Crimes* (2002), Art. 8 (2) (b) (xxi), and 8 (2) (c) (iv), Element 2.

40. See also *Declaration on the Protection of All Persons from Enforced Disappearance* (1992), Article 17; *International Convention for the Protection of All Persons from Enforced Disappearance* (2006), preamble, Articles 8, 24.

41. ICC, *Rome Statute* (1998), Articles 7.1(i), 7.2(i).
42. ICC, *Rome Statute* (1998), Articles 8.2(b)(ix), 8.2(e)(iv).
43. ICC, *Rome Statute* (1998), preamble.
44. "International Criminal Court Judges Embody 'Our Collective Conscience' Says Secretary-General to Inaugural Meeting in The Hague" (press release SG/SM/8628–L/3027) (2003).
45. *Reports of International Arbitral Awards: Opinion in the Lusitania Cases (November 1, 1923)*, volume 7, 32–44 (quote on 35). For its present use, see *Draft Articles on Responsibility of States for Internationally Wrongful Acts, with Commentaries* (2001), art. 36, § 18.
46. UN, *Declaration of Basic Principles of Justice for Victims of Crime and Abuse of Power* (1985), Principles 1–2 (and 12b). See also UN, *Declaration on . . . Enforced Disappearance* (1992), Article 19.
47. ICC Judge Hans-Peter Kaul in *Case of the Prosecutor v. Jean-Pierre Bemba Gombo*: Fourth Decision on Victims' Participation (Pre-Trial Chamber III) (ICC-01/05-01708) (2008), §§ 40, 46.
48. See De Baets (2009b, 2011).
49. *Basic Principles and Guidelines on the Right to a Remedy and Reparation for Victims of Gross Violations of International Human Rights Law and Serious Violations of International Humanitarian Law* (UN Doc. A/RES/60/147) (2006), Principles 18–23, especially 22. See also *Impunity Principles*, Principles 31–38; UN Human Rights Committee, *General Comment No. 31: The Nature of the General Legal Obligation Imposed on States Parties to the Covenant* (UN Doc. CCPR/C/21/Rev.1/Add. 13) (26 May 2004), § 16. For background, see Grosman (2018) and International Commission of Jurists (2018: 207–213). ICC Statute, Article 75, only distinguishes restitution, compensation, and rehabilitation. Some other forms of reparation, however, can be found under Article 93.1(a) (identification and whereabouts of persons or the location of items) and (g) (examination of places or sites, including the exhumation and examination of gravesites).
50. Article 37 of the *Draft Articles on Responsibility of States for Internationally Wrongful Acts* (2001) provides that "2. Satisfaction may consist in an acknowledgement of the breach, an expression of regret, a formal apology or another appropriate modality. 3. Satisfaction shall not be out of proportion to the injury and may not take a form humiliating to the responsible State."
51. *Impunity Principles*, Principles 1–5, 14, 24.
52. See also Boel et al. (2021).
53. Human Rights Council, *Report on Best Practices in the Matter of Missing Persons* (UN Doc. A/HRC/AC/62) (2010), § 88.

References

Barkan, E. and R. Bush (eds.) (2002). *Claiming the Stones, Naming the Bones: Cultural Property and the Negotiation of National and Ethnic Identity*. Los Angeles, CA: Getty Publications, pp. 201–223.

Barker, A. (2020). The Predatory Present (Presidential Address 118th Annual Meeting American Anthropological Association, 2019). *American Anthropologist* **122**(2): 250–258.

Boel, J., Canavaggio, P., and González Quintana, A. (eds.) (2021). *Archives and Human Rights*. London: Routledge.

Brown, D. (1991). *Human Universals*. New York: McGraw-Hill.
Cholbi, M. (2021). *Grief: a philosophical guide*. Princeton and Oxford: Princeton University Press.
Cotkin, G. (2008). History's moral turn. *Journal of the History of Ideas* **6**(2): 293–315.
De Baets, A. (2004). A declaration on the responsibilities of present generations toward past generations. *History and Theory* **43**(4): 130–164.
De Baets, A. (2007). A Successful Utopia: the doctrine of human dignity. *Historein* **7**: 71–85.
De Baets, A. (2009a). *Responsible History*. New York, Oxford: Berghahn Books.
De Baets, A. (2009b). The Impact of the Universal Declaration of Human Rights on the Study of History. *History and Theory* **48** no. 1: 20–43.
De Baets, A. (2011). Historical imprescriptibility. *Storia della Storiografia* **59–60**: 128–149.
De Baets, A. (2021). Memory and tradition as limits to free expression about the past. *Storia della Storiografia* **79**(1): 19–42.
De Baets, A. (2022). The View of the Past in International Humanitarian Law (1860–2020). *International Review of the Red Cross* **104**, (920–921): 1586–1620.
Dörmann, K. (2003). *Elements of War Crimes under the Rome Statute of the International Criminal Court: Sources and Commentary*. Cambridge: Cambridge University Press.
Eser, A. (2002). Mental elements – mistake of fact and mistake of law. In: *The Rome Statute of the International Criminal Court: A Commentary* (eds. A. Cassese, P. Gaeta, and J. Jones). Oxford: Oxford University Press.
Feinberg, J. (1985). *Offense to Others*. New York and Oxford: Oxford University Press.
Genocide Network (2018). *Prosecuting War Crimes of Outrage upon Personal Dignity Based on Evidence from Open Sources – Legal Framework and Recent Developments in the Member States of the European Union*. The Hague: Eurojust.
Grosman, L. (2018). Principle 34: Scope of the Right to Reparation. In: *The United Nations Principles to Combat Impunity: A Commentary* (eds. F. Haldemann and T. Unger), 369–379. Oxford: Oxford University Press.
Gross, L., Katz, J.S., and Ruby, J. (eds.) (1988). *Image Ethics: The Moral Rights of Subjects in Photographs, Film, and Television*. New York and Oxford: Oxford University Press.
Hutton, P. (1993). *History as an Art of Memory*. Hanover NH and London: University Press of New England.
International Commission of Jurists (2018). *The Right to a Remedy and Reparation for Gross Human Rights Violations: A Practitioners' Guide*. Geneva: ICJ.
Krznaric, R. (2020). *The Good Ancestor: How To Think Long Term in a Short-Term World*. London: W.H. Allen.
Luper, S. (2019). Death. In: The Stanford Encyclopedia of Philosophy (ed. E. Zalta). Stanford: Stanford University.
Madoff, R. (2010). *Immortality and the Law: The Rising Power of the American Dead*. New Haven and London: Yale University Press.
Meyer, L. (2021). Intergenerational justice. In: The Stanford Encyclopedia of Philosophy (ed. E. Zalta). Stanford: Stanford University.
Parfit, D. (1984). *Reasons and Persons*. Oxford: Clarendon Press.
Parfit, D. (2011). *On What Matters*. Oxford: Oxford University Press.
Partridge, E. (1981). Posthumous interests and posthumous respect. *Ethics* **91**(2): 243–264.
Petrig, A. (2009). The war dead and their gravesites. *International Review of the Red Cross* **91**(874): 341–369.
Prior, A. (1978). Past, Present and Future. Oxford: Clarendon Press.

Rosenblatt, A. (2010). International forensic investigations and the human rights of the dead. *Human Rights Quarterly* **32**(4): 922–951.

Schauer, F. (1992). Speaking of dignity. In: *The Constitution of Rights: Human Dignity and American Values* (eds. M. Meyer and W. Parent). Ithaca and London: Cornell University Press.

Scruton, R. (1994). *Modern Philosophy: An Introduction and Survey*. London: Pimlico.

Smilansky, S. (2018). Punishing the dead. *Journal of Value Inquiry* **52**: 169–177.

Soll, I. (1998). On the purported insignificance of death. In: *Death and Philosophy* (eds. J. Malpas and R. Solomon). London/New York: Routledge.

Toshiko, K. and Haub, C. (2020). How Many People Have Ever Lived on Earth? Washington, D.C.: Population Reference Bureau.

UNESCO (1997). *Declaration on the Responsibilities of the Present Generations towards Future Generations*. Paris: UNESCO.

White, A. (1984). *Rights*. Oxford: Clarendon Press.

Winter, S. (2010). Against posthumous rights. *Journal of Applied Philosophy* **27**: 186–199.

Zhao, B. (2011). Public figures and their posthumous reputation. *Storia della Storiografia* **59–60**: 84–105.

Zhao, B. (2014). Legal cases on posthumous reputation and posthumous privacy: history censorship, law, politics and culture. *Syracuse Journal of International Law and Commerce* **42**(1): 39–122.

Zhao, B. (2016). Posthumous defamation and posthumous privacy cases in the digital age. *Savannah Law Review* **3**(1): 15–35.

CHAPTER 3

Continuing bonds and social memory: absence–presence

Avril Maddrell

Department of Geography and Environmental Science, University of Reading, UK

3.1 What are continuing bonds and how are they experienced and expressed?

"Continuing bonds" are expressions of ongoing attachment and relation to a significant other person after their death. It is also a conceptual framework used by scholars of bereavement, which centers on understanding the relationship between the living and the dead, which has gained traction within scholarship on bereavement and the clinical, spiritual, and social care of mourners. Attention to continuing bonds emerged in multiple studies in the 1990s, especially interviews with bereaved and adoptive families, as explored in the influential collection *Continuing Bonds* edited by Klass, Siverman, and Nickman (1996). Understanding continuing bonds includes attention to both the context of religious belief systems and secular experiences of ongoing attachment to the dead. Ongoing attachment is often strongly felt and expressed in association with child, parental, and spousal bereavement, reflecting strength of attachment (O'Connor 2017) and social networks (or convoys) in life (Stemen 2020).

The idea of continuing bonds stood in contrast to dominant Western clinical models, which, grounded in Freud's (1917/1961) work *Mourning and Melancholia* and Bowlby on Attachment and Loss (1969–1980), focused on the need for emotional and psychological separation of the bereaved from the dead, often presented in popular discourse as "closure." Related counseling frameworks sought to facilitate that separation and restore personal autonomy for the bereaved, which was thought to be a necessary prerequisite for making future attachments. Further, those who expressed continued attachment after death to those who had been significant in their lives were often deemed to be presenting

Anthropology of Violent Death: Theoretical Foundations for Forensic Humanitarian Action, First Edition. Edited by Roberto C. Parra and Douglas H. Ubelaker.

pathological symptoms of unresolved or complicated grief or hysteria (a gendered diagnosis usually given to women). It has been noted that Freud's published ideas, so dominant in Western conceptualizations of healthy grieving, did not match his own experience of subsequent bereavement, as evident in his response to the deaths of his daughter and grandson, which he expressed as ongoing love which he did not want to let go (Freud 1961, cited by Silverman and Klass 1996, p. 6). Rather than essentially pathological, continuing bonds with the dead are a common phenomenon across time and cultures (Walter 2018), and numerous researchers and clinicians have found a sense of continuing bonds to the deceased to be evident in many contemporary accounts of the bereaved in varied national and cultural settings. This suggests a blind spot in conceptualizing and understanding bereavement, and in providing the best therapeutic treatment for the bereaved (Klass et al. 1996): "The expectation that they [the bereaved] can and should reach the end of their grief is based on a misunderstanding of normal grieving and does them a disservice" (Rosenblatt 1996, p. 45).

While debate about the definition and parameters of continuing bonds persists (Root and Exline 2014), the core concept has been widely incorporated into psychological models of grief in the twenty-first century (Klass and Steffen 2018). This has included extensive further research on the subject, using both qualitative and quantitative methods. This wider scholarship on the subject has yielded important insights for scholarship and relevant clinical practice, including more nuanced understanding of different expressions and experiences of continuing bonds, in relation to personal, cultural, and religious contexts, and how these different expressions and experiences may or may not relate to clinical concerns. Findings from different types of study need to be evaluated in their wider context and triangulated in relation to other settings and methods, e.g. gender-balanced samples, small cohort long-term in-depth vs. large-scale short-term studies, and ethnically homogenous vs. culturally diverse participants, local vs. international studies. Further research on mapping neural responses to the intensity of continuing bonds would also be of interest (O'Connor 2017). Nonetheless, the findings of both in-depth qualitative and large-scale quantitative studies to date indicate that for many, both those with and without a religious faith, continuing bonds with the deceased are a significant part of the experience of grief and adjustment to bereavement.

An ongoing sense of relationship is at the heart of varied expressions of continuing bonds with the deceased: "many bereaved people continue to experience a strong sense of the presence of the absent deceased in their lives, and work to give, mark, and insist on, the presence of the deceased in ongoing wider social relations, the material topography of the home and the wider environment" (Maddrell 2013, p. 505). This paradoxical relationship between the living and the dead, which is the essence of continuing bonds, is captured in various publication titles, such as *Dead but not Lost* (Goss and Klass 2005), *Rebirth of the Dead* (Howarth 2007), "Living with the deceased" (Maddrell 2013), and "They are in my heart, mind, and cells" (Stemen 2020). The latter highlights the possibility of genetic continuity in addition to ongoing emotional attachment and the role of social memory in keeping the dead "alive." Understandably, this continued sense of attachment is most commonly experienced in relation to those with whom strong bonds have been established in life, notably parents, children, spouses, and siblings (Conant 1996; Silverman and Klass 1996; Field et al. 2003), but may also be experienced and expressed by friends, colleagues, and others within the sphere of influence of the deceased. As noted above, religion is a crucial factor in determining beliefs, experiences, and expressions of continuing bonds.

Many religions include beliefs of an afterlife, whereby the spirit of the deceased continues, for example through reincarnation, as an elevated ancestor spirit, restless ghost, or as a resurrected soul in heaven. For those holding such beliefs, a sense of continued relation to the deceased is often a natural extension of their understanding about the ongoing existence and/or agency of the dead. This is particularly clear in belief systems which center on a form of spiritualism, and those where obligations for the wellbeing of the dead continue through ritual observances, such as Hindu prayers and *Pindas* (rice ball offerings); the performance of *Ghusl* and *Janazah* (body washing and funeral prayers) for Muslims; and Roman Catholic requiem mass. Some religions also ascribe the status of the "sacred dead" to important figures such as saints or gurus who play a key role in wider religious teachings and narratives.

Despite a taboo around talking about death, filial piety in Confucian traditions extends from family-centered social bonds in life into the afterlife, whereby "the traditional practice of ancestor worship fosters the concept of a continued bond with the deceased and with life after death"; moreover, the dead as spirits have influence over the lives of survivors and descendants (Hsu et al. 2009, p. 155). As Klass (2014, p. 99) notes, "In most times and places, the focus of continuing bonds is on the wellbeing and activity of the dead that are linked to the wellbeing and activity of the living." The relationship between the living and the dead is particularly interesting in cultures where there is syncretism, incorporating traditional and institutional religious beliefs. The Acholi in northern Uganda are typically members of the Roman Catholic church but practice traditional burial rituals within their compounds in order to appease the spirits of the dead: "the day-to-day interaction between the living and the dead does not cease at the point of death; indeed, it continues as they proceed to share the same space" (Seebach 2019, p. 166).

However, belief in an afterlife and continuing bonds are not synonymous. Not all religions which profess an afterlife, espouse belief in or encourage continued interaction and relationship with the dead. This can be seen in Protestant Christian beliefs which prohibit intercession for the dead and other belief systems which associate the dead with pollution and a need for absolute separation of the living from the dead, e.g. Hopi Americans (see Silverman et al. 1992). Further, experiences of continuing bonds are not exclusive to those professing religious beliefs in an afterlife, they are also reported by those holding looser informal spiritual beliefs *and* those who have no religious belief in life after death. Some cultural and political movements also have secular equivalents to saints (Goss and Klass 2005), as seen in cases where founders are mythologized. Moreover, on a personal level, many people continue to feel a sense of attachment to, or a sense of the presence of, the deceased. Understanding what is meant by, and the significance of, such varied expressions of continuing bonds as a response to bereavement necessitates placing the loss and meaning-making processes in situated personal and cultural contexts (Klass et al. 1996; Maddrell 2013, 2016; Klass 2014).

Clearly, there is a wide range of expressions of continuing bonds, which can include the continuous spirit presence of the now dead; the occasionally accessible temporally or spatially confined spirit dead; those whose spirit or souls are located in heaven or in a similar spiritual arena; the reincarnated, ghosts and ghost-like presences; utterances, appearances, or interventions by the deceased; the living consulting the dead; messaging, talking, writing, or singing to the dead; practically and/or spiritually caring for the dead via grave or shrine tending and rituals; an ephemeral sense of the presence of the dead; a sense of ongoing feelings for the deceased; and through acting as a mouthpiece or delegate for the dead, either literally or symbolically through continuing/representing their family, social, cultural, or political roles, agenda, or values. Efforts to codify these expressions and practices of continuing bonds include grouping and distinguishing between communication, continuity, and reciprocity between the living and the dead (Stemen 2020) and relation to the family dead, hostile dead, and political dead (Klass 2014). Parasocial grief for dead celebrities and other influential figures is also common in Western society (O'Connor 2017), and this can morph into continuing bonds, as exemplified by some fans attending vigils for Elvis at Graceland, Tennessee.

Both spaces and material objects can function as linking objects between the living and the dead. For example, graves or personal items have been shown to reinforce a sense of continuing bonds in the early phase of bereavement (Goss and Klass 2005). Specific events and practices, such as festivals and anniversaries, and both physical and virtual spaces, are identified as sites of memory, practice, and ongoing connection, with the capacity to trigger mourning and/or consolation (Maddrell 2012, 2016; Jedan et al. 2019). Various types of memorialization can communicate a sense of the vitality of the dead; this includes "living memorials," such as trees, but this animation is also especially evident in burgeoning commercial online memorial pages and informal remembrance via social media sites and gaming platforms (Maddrell 2012). Many of these sites accommodate and facilitate shared memories and continued communication with the deceased, which is particularly evident in the early stages of bereavement and on significant days, such as birthdays and holidays (Kasket 2012; Maddrell 2012; Blower and Sharman 2021). Posting memories and collective reminiscing about the deceased can be a source of new insights into the life of the deceased, but they can also help to "maintain and transform a connection to the deceased person, who for some participants was 'still there' on Facebook" (Akinyemi and Hassett 2021, p. 1). This underscores a sense of ongoing connection that can occur between the living and the dead, a simultaneously relational absence–presence, i.e. the dead are materially absent, but mourners still feel emotionally connected to them and/or a sense of their presence. These continuing bonds can be mediated within particular sites and practices, in this case, through posting in the virtual space of social media, which may also overlap other more materialized expressions, such as tending a grave or altar for the deceased, or symbolic lobbying or practical fundraising for a cause associated with the deceased (Maddrell 2013).

3.2 Continuing bonds and the well-being of mourners

Studies evidence that, as with any relationship, the intensity of expression and experience of continuing bonds may vary over time (Silverman and Nickman 1996), but although some bonds may weaken over time, some may simply recede only to reappear strongly in response to particular stimuli, and some may persist strongly, as shown in a study of widows, the majority of whom reported strong continued attachment to their late husbands, even after the passing of decades and/or remarriage (Dekel et al. 2021). Ongoing attachment to the dead who have been significant in life is generally presented as a psychologically positive experience, for example, bereaved children benefit emotionally from a continued sense of attachment to their deceased parents (Silverman and Nickman 1996); bereaved parents reported perceiving their deceased children as bridges to the transcendental world and/or "guides to right living" (Goss and Klass 2005, p. 267). Therefore, rather than symptomatic of pathology, a sense of continuing bonds can facilitate healthy adaptation to grief (Stroebe et al. 2010; Field et al., 2005; Field and Filanosky, 2010).

Stroebe et al. (2010) argued that a positive relationship with a significant other person is based on secure attachment, and secure vs. insecure attachment in life is strongly correlated with the quality of continuing bonds and degree of grief resolution. Thus, "persons with secure attachment styles will be able to retain attachment to a deceased person to use a continued connection to the deceased to work toward acceptance of loss" (Stroebe et al. 2010, p. 263). By contrast, those who had a clingy (Insecure-preoccupied), or uncertain (Insecure-disorganized/fearful) relationship with the deceased are likely to experience unhelpful continuing bonds over a prolonged period (Stroebe et al. 2010). This approach links quality of attachment to quality of continuing bonds, and the quality of continuing bonds to risk factors for clinically defined complicated grief or prolonged grief disorder, i.e. grief which is considered exaggerated and "unresolved" relative to what is culturally defined as "normal." Thus, not all experiences of continuing bonds are positive.

For some of the bereaved, bad relations with a significant person in their lifetime may be perceived as persisting after the death of that person, evidenced for example in a continued negative internal dialogue with a critical parent or abusive partner. Alternatively, poor health and other misfortunes for the living can be interpreted as caused by or linked to the spirit dead, e.g. a hungry ghost in Chinese, Tibetan, Japanese, and Vietnamese Buddhism or vernacular religion. An ancestor may become a hungry ghost because the whole family has been killed or some other cause of a lack of filial veneration. Some religious beliefs about an afterlife can therefore offer consolation to the dying and the bereaved, but other beliefs and practices may reinforce a sense of continuing bonds, but these may be experienced negatively as a continued reminder of loss or critical presence (Seebach 2019), or as an onerous burden of obligation (Goss and Klass 2005). Regardless of religious beliefs, the cause of death and any sense of guilt or failure on the part of the survivor can also contribute to negative continuing bonds, e.g. feelings of recrimination from the dead or recurring nightmares about the death. Various studies have shown that these factors, quality of relationship/attachment and cause of death/quality of death, are pivotal to the nature of any experience of continuing bonds, the associated impact of bereavement, and the longevity of acute symptoms of grief. Therefore, the nature of any continuing bonds with the dead has implications for the mental, emotional, and spiritual well-being of their mourners.

A large-scale survey of college students suggested that increased continuing bonds caused prolonged grief (Balk 1996). While this evidenced different findings from contiguous qualitative studies, it also raised questions about contextual factors and the duration of the study. Building on the attachment model and a large-scale survey with 502 participants, Field and Filanosky's (2010) study focused on the type of continuing bond expression and risk factors for bereavement adjustment and complicated grief. Using Stroebe et al.'s (2010) distinction between what they described as internalized vs. externalized continuing bonds and other indicators of depression and grief intensity, Field and Filanosky argued that insecure or anxious attachment in life tended to result in unhelpful externalized expressions of continued bonds, such as hallucinations of the deceased or retention of all of the deceased's belongings. In contrast, those who had a secure base of attachment during life tended to experience and express more positive internalized continuing bonds with the dead, such as reliving memories and referring to the deceased as reference point or role model, which supported personal growth, including mechanisms for integrating bereavement and loss into ongoing lives (Field and Filanosky 2010). However, there is a gray area between the categories described, for example, those who continue to feel emotionally dependent on, talk to, and feel they receive guidance from the dead, as reported widely in studies of parental and spousal death (Conant 1996). Importantly, Field and Filanosky also found that the type/cause of death, particularly violent death, was a crucial factor in both the experience of continuing bonds and grief resolution. Unanticipated deaths, such as death by suicide or homicide, or as a result of an accident, are all associated with complicated grief, as are deaths where the bereaved feels a sense of responsibility for the death, for example, as the driver in a road traffic accident which resulted in death. In such cases, even secure attachment in life and an expectation of positive continuing bonds may be overridden by trauma, resulting in negative experiences of continuing bonds, such as difficulty in accepting the death and long-term retention of all of their possessions. After a traumatic death, the bereaved may be less likely to evoke memories of the deceased in order to avoid unwanted reminders of the nature of their death (Field and Filanosky 2010). This blocking of memories also blocks positive continuing bonds, and while this may constitute a short-term coping mechanism, in the longer term it may indicate psychological challenges.

It is notable that in contrast to smaller in-depth qualitative studies, Field and Filanosky's (2010) large-scale study also seemed to confirm Balk's (1996) identification of a correlation between ongoing attachment to the deceased (including *positive* internalized continued bonds) and *poorer* health as measured by grief scores. However, they noted the obvious connection between the closeness of the relationship with the deceased and what is defined as severe grief on the comparative grief scale; hence, those who were particularly attached to the deceased might naturally experience intense grief for a significant length of time, and this may be coupled with a sense of ongoing attachment expressed as continuing bonds. Overall, they concluded: "The positive relationship found between internalized continuing bonds and personal growth suggests that this type of continuing bond may serve as an important resource in facilitating integration of the loss" (Field and Filanosky 2010, p. 25). Ongoing studies are increasingly identifying more nuanced understandings of different types and intensities of continuing bonds. For example, one recent large cohort study using a multidimensional continuing bonds scale, identified post-bereavement meaning reconstruction as a crucial mediating factor between continuing bonds and symptoms of grief (Keser and Işıklı 2022). Another study with bereaved young people in Poland distinguished between concrete negative continuing bonds reflecting mostly externalized presencing of the dead, reflecting attachment anxiety and unresolved grief, relative to symbolic continuing bonds which incorporated both acceptance of the death and ongoing attachment to the deceased, reflecting greater security of attachment and grief resolution (Sekowski 2021). Crucially, findings in this study also showed an overlap of concrete and symbolic continuing bonds is possible and that this can result in prolonged experiences of intense grief, as well as highlighting the need for more international studies (Sekowski 2021).

3.3 Implications for professional service providers

Regardless of the ontological status of continuing bonds, ongoing attachment to the dead on the part of the living has *effects* (Klass 2014) and *affects* (Maddrell 2013). Consequently, there is a strong case for professionals dealing with the bereaved to be aware of, and sensitive to, a bereaved person's or community's sense of continuing bonds to the deceased. This most obviously applies to those overseeing death care and rituals (Silverman and Nickman 1996; Hsu et al. 2009), including the medical, mortuary, forensic, funeral, cemetery, and crematoria professionals dealing directly with the remains of the dead (Maddrell 2013; Maddrell et al. 2021). It is also significant to the work of grief counselors and psychotherapists (Field and Filanosky 2010; Keser and Işıklı 2022), gerontologists (Stemen 2020), adoption agencies (Silverman and Klass 1996), and marriage guidance counselors (Moss and Moss 1996; Dekel et al. 2021).

Sensitivity to particular understandings of continuing bonds requires emotional intelligence and multifaith religious literacy, for example, understanding different religious beliefs about the location and needs of a spirit or soul, the status of the corpse and any requirements for its preparation (and gender roles associated with this), and the religious imperative for prompt burial or cremation. It is also important that professionals accommodate bereaved people's continuing bonds in ways that do not stigmatize the bereaved for their beliefs (Hsu et al. 2009); likewise respectful consideration of ongoing emotional attachment to and concern for the absent-yet-present dead. A wealth of studies also evidence that whether based on religious beliefs or not, many have a particular sense of strong emotional attachment and other continuing bonds with the dead in the first phase of bereavement, but ongoing attachment may be long-lasting, even if the intensity varies. Ongoing feelings of grief and loss are a natural part of life and "after one's first major loss, one will never be completely free of grieving" (Rosenblatt 1996, p. 54). While a sense of even lifelong continuing bonds with the deceased may be positive and contribute to the adaptation of living with loss, they may be problematic for the bereaved, triggering the need for professional support.

References

Akinyemi, C. and Hassett, C. (2021 online first). "He's Still There": how facebook facilitates continuing bonds with the deceased. Omega: Journal of Death and Dying: 1–18.

Balk, D. (1996). Attachment and the reactions of bereaved college students: a longitudinal study. In: Continuing Bonds. New Understandings of Grief (eds. D. Klass, P.R. Silverman, and S.L. Nickman), 311–328. London: Routledge.

Blower, J. and Sharman, R. (2021). To grieve or not to grieve (online)? Interactions with deceased Facebook friends. Death Studies **45**(3): 167–115. doi: 10.1080/07481187.2019.1626937.

Conant, R.D. (1996). Memories of the death and life of a spouse: the role of images and sense of presence in grief. In: Continuing Bonds. New Understandings of Grief (eds. D. Klass, P.R. Silverman, and S.L. Nickman), 179–196. London: Routledge.

Dekel, R., Shorer, S., and Nuttman-Shwartz, O. (2021). Living with spousal loss: continuing bonds and boundaries in remarried widows' marital relationships. *Family Process* **00**: 1–15. doi: 10.1111/famp.12687.

Field, N.P. and Filanosky, C. (2010). Continuing bonds, risk factors for complicated grief, and adjustment to bereavement. *Death Studies* **34**(1): 1–29. doi: 10.1080/07481180903372269.

Field, N.P., Gal-Oz, E., and Bonanno, G.A. (2003). Continuing bonds and adjustment at 5 years after the death of a spouse. *Journal of Consulting and Clinical Psychology* **71**(1): 110.

Goss, R.E. and Klass, D. (2005). Dead but Not Lost. Grief Narratives and Religious Traditions. Walnut Creek, CA: Alta Mira Press.

Howarth, G. (2007). The rebirth of death: continuing relationships with the dead. In: *Remember Me: Constructing Immortality – Beliefs on Immortality, Life, and Death* (ed. M. Mitchell), 19–34. London: Routledge.

Hsu, C., O'Connor, M., and Lee, S. (2009). Understandings of death and dying for people of Chinese origin. Death Studies **33**(2): 153–174. doi: 10.1080/07481180802440431.

Jedan, C., Maddrell, A., and Venbrux, E. (2019). Introduction: from deathscapes to consolationsaceps: spaces, practices and experiences of consolation. In: *Consolationscapes in the Face of Loss* (eds. C. Jedan, A. Maddrell, and E. Venbrux), 1–13. London: Routledge.

Kasket, E. (2012). Continuing bonds in the age of social networking: Facebook as a modern day medium. Bereavement Care **31**(2): 62–69. doi: 10.1080/02682621.2012.710493.

Keser, E. and Işıklı, S. (2022). Investigation of the relationship between continuing bonds and adjustment after the death of a first-degree family member by using the Multidimensional Continuing Bonds Scale. *Journal of Clinical Psychology* **78**: 218–232. doi: 10.1002/jclp.23210.

Klass, D. (2014). Continuing bonds, society, and human experience: family dead, hostile dead, political dead. *Omega* **70**(1): 99–117.

Klass, D. and Steffen, E.M. (2018). *Continuing Bonds in Bereavement: New Directions for Research and Practice.* Milton: Taylor and Francis.

Klass, D., Silverman, P.R., and Nickman, S. (1996). Continuing Bonds: New understanding of Grief. New York: Taylor & Francis.

Maddrell, A. (2012). Online memorials: the virtual as the new vernacular. *Bereavement Care* **31**(2): 46–54.

Maddrell, A. (2013). Living with the deceased: absence, presence and absence-presence. *Cultural Geographies* **20**(4): 501–522.

Maddrell, A. (2016). Mapping grief: a conceptual framework for understanding the spatialities of bereavement, mourning and remembrance. *Social and Cultural Geography* **17**(2): 166–188 [Open Access].

Maddrell, A., McNally, D., Beebeejaun, Y., McClymont, K., et al. (2021). Intersections of (infra)structural violence and cultural inclusion: the geopolitics of minority cemeteries and crematoria provision. *Transactions of the Institute of British Geographers*. doi: 10.1111/tran.12437.

Moss, M.S. and Moss, S.Z. (1996). Remarriage of widowed persons: a triadic relationship. In: Continuing Bonds. New Understandings of Grief (eds. D. Klass, P.R. Silverman, and S.L. Nickman), 163–178. London: Routledge.

O'Connor, A. (2017). Undertanding Transitions in the early Years: Supporting Change through Attachment and Resilience, 2 e. London: Routledge.

Root, B.L. and Exline, J.J. (2014). The role of continuing bonds in coping with grief: overview and future directions. *Death Studies* **38**(1–5): 1–8. doi: 10.1080/07481187.2012.712608.

Rosenblatt, P. (1996). Grief that does not end. In: Continuing Bonds. New Understandings of Grief (eds. D. Klass, P.R. Silverman, and S.L. Nickman), 46–58. London: Routledge.

Seebach, S. (2019). Love the dead, fear the dead: creating consolationscapes in post-war Northern Uganda. In: *Consolationscapes in the Face of Loss* (eds. C. Jedan, A. Maddrell, and E. Venbrux), 166–180. London: Routledge.

Sekowski, M. (2021). Concrete and symbolic continuing bonds with a deceased person: the psychometric properties of the continuing bonds scale in bereaved surviving family members. *Journal of Social and Personal Relationships* **38**(5): 1655–1670. doi: 10.1177/02654075211001574.

Silverman, P.R. and Klass, D. (1996). Introduction: what's the problem? In: Continuing Bonds. New Understandings of Grief (eds. D. Klass, P.R. Silverman, and S.L. Nickman), 3–27. London: Routledge.

Silverman, P.R. and Nickman, S.L. (1996). Concluding thoughts. In: Continuing Bonds. New Understandings of Grief (eds. D. Klass, P.R. Silverman, and S.L. Nickman), 349–355. London: Routledge.

Silverman, P.R., Nickman, S., and Worden, J.W. (1992). Detachment Revisited. *American Journal of Orthopsychiatry* **62**(4): 494–593.

Stemen, S.E. (2020). They're in my heart, mind, and cells: what continuing bonds reveal about social networks. *The Gerontologist* **60**(6): 1085–1093. doi: 10.1093/geront/gnz188.

Stroebe, M., Schut, H., and Boerner, K. (2010). Continuing bonds in adaptation to bereavement: toward theoretical integration. *Clinical Psychology Review* **30**(2): 259–268. doi: 10.1016/j.cpr.2009.11.007.

Walter, T. (2018). How continuing bonds have been framed across millennia. In: *Continuing Bonds in Bereavement: New Directions for Research and Practice* (eds. D. Klass and E.M. Steffen), 43–55: Taylor and Francis Group.

CHAPTER 4

The archaeology of disappearance

Alfredo González-Ruibal

Instituto de Ciencias de Patrimonio (INCIPIT), Consejo Superior de Investigaciones Científicas (CSIC), Madrid, Spain

4.1 Introduction

The disappearance of people has defined political violence during the twentieth and twenty-first centuries. My intention in this chapter is twofold: I would like both to reflect on the wider political economy of disappearance in the context of supermodernity and to explore the possibilities offered by archaeology to reveal the functioning of such economy. I believe that archaeology as a discipline can contribute not only to the recovery of the remains of the disappeared but also to three things: first, the technologies of disappearance, understood at the same time in Foucauldian perspective and in a strictly material way; second, the material context of disappearance (that is, the relations between different forms of disappearance: human and non-human); and third, the disappearance of disappearance – the erasure of the traces of the technologies employed in annihilation.

In relation to the first question, archaeology can reveal the practices of disappearance: the stages, the objects, the spaces employed in each of these stages, and perhaps the most characteristic from an archaeological point of view, the traces, detritus, and remains left by each of the stages of the technical process. Paraphrasing Foucault (1997, p. 26), it could be argued that the point is not so much to "try to grasp subjection in its material instance as a constitution of subjects", but annihilation in its material instance as a dissolution of subjects. In the same way that "new techniques appear through which the individual can be integrated in the social entity" (Foucault 2000, p. 410), new techniques also appeared from the late nineteenth century onward to disintegrate individuals (concentration and extermination camps, racial science, and nuclear bombs). Indeed, during the last century and a half, power has not simply devoted itself to constitute subjects but also to deconstitute them, expelling them from the social body or disintegrating

Anthropology of Violent Death: Theoretical Foundations for Forensic Humanitarian Action, First Edition.
Edited by Roberto C. Parra and Douglas H. Ubelaker.

them completely: the shadows of human bodies left on walls by the explosion of the atomic bomb in Hiroshima are the most obvious manifestation of this new form of necropolitics that obliterates human life (Foucault 2000, p. 416; Mbembé 2003), the negative of biopolitics. Like biopolitics, necropolitics is also "embodied in techniques, and has equipped itself with instruments and eventually even violent means of material intervention" (Foucault 1997, p. 25). What will be discussed here is not just a Foucauldian (that is, metaphorical) archaeology but also a literal one: the study of the materiality of *chaînes operatoires* of disappearance (González-Ruibal 2016; Lemonnier 1992). In archaeology and anthropology, a *chaîne operatoire* is a series of operations that transform raw material into a finished product. In the case of biopolitics, *chaînes operatoires* include spaces and artifacts that make a person into a useful, law-abiding citizen (such as the school and the factory). In the case of necropolitics, the idea is to make a person into nothing (a non-citizen first, and subsequently a non-human, a corpse, and a bunch of ashes), and this is usually a process that requires different spaces and artifacts as well: it can be the transit camp, the concentration camp, the extermination camp or the prison, the place of execution, and the mass grave.

To better understand the political economy of disappearance, it is useful to understand its wider material context. I start from the idea that the notion of disappearance is not something exclusively related with the extermination of political opponents, although this is its most extreme manifestation. Absolute annihilation (which entails physical destruction, the erasure of the traces of such destruction, and the deletion of the memory of what has been annihilated) is a recurring phenomenon in a variety of regimes during the twentieth and twenty-first centuries. The disappearance of political opponents does not represent just one option among many at the disposal of dictatorships or a solution to specific problems or a manifestation of a particular form of sadism, although it is all this as well. An archaeological approach, which focuses on ruins and material remnants left by different forms of annihilation of human and non-human life, can be useful to better comprehend the wider logic of the political economy of disappearance. Disappearance and annihilation can be understood together as one of the foundations of supermodern metapolitics. By metapolitics, I refer to a political worldview that goes beyond specific ideologies and regimes of power; thus, the politics of nature of real socialism, fascism, and liberal democracies were very similar during the twentieth century – nature seen as an external entity to be relentlessly exploited for the economic benefit of human society. As for the notion of the supermodern, I start from Marc Augé's concept of *surmodernité* (Augé 1992), who understands contemporary times as an excessive version of modernity, which is manifested in space, temporality, and self. If we factor in the material and political dimensions – more specifically necropolitics (Mbembé 2003) – we can speak of supermodernity from as early as the transition between the nineteenth and twentieth centuries and without any doubt from the First World War onward (González-Ruibal 2008; González-Ruibal 2019). From the point of view of the political economy of disappearance, it is precisely in those dates when two key phenomena emerge: total war and planned genocide.

Finally, archaeology can do more than study the technologies and material logic of disappearance; it can also explore the ways in which the traces of the crimes are erased, that is, how disappearance disappears. Archaeologists have always studied postdepositional phenomena and the formation processes of the archaeological record (Schiffer 1987), that is, all those elements – anthropogenic and biogeochemical – that alter a specific site. When applied to cases of human rights violations, the archaeological study of the afterlife of places can explain not just what happened at a specific site while in use but also the operations undertaken to erase all traces of what happened: the disappearance of disappearance.

Starting from these three points, in the following sections, I will describe first the modes in which power disappears in supermodernity (concealment, dispersal, and virtualization); I will then explore the forms of continuity between material and human disappearance and what this reveals of supermodern rationality. In the last section, I will examine the elimination of the traces of annihilation.

4.2 Disappearance and power: concealment, dispersal, and virtualization

Supermodenrity has transformed into an ordinary activity what had previously been extraordinary: total disappearance. It can be the annihilation of entire human groups, as in the Holocaust or the Rwandan genocide; the devastation of the environment – the deforestation of the Chaco for soya cultivation, for instance (Gordillo 2014) – or the systematic destruction of the built environment. The latter does not necessarily occur in the context of armed conflict: the annihilation of Shanghai under the effects of advanced capitalism is greater than that provoked by any war in a megalopolis (Ren 2014). Disappearance, thus, becomes one of the many techniques at the disposal of governmentality to establish "the correct disposition of things" (Foucault 2000, p. 208). In some cases, total annihilation is the only way of achieving such disposition. Disappearance has a transitive and intransitive dimension in relation with supermodern power: power makes disappear and power itself disappears. On the one hand, it eliminates everything that is burdensome and uncomfortable or that does not fit a specific idea of the correct disposition of things or that hampers elimination. On the other hand, power itself becomes less physical. "All power will be secret or will not be, since all visible strength is threatened", writes Virilio (1988, p. 24) following Balzac.[1] We can even conclude that to make something or somebody disappear is possible only by disappearing oneself, in the same way that hunting is possible only by camouflaging oneself in the landscape, becoming invisible. In the case of crimes against humanity, resorting to invisibility is dictated by both practical and political efficaciousness.

The work of disappearance implies simultaneously three phenomena: concealment, virtualization, and dispersal. Concealment is one of the great obsessions of supermodernity and works at all levels. Power disappears while annihilating and makes the traces of its annihilation disappear as well. This process of concealment has wider ramifications and can be traced back to the origins of modernity itself. During the late fifteenth century, the spread of artillery led to the design of low fortifications that became less and less conspicuous. By the eighteenth century, most forts did not stand out in the landscape at all. This was taken a step further during the early twentieth century: available fire power leads to the construction of underground fortifications, which are both difficult to locate and to destroy. The general staff and the governments that directed the Second World War in Europe (and its respective exterminations) did so largely underground. At the same time, the colorful uniforms typical of the armies of the eighteenth and nineteenth centuries were replaced by dull ones, allowing soldiers to blend with the landscape (Virilio 1988, p. 104). Techniques of concealment had not stopped growing and becoming more complex: from submarines to aircraft undetectable to radars.

Supermodern power does not disappear only at the moment of delivering the blow. The idea is also not to be seen later. This double concealment is also typical of our era: Assyrians or Romans were not very concerned with their own massacres and destructions. Rather the opposite: if anything, they went great lengths to make them visible and public. They were even immortalized in stone and narrated them in verse and prose. This is just the opposite of what happens in the contemporary era. It is not surprising that recovering evidences of crimes against humanity committed by the state or state actors very often requires digging or at least looking underground: from the location of mass graves using georadar to their exhumation or the excavation of concentration camps. All efforts are made to invisibilize crimes, to put them below the "threshold of detectability" (Weizman 2017, pp. 69–71), a thin space in which things move between the possibility of being and not being identified. This is the case with the chimneys of the crematorium and the columns of prisoners in Auschwitz, which are on the limit of the technically discernible in the aerial photographs taken by the Allies during the war. With current technology, the threshold of detectability could be irrelevant, given the enormous precision of satellite imagery. However, those that are made public have a resolution limited to 0.5 m per pixel for political and military reasons, thus concealing key details for any forensic investigation

(Weizman 2017, pp. 74–75), which means that large regions in the world become disappeared zones, impregnable to public scrutiny: the "pixel", writes Weizman, "has become a sort of ex-territorial zone" (Weizman 2017, p. 79). Pixel manipulation is the virtual equivalent to physical destruction of mass graves or extermination camps: the idea is to eliminate incriminatory evidence, to erase the erasure. It is meaningful that this proliferation of mechanism of disappearance (physical as well as virtual) deployed by power began with the rise of what Virilio (2005, p. 13) has called the "Era of Illusion", that is, a period – coinciding with supermodernity as defined here – in which politics are mediated by technologies of mass deception: from cinema to media and special effects.

However, concealment has deeper roots. The way in which power emerged in the transition from the seventeenth to eighteenth centuries and that replaced the previous sovereign power is a disciplinary regime in which coactions are "concealed as an effective exercise of power" (Foucault 1997, p. 33). The baroque spectacle of sovereignty was replaced by a practice of power much less visible, which was materialized in spaces, instruments, and forms of knowledge. Instead of the law legitimizing sovereign power, we now have the natural rule, that is, the norm, which is based not so much in jurisprudence as in science (Foucault 1997, p. 34). The dangers of this new regime of power are evident; on the one hand, they create a "society of normalization" (Foucault 2000, p. 328), in which deconstructing the discourse of power becomes more difficult; on the other, the rationalization of political power leads more easily to excess, while the power structures remain in the darkness. The invisible annihilations of the twentieth century were doubtless made possible because they were founded on this kind of sovereignty. Sovereign power in the Ancien Régime would have been incapable of carrying out successfully the extermination of entire groups, for both practical and ethical questions: thus, order during the mass execution of Jews during the Holocaust was maintained by deceiving the victims as to their final fate, whereas displacing, concealing, and sanitizing the massacre avoided the problems caused by the instinctive refusal of spontaneous and physical violence typical of pogroms (Bauman 2000, pp. 99–100).

As for dispersal, this is a Foucauldian theme par excellence: the microphysics of power. When we talk about technologies of disappearance, Foucauldian concepts – such as micromechanics, capillarity of power, material operators, or local systems – take a more concrete and physical aspect. Disappearance at a large scale requires a wide and complex institutional materialization, an infrastructure at the same time physical and bureaucratic. Thus, in the collective imagination, the Nazi genocide was perpetrated in half a dozen extermination centers. However, the working of these centers would have been impossible without a dense network of camps and sub-camps dispersed throughout Europe, without the related infrastructures (ghettoes, railways, roads, mass graves, barracks, administrative buildings) and a multitude of people (from Gauleitern to guard-rails). Archaeology contributes to understanding this dispersal of genocidal infra-structures by paying attention to often small, ephemeral, and transit spaces (Sturdy Colls 2015, pp. 199–233), which were crucial in both the logistics of annihilation and making them inconspicuous. The case of the Holocaust is extreme for its spatial reach, its effectiveness, and the number of victims. But in fact, all contemporary systems of disappearance are based on similar systems of capillarity.

Thus, in the case of the Spanish Civil War, the reuse of buildings, such as clandestine detention centers, makeshift prisons, and concentration camps, blurred the difference between everyday space and space of repression, the distinction between inside and outside (Colombo 2011), an indeterminacy that, as in the case of the Soviet Union, imposed an atmosphere of paralyzing terror that facilitated the process of disappearance of the victims (González-Ruibal 2016). Something similar happened in the case of Latin American dictatorships (Salerno et al. 2012; Santos Herceg 2016) and even under liberal regimes: a good case in point is the internment of Japanese-Americans during the Second World War (Camp 2016). Here, the objective was not the physical disappearance of a collective, but its social disappearance. The elements, spaces, and steps that were part of the *chaîne operatoire* of social disappearance were, however, not too different from those employed in genocide: control stations, transit centers, and internment camps (Lau-Ozawa 2021). Control stations were dispersed throughout the United States and always reused extant buildings, which again makes the process smoother and more acceptable. The concept of "landscape" as commonly employed in archaeology (Sturdy Colls 2015; Camp 2016) is useful to grasp the spatiality of disappearance, its dispersal, and capilarity.

Dispersal can take other forms: mass graves are often destroyed and the human remains removed, displaced, and reburied, often far away from the original grave, as happened in the case of the former Yugoslavia (Skinner et al. 2002). In Argentina, bodies and body remains were dispersed through the landscape, including the sea.

Finally, virtualization is tightly linked to the two phenomena described so far – concealment and dispersal. The term is used by Olivier Razac (2015) to describe how supermodern power requires fewer material investments to achieve its goals. Following his argumentation, the stone walls of premodern and early modern regimes of power were replaced by barbed wire in the late nineteenth century, itself replaced by electronic surveillance. Each stage implies a material lightening that does not detract from technical efficaciousness; rather the opposite: virtualization leads to greater control. The greater imaginable control (chips implanted under the skin that permit the geolocalization of a person wherever she goes) is the most effective and at the same time the most visible; power achieves fully the fantasy of disappearance. Virtualization, as dematerialization, has another meaning and another purpose. Concentration camps, which can be considered a dematerialization of the classic nineteenth-century prison, differ from them in the way they annihilate space-time. This is achieved, among other things, through material disinvestment; concentration camps have a very basic layout, with a barbed wire fence and barracks and sometimes not even barracks. Daily life and daily routines, which are crucial for the maintenance of ontological security and the self, disappear in these underregulated spaces. Material disinvestment is shared by Nazi camps (Sofsky 2013), Francoist concentration camps in Spain (González-Ruibal 2016, 2020), and clandestine detention centers in Argentina during the last dictatorship (Colombo 2011). A prison is, in many ways, the opposite of a concentration camp, inasmuch as it is an overregulated and overbuilt structure: there are cells, corridors, refectories, workshops, and yards, and the occupation of each space is perfectly scheduled. Concentration camps, instead, are usually characterized by a minimal number of material markers: it can be a simple space delimited by barbed wire as in Spain in 1939–1940; it can be a tiny cubicle (as in Argentina in the 1970s). Material disinvestment helps dehumanize the victims of the repressive machine, but it has another, more practical end: camps and detention centers can be easily and quickly assembled and disassembled, leaving no trace (or this is what perpetrators think; see below). The work of sovereign power in the Ancien Régime was easily seen and targeted: the example of the Bastille destroyed by revolutionaries in 1789 is perhaps the most eloquent. In a constellation of ephemeral detention centers, transit camps, and sites of extermination, necropolitical power is both dispersed and dematerialized. As Colombo notes for the case of Argentina, the way in which corpses are kidnapped, imprisoned, killed, and disappeared produces the impression of taking place "nowehere" (Colombo 2011, p. 642). Is there a more radical virtualization/dematerialization than the annihilation itself of place?

4.3 Material disappearance, human disappearance

"The evolution of culture resembles the march of an army constituted mainly by stragglers. Perhaps I live in 1913, but a neighbor of mine lives in 1900, and another, in 1880. . . The peasants of the upper valleys of Tyrol live in the twelfth century . . . Happy the country free from stragglers and marauders", writes Adolf Loos (apud Virilio 1988, p. 105), father of architectural rationalism. His desire of a pure architecture, devoid of adornment, strictly functional and homogeneous is nothing but the modern aspiration to a social space equally clean and homogeneous. Under a liberal regime, disappearance is achieved through a mixture of control, repression, and education – the "police" (Foucault 2000, pp. 318–319) – that is, through biopolitics. Under a totalitarian regime, cleansing takes the shape of annihilation, that is, necropolitics (Mbembé 2003). Yet the hygienic element remains and thus the concept of "ethnic cleansing" to refer to genocide or "rear-guard cleansing operation" to describe the extermination of partisans, political dissidents, and civilian sympathizers.

That disappearance goes beyond dispossession, and the elimination of political rivals and their bodies is demonstrated in a particularly obvious way in those cases in which mass assassinations have come hand in hand with processes of systematic destruction of the landscape. In the Soviet Union, during the year of the Stalinist purges (1936–1938), hundreds of thousands of people were made to disappear, while the capital of the USSR was physically and symbolically annihilated, along with the pre-revolutionary landscape more generally: "the old hamlet with its church in the most conspicuous church, with the best houses in the foreground, those of the guard, the pope, the kulak, with its half-ruined huts of the peasants in the background: all this is now beginning to disappear", wrote Stalin (apud Schlögel 2014, p. 353). It is all part of the same technology of desubjectivation: it is not enough with exterminating people; it is necessary also to annihilate the material presence of the old order. The same double extermination, human and material, took place in the territories devastated by the Nazis: while the Jews were being murdered, synagogues were destroyed and the tombs desecrated and the tombstones used to pave the streets (Bartov 2007). In turn, after the end of the war, German cultural landscapes in Eastern Europe were razed to the ground as part of the ethnic cleansing conducted by Russians, Polish, and Czechs (Glassheim 2006). Although murders were indeed committed, in this case it was the landscape, rather than people, that was annihilated.

What has to disappear is often associated with garbage. This is what has happened with one of the main victims of supermodern politics: traditional societies and material cultures. Authoritarian modernity has often implied the destruction of entire cultural landscapes and livelihoods, including those of peasant and indigenous communities. They are seen as backward and out of place in the modern world and are dealt with accordingly: the result is vast landscapes of ruins, of old agrarian systems, villages, and forests (Gordillo 2014; Witmore 2020; González-Ruibal 2021). Sociologist Gatti (2008) writes about the materiality of proper and improper identities in modernity. Proper identities are solid, homogeneous, and clean – like those to which totalitarian or fundamentalist regimes aspire. According to Gatti, their model of materialization is heritage, but we could also talk of monuments, development programs, and public architecture. Instead, improper identities are dirty and fragmentary – those of the subaltern, marginalized and expelled from the dominant system – and have as material correlate garbage, with which they are identified in the hegemonic narrative.

Waste is, in fact, essential to understand the political economy of disappearance. It has been often pointed out that eliminationism (Goldhagen 2010) is predicated on the dehumanization of the Other (Bauman 2000; Haslam 2006; Kelman 1973). This dehumanization is usually understood as animalization (there are manifold comparisons with cattle, vermin, dogs, rats, etc.), but it would perhaps be more precise to talk of reification. Thus, Haslam (2006) distinguishes between animalist and mechanicist forms of dehumanization. Reification, however, consists of something more than the transformation of the Other in an inanimate thing, because things are not treated as the victims of genocidal violence. Eliminationism transforms the Other in refuse, which is the lowest scale of existence; it is an inanimate matter (and thus inferior to any living being, notwithstanding its biological simplicity) and also an amorphous matter – not object but pure thing, useless – and dangerous, the degradation of the thing. Rubbish is "the necessary opposite of identity", the place of "various monsters" (Gatti 2008, p. 5). It is also an abject matter, which attacks our senses. We try to get rid of it as soon as possible; we put it out of our sight; we burn it or bury it so that there are no traces of it.

Rubbish disgusts us because it is a sensorial affront but also because in the last instance, we recognize ourselves in it; we know that it is part of us, in the same way that the Nazis recognized it in their prisoners, and this recognizance increased their hatred and violence. We find ourselves in our refuse and are ashamed of them because rubbish, as Canetti (2010, p. 325) said, is also the proof of all our crimes. In the case of domestic refuse, it can be part of an unhealthy diet or excessive and irresponsible consumerism (Rathje and Murphy 1992). In the case of human refuse produced by eliminationism, it is the stain of a necessary but excessive action that has transgressed all moral limits – thus the remorse and shame that are so common among perpetrators after the end of an eliminationist cycle (Goldhagen 2010). In the case of cultural refuse – traditional landscapes destroyed by authoritarian high modernity (Scott 1998) – it is the price that has to be paid to achieve progress. In all cases, we would like that things and humans disappeared leaving no trace behind, so as to feel free of guilt, as if they had never occurred.

"Dirt is matter out of place . . . Where there is dirt, there is a system", wrote Mary Douglas (2004, p. 44). This is the case irrespective of whether dirtiness is material or human. What is out of place can be organic remains, broken and useless artifacts, people, societies, ecosystems; meaningfully, the primeval forest (wrongly equated with "jungle", secondary-growth forest) has been commonly associated with disorder. In any of those cases, authoritarian modernity has resorted to disappearance, which is not incompatible with recycling: the "internalization of garbage" (Gatti 2008, p. 10). The hair, fat, and ashes of those massacred in the gas chambers were reused in multiple ways. Ashes, for instance, as fertilizers or to pave roads (Dziuban 2017, p. 266). Tropical forests are transformed into wood or sawdust. Dirt is an offense to order: "eliminate it is not a negative act, but a positive effort to organize the environment" (Douglas 2004, p. 2). This returns us to Foucault and his concept of governmentality as a way of correctly arranging things. Disappearance, therefore, is, in the last instance, a fulfillment of a fantasy of order, the price to be paid to achieve a homogeneous and clean identity. The goals are not only symbolic but economic as well; the disappearance of Jews and slaves in Eastern Europe was the previous stage to the colonization of the territory by productive German farmers, whereas the annihilation of the forest represents less an objective per se than the desire to make productive a space perceived as unproductive. Irrespective of the intentions, the destructive operations of supermodernity justify identifying our era as the Age of Devastation (Olivier 2013a, 2013b), and it is within this age that we have to understand the political economy of disappearance that affect humans and nonhumans alike.

4.4 The disappearance of disappearance

If annihilation is one of the signs of supermodernity, another is the disappearance of its traces. Never in human history did rulers invest so much in erasing the evidence of their crimes. At the same time, it is also truth that never in history was so huge the divergence between ethics, technology, and politics. The era of genocide and disappearance is also the period in which the assassination of civilians is more widely seen as morally reprehensible, when *Habeas Corpus* becomes generalized, the age of international humanitarian law, universal justice, and human rights. The economy of disappearance can exist only in the shadows. The Nazis blew up the four Polish camps created with the sole purpose of extermination during the second half of 1943. The soil was plowed, pine trees were planted, and farms were constructed to eliminate all trace of their existence (Gilead et al. 2010). Similar actions of erasure were undertaken in other camps and mass graves (Karski and Kobiałka 2021; Kobiałka 2022). In Chile, clandestine centers of detention were burnt down and demolished after use, during the dictatorship (Santos Herceg 2016). The same process of erasure is found in uncomfortable conflicts. Writer Jonathan Littell visited Chechnya as a member of an NGO during the two wars that razed the region between 1999 and 2005. Three years after the end of the conflict, he returned to Grozni, the capital, which had been reconstructed by Russian authorities. He could barely recognize the city: "It could be stated, without exaggeration, that Paris preserves more traces of the Second World War on the limestone walls of its ministries and museums, than Grozni of its two wars" (Littell 2014, p. 258). The goal of such a quick and systematic reconstruction was to allow people to reoccupy the city and to compensate a region and a people punished by violence exercised by the same country now doing the reconstruction. But it is obvious that it was also a way of erasing the past, making it disappear as if it had never happened. An SS says as much in the first page of Primo Levi's *The saved and the drowned*:

> "No matter how this war ends, we have won the war against you; none of you will survive to bear witness, but even if somebody does escape, the world would not believe him. There might be suspicions, discussions, research by historians, but there will be no certitude, because the proofs will be destroyed with you" (Levi 1986, p. 3).

Referring to the dismantling of Chilean detention centers, Santos Herceg (2016, p. 260) writes: "The type of destruction is generally total and definitive". In a similar way, Olivier Razac (2015, p. 72) writes: "A wall leaves a trace, a fence of barbed wire, does not". This reasoning explains in part the systematic use of ephemeral structures made of wire, metal sheet, and wood in concentration and extermination camps, from the Nazi period to our times. The point is both to save money and fasten the construction and disassembly, as noted above, but also to facilitate the erasure of the traces of the crimes. The fantasy of absolute disappearance has absolute faith in the materials that make it possible. But such faith is unfounded.

If archaeology can contribute something is to expose the strategies of disappearance of disappearance developed by dictatorial political regimes. The mere destruction of evidence is an incriminating element. Archaeological research in Nazi extermination camps has been documenting both traces of what happened in them and attempts to conceal the crimes. The use of conventional excavation techniques and new geophysical survey methods is enabling the identification of traces that were hitherto invisible (Gilead et al. 2010; Kola 2000; Pawlicka-Nowak 2004; Sturdy Colls 2015; Theune 2018; Karski and Kobiałka 2021). The structures that the Nazis put more effort into eliminating were precisely those that made people disappear: the gas chambers and crematoria. In the case of Mauthausen, the Nazis sealed a hole on the wall of the room where the machine that pumped the gas was located. However, the geophysical examination of the wall and the detailed typological analysis of the tiles allowed for an identification and reconstruction of the sequence of construction, use, and sealing. The geophysical survey, in turn, offered a precise image of the orifice through which the toxic substance was pumped (Theune 2018, pp. 83–84). In Sachsenhausen, the excavation of the paved way leading to the gas chamber yielded several dental prostheses and other small objects embedded amid the stones (Theune 2018, p. 80). Artifacts related to the Jewish victims of Chelmno were also discovered in the basement of the corridor that the naked prisoners had to cross in their way to the gas truck (Pawlicka-Nowak 2004). Even in the absence of structures, activities related to annihilation can be detected in small finds. Not only that: those small finds counteract, in their very humanity and singularity, the perpetrators' willingness to leave no trace of individual and collective existences.

We have archaeological examples of internment centers in other contexts that were exhaustively dismantled. In Argentina, the demolition of the Club Atlético was followed by the construction of a highway over the remains, which was, however, unable to prevent the archaeological excavation of the building's basement, which revealed remains of the elevators, three isolation cells, the infirmary, toilets, and operating rooms (Salerno et al. 2012). In another center, Mansión Seré, the military provoked an explosion and burnt down the building to erase evidence of its use, but again archaeology exposed the structure of the building, showing the internal distribution and numerous objects related to the period of repressive use (Salerno et al. 2012). In Spain, the concentration camp of Castuera (Badajoz) was active between April 1939 and April 1940, immediately after the Spanish Civil War (González-Ruibal 2020, pp. 281–296). Archaeological work yielded abundant evidence of the dismantling of the camp (metal sheet, nails, asbestos cement, and zinc washers) and the barbed wire fence (the wire itself and the pickets to fix it). It was also discovered that the living quarters of the camp guards had been reused by the last inmates in charge of dismantling the camp: discarded construction material was found, tin cans and hearths indicating the places where the prisoners rested and ate, including the latrine. This building was also demolished and backfilled with rubble after the abandonment of the camp.

While the demolition of an internment center can hamper the interpretation of the remains, it can hardly conceal its nature. The presence of hundreds or thousands of human beings in many cases has left an enormous volume of buried artifacts. It is calculated that in the transit camp of Westerbork (the Netherlands), there may be as many as 5.2 million objects left (Schute 2018, p. 604). In Buchenwald, in an area of just 32 m^2, 6500 artifacts were found, including 4000 buttons (Theune 2018, p. 79). In addition to offering material testimony on the quantity of people victim of extermination, artifacts are evidence of the process of desubjectivation – the dissolution of the subject – in which many objects and events participate including cattle wagons, barbed wire, the dispossession of personal objects, nakedness, mass assassination, cremation, and the discarding of ashes. Meaningfully, of the whole mass of artifacts recorded in Nazi camps, only a small percentage belongs to personal objects (Starzmann 2014), and there are even less that can be directly related with specific individuals (Schute 2018, p. 604). It is not only in extreme cases of genocide where people are stripped away of things and clothes: Márcia Lika Hattori (2020) has shown how the unclothing of corpses in Brazil both under dictatorship and democracy is a way of preventing people from being identified and therefore an effective way of making them disappear.

Objects are indeed a crucial part of our constitution as persons (Webmoor and Witmore 2008). Depriving people of their possessions is the first step in the annihilation of a subject. And it can also be the first step in the reconstruction of annihilated subjecthood. In the case of extermination camps, it is extremely difficult to retrieve the individual identity of the victims in the usual forensic way (that is, to put together names and human remains), but it is indeed possible to recover both collective identities from lost objects and individual traits of personality – an adornment, an identification tag, a prosthesis, and an object with a name inscribed in it. Besides, special emphasis has been put on the recovery of individuals, which fits well modern forms of subjectivity, but in the case of those killed for political reasons, it should be no less important to identify collective subjects: Jews, women, kulaks, communists, or wage laborers. Thus, in the case of the mass graves of the Spanish Civil War, it is possible to identify collectives of workers through specific artifacts: for example, railway workers, who were killed en masse during the early months of the war for their leftists sympathies (González-Ruibal 2020, p. 34). In fact, it was group solidarity that often led victims to the mass grave or the extermination camp.

The most powerful image of total annihilation is the smoke leaving from the chimneys of the crematoria of the Nazi extermination camps. However, even cremation leaves a trace of ash. As I have pointed out, the Nazis (and the Polish) reused the ashes in construction works and as fertilizer. However, large deposits of ashes are still being documented in the concentration and extermination camps, often associated with small fragments of human bones (Sturdy Colls 2015). In the excavations of Sachsenhausen, a container with ashes related to the crematorium was recently found (Theune 2018, fig. 6.9). When the container was full, the ashes were transferred to the large pits dug in the vicinities of the crematorium. In other extermination camps, such as Chelmno, Sobibor, and Belzec, the presence of large mass graves has been verified with enormous amounts of ashes, bones, and even human hair and fat (Kola 2000; Pawlicka-Nowak 2004). Ashes, writes Dziuban (2017, p. 285), are witness to the "complete and irrevocable destruction of what is no more, but also the reality of something that persists, that is there, as the only thing that has survived incineration".

In more recent crimes, other forms of erasing traces have been documented: in the case of the former Yugoslavia, as noted above, mass graves were emptied and the remains dispersed in other graves. Osteological and DNA analyses have enabled the connection of bones belonging to the same individuals dispersed in different pits (Skinner et al. 2002). In Uruguay, "Operation Carrot" was carried out by the military between 1983 and 1985 with the aim of eliminating evidence of the existence of mass graves with remains of political dissidents. Although many disappeared, archaeological work managed to identify stratigraphic anomalies, fragments of bones, and traces of heavy machinery employed in the destruction of the graves (López Mazz 2017), which confirms at the same time the existence of the graves itself and the operation to make them disappear: two crimes instead of one. In Spain, exhumations in the mass graves of Mérida (Badajoz) exposed a triple annihilation: the graves originally had the bodies of hundreds of soldiers and civilians killed by the Nationalist army at the beginning of the Spanish Civil War. However, the excavation could recover only tiny and scattered remains of bones, buttons, clasps, and other small objects. This shows that the mass graves were emptied at some point during the postwar period. Besides, traces of burning were recorded, which means that the bodies were incinerated during the war (Muñoz Encinar 2016, pp. 157–158). Thus, people were first unlawfully killed, then the bodies incinerated and buried in unmarked graves, and the graves themselves later destroyed. Despite this systematic process of erasure, archaeology was still able to find incriminating evidence both of the massacres and of the attempts to erase the traces.

4.5 Concluding Remarks

The political economy of disappearance is one of the distinctive features of our era. At first sight, it may seem that the annihilation of human beings from another ethnic group, the disposal of rubbish in landfills, and the devastation of the rainforest by agribusiness have nothing to do with each other. Yet they all belong, in the last instance, to the same order of rationality. What lies underneath is a similar desire to attain a clean and homogeneous identity in a space equally clean and homogeneous. Cleansing is not enough, however: it is also necessary to forget that we have cleansed, so that it is not just space and time that remain immaculate but also our conscience. Thus, something as innocuous as the elimination of garbage is not devoid of political connotations. The daily disappearance of garbage from our households allows us to continue consuming in an unsustainable manner, part of the postmnemonic regime of modernity (Connerton 2009). That the most polluting landfills are located further and further away, far from the sight of the rich part of the world, in Sub-Saharan Africa or South-East Asia is also part of the political economy of disappearance.

In this chapter, I have approached the phenomenon of disappearance from an archaeological perspective. Archaeology has important limitations when it comes to producing knowledge, but it also offers some advantages, mainly when it comes to investigating what has been concealed, consciously or unconsciously: if the supermodern authoritarian regimes work within an economy of disappearance, archaeology works within an epistemology of appearance or revelation, inasmuch as its objective is to discover things, bring them to light and unearth them literally: the remains of the killed in a concentration camp, the refuse of homeless people. This process is carried out in public (Moshenska 2009), which again runs against the attempts of concealment characteristic of the politics of disappearance. Furthermore, it is possible to document archaeologically not just the strategies of disappearance but also the way in which disappearance is made to disappear, that is, how the traces of extermination are erased. Finally, the abject is part of the matter with which archaeology works (Shanks et al. 2004), be it garbage or human remains. In this chapter, emphasis has been put on the relevance of abjection to understand the processes of disappearance in supermodernity, in which garbage and people are equated, and both are given similar treatments.

Note

1. The author of this chapter has been unable to locate Balzac's quote. It is possible that Virilio has paraphrased feely.

References

Augé, M. (1992). *Non-lieux. Introduction à une anthropologie de la surmodernité*. Paris: Le Seuil.

Bartov, O. (2007). *Erased: Vanishing Traces of Jewish Galicia in Present-Day Ukraine*. Princeton, NJ: Princeton University Press.

Bauman, Z. (2000). *Modernidad y holocausto*. Barcelona: Sequitur.

Camp, S.L. (2016). Landscapes of Japanese American Internment. *Historical Archaeology* **50**(1): 169–186.

Canetti, E. (2010). *Masa y poder*. Barcelona: DeBolsillo.

Colombo, P. (2011). Espacio y desaparición: los campos de concentración en Argentina. *Isegoría* **45**: 639–652.

Connerton, P. (2009). *How modernity forgets*. Cambridge: Cambridge University Press.

Douglas, M. (2004). *Purity and Danger: An Analysis of Concepts of Pollution and Taboo*. London: Routledge.

Dziuban, Z. (2017). Between subjectification and objectification. Theorizing ashes. In: *Mapping the Forensic Turn* (ed. Z. Dziuban), 261–288. Viena: New Academic Press.

Foucault, M. (1997). *«Il faut défendre la société» Cours au Collège de France, 1976*. Paris: Seuil.

Foucault, M. (2000). The subject and power. In: *Ethics Subjectivity and Truth. The Essential Works of Michael Foucault* (ed. P. Rabinow). New York: New Press.

Gatti, G. (2008). *Identidades (de la) basura. La materialidad de la identidad*. San Sebastián: Hariadna.

Gilead, I., Haimi, Y., and Mazurek, W. (2010). Excavating Nazi Extermination Centres. *Present Pasts* **1**(1) https://www.presentpasts.info/1/volume/1/issue/1/.

Glassheim, E. (2006). Ethnic cleansing, communism, and environmental devastation in Czechoslovakia's Borderlands, 1945–1989. *The Journal of Modern History* **78**(1): 65–92.

Goldhagen, D.J. (2010). *Peor que la guerra: genocidio, eliminacionismo y la continua agresión contra la humanidad.* Madrid: Taurus.
González-Ruibal, A. (Ed) (2008). Arqueologia de la Guerra Civil Española. *Complutum,* 19 (2). Universidad Complutense de Madrid, Madrid. España.
González-Ruibal, A. (2016). Beyond the mass grave: producing and remembering landscapes of violence in Francoist Spain. In: *Legacies of Violence in Contemporary Spain,* 111–136. London: Routledge.
González-Ruibal, A. (2019). *An archaeology of the contemporary era.* Abingdon: Routledge.
González-Ruibal, A. (2020). *The archaeology of the Spanish Civil War.* Abingdon: Routledge.
González-Ruibal, A. (2021). Lessons from a peasant ecology. In: *Heritage Ecologies* (eds. T. Rinke-Bangstad and T. Pétursdóttir), 246–263. Abingdon: Routledge.
Gordillo, G. (2014). *Rubble. The Afterlife of Ruins.* Durham, NC: Duke University Press.
Haslam, N. (2006). Dehumanization: an integrative review. *Personality and Social Psychology Review* **10**(3): 252–264.
Hattori, M.L. (2020). Undressing corpses–an archaeological perspective on state violence. *Journal of Contemporary Archaeology* **7**(2): 151–168.
Karski, K. and Kobiałka, D. (2021). Archaeology in the shadow of Schindler's list: discovering the materiality of Plaszow Camp. *Journal of Contemporary Archaeology* **8**(1): 89–111.
Kelman, H.G. (1973). Violence without moral restraint: reflections on the dehumanization of victims and victimizers. *Journal of Social Issues* **29**(4): 25–61.
Kobiałka, D. (2022). The devil burns gold there: the heritage of Nazi Germany Crimes in Death Valley, Chojnice, Poland. *International Journal of Historical Archaeology* **26**: 359–378.
Kola, A. (2000). *Bełżec: the Nazi camp for Jews in the light of Archaeological Sources: Excavations 1997–1999.* The Council for the Protection of Memory of Combat and Martyrdom, Warsaw.
Lau-Ozawa, K. (2021). Conglomerate infrastructures: ordinary sites used for extraordinary regimes of power. *World Archaeology* **53**(3): 486–501.
Lemonnier, P. (1992). *Elements for an Anthropology of Technology.* Anthropological Papers, Museum of Anthropology, 88. University of Michigan, Ann Arbor, MI.
Levi, P. (1986). *I sommersi e i salvati.* Turin: Einaudi.
Littell, J. (2014). Chechnya album. In: *Forensis. The Architecture of Public Truth* (eds. (ed. Forensic Architecture), 242–263. Berlin: Sternberg Press.
López Mazz, J.M. (2017). Cuando la historia se escribe con una pala. In: *Después de la violencia. El presente político de las dictaduras pasadas* (eds. J. López Mazz, E. Anstett, and D. Merklen), 121–131. Montevideo: Banda Oriental.
Mbembé, J.A. (2003). Necropolitics. *Public Culture* **15**(1): 11–40.
Moshenska, G. (2009). Beyond the viewing platform: excavations and audiences. *Archaeological Review from Cambridge* **24**(1): 39–53.
Muñoz Encinar, L. (2016). *De la exhumación de los cuerpos al conocimiento histórico. Análisis de la represión irregular franquista a partir de la exhumación de fosas comunes en Extremadura (1936-1948).* PhD Dissertation, Departamento de Historia, Universidad de Extremadura.
Olivier, L. (2013a). The business of archaeology is the present. In: *Reclaiming Archaeology. Beyond the Tropes of Modernity* (ed. A. González-Ruibal), 133–145. London: Routledge.
Olivier, L. (2013b). Nous sommes à l'âge de la dévastation. In: *Destruction: Archaeological, Philological and Historical Perspectives* (ed. J. Driessen), 27–36. Leuven: UCL Press.
Pawlicka-Nowak, Ł. (ed.) (2004). Chełmno Witnesses Speak. The Council for the Protection of Memory of Combat and Martyrdom in Warsaw, The District Museum of Konin, Konin and Łódź.

Rathje, W.L. and Murphy, C. (1992). *Rubbish!: The Archaeology of Garbage*. New York: HarperCollins.
Razac, O. (2015). *Historia política del alambre de espino*. Santa Cruz de Tenerife: Melusina.
Ren, X. (2014). The political economy of urban ruins: redeveloping Shanghai. *International Journal of Urban and Regional Research* **38**(3): 1081–1091.
Salerno, M.A., Zarankin, A., and Perosino, M.C. (2012). Arqueologías de la clandestinidad: una revisión de los trabajos efectuados en los centros de detención clandestinos de la última dictadura militar en Argentina. *Revista Universitaria de Historia Militar* **2**: 49–84.
Santos Herceg, J. (2016). Los centros de detención y/o tortura en Chile: su desaparición como destino. *Izquierdas* **26**: 256–275.
Schiffer, M.B. (1987). *Formation Processes of the Archaeological Record*. Albuquerque, NM: University of New Mexico Press.
Schindel, E. (2019). Desiertos, mares, islas: geografías de intemperie como espacios de desaparición en contextos migratorios. Paper presented at the Seminario 'Nuevas desapariciones, nuevos espacios'. Universidad del País Vasco, Bilbao.
Schlögel, K. (2014). *Terror y utopía. Moscú en 1937*. Madrid: Acantilado.
Schute, I. (2018). Collecting artifacts on holocaust sites: a critical review of archaeological research in Ybenheer, Westerbork, and Sobibor. *International Journal of Historical Archaeology* **22**(3): 593–613.
Scott, J.C. (1998). *Seeing Like a State: How Certain Schemes to Improve the Human Condition have Failed*. New Haven: Yale University Press.
Shanks, M., Platt, D., and y Rathje, W.L. (2004). The perfume of garbage: modernity and the archaeological. *Modernism/Modernity* **11**(1): 61–83.
Skinner, M., York, H.P., and Connor, M.A. (2002). Postburial disturbance of graves in Bosnia-Herzegovina. In: *Advances in Forensic Taphonomy: Method, Theory, and Archaeological Perspectives* (eds. W.D. Haglund and M.H. Sorg), 293–308. Boca Raton: CRC.
Sofsky, W. (2013). *The Order of Terror: The Concentration Camp*. Princeton: Princeton University Press.
Starzmann, M.T. (2014). Excavating tempelhof airfield: objects of memory and the politics of absence. *Rethinking History* **18**(2): 211–229.
Sturdy Colls, C. (2015). *Holocaust Archaeologies: Approaches and Future Directions*. New York: Springer.
Theune, C. (2018). *A Shadow of War. Archaeological Approaches to Uncovering the Darker Sides of Conflict from the 20th Century*. Leiden: Sidestone Press.
Virilio, P. (1988). *Estética de la desaparición*. Barcelona: Anagrama.
Virilio, P. (2005). *Desert Screen. War at the Speed of Light*. London: Verso.
Webmoor, T. and Witmore, C.L. (2008). Things are us! A commentary on human/things relations under the banner of a 'social'archaeology. *Norwegian Archaeological Review* **41**(1): 53–70.
Weizman, E. (2017). Violence at the Threshold of Detectability. In: *Mapping the Forensic Turn* (ed. Z. Dziuban), 63–88. Vienna: New Academic Press.
Witmore, C. (2020). *Old lands: A chorography of the Eastern Peloponnese*. Abingdon: Routledge.

CHAPTER 5

Bioarchaeology of violent death

Anna Osterholtz[1], Debra Martin[2] and Ryan Harrod[3]

[1]*Department of Anthropology and Middle Eastern Cultures, Mississippi State University, Mississippi, MS, USA*
[2]*Department of Anthropology, University of Nevada, Las Vegas, NV, USA*
[3]*Academic Affairs, Garrett College, McHenry, MD, USA*

5.1 Introduction and background

This chapter specifically examines the concept of violent death, and so the topics focused upon revolve around perimortem indicators of death and peri- and postmortem processing that is indicative of violence. The topic of violence in bioarchaeology has been explored with a multitude of approaches, and the authors of this chapter have previously highlighted the importance of studying antemortem trauma as indicators of lived experience and the social role of violence within identity formation (e.g. Martin and Osterholtz 2012; Martin et al. 2010, 2012b; Martin and Harrod 2015; Harrod et al. 2012a, 2012b, 2013; Baustian et al. 2012; Martin and Harrod 2012; Martin and Frayer 1997; Pérez-Flórez and Harrod 2021).

Here, we focus on the contributions of bioarchaeology to understand how perimortem trauma can reveal violent death, or deaths caused by direct violent actions, at either intra- or inter-group scales. Central to this discussion will be explorations of four different categories of violent death: (i) Massacres; (ii) kretaphenous violence (witch destruction) and ritualized murder; (iii) Captives, captivity, and the enslaved; and (iv) raiding and warfare. These categories do not encompass all the elements of violent death, but we specifically exclude interpersonal violence (homicides, domestic partner abuse, child endangerment, and abuse). This is not to downplay the importance of that kind of violence or those deaths. The entire range of violent death simply cannot be encompassed within a single chapter, and so we focus here on group-level violent interaction resulting in death.

Anthropology of Violent Death: Theoretical Foundations for Forensic Humanitarian Action, First Edition.
Edited by Roberto C. Parra and Douglas H. Ubelaker.

All of the types of violent death discussed here are on some level socially legitimized and sanctioned, from witch execution to warfare. These are found cross-culturally and across all temporal periods as distinctive and culturally specific forms of communication and cultural expressions that are "encoded with intricate cultural meaning" (Martin et al. 2013, p. 75). In this chapter, we take the view that violence, particularly group-level violence, can be seen as a form of social communication (Osterholtz 2012) that becomes embodied in skeletal assemblages with varying demographic profiles, types and locations of traumatic lesions, and archaeological contexts. "To ignore these cultural expressions or, worse yet, suggest they do not exist, minimizes our understanding of violence as a complex expression of cultural performance" (Martin et al. 2013, p. 75). Using this approach draws on social theory and methods from a range of disciplinary approaches and represents a non-reductionist and non-stereotypic way of understanding violent behavior in the past.

Another reason to focus on group-level violent death is that determining the cause of death based solely on skeletal remains is difficult and very often equivocal (Seidel and Fulginiti 2014). By building on patterns visible in multiple individuals, violent death can be both identified and contextualized within larger social structures. For example, internationally known massacre theorist Klusemann (2012, p. 479) writes that massacres should be viewed as a process or as an unfolding of nonrandom patterns or a chain of events that preceded the massacre itself and continue long after. Bioarchaeologists Anderson and Martin (2018, p. 1) have used this perspective to demonstrate that for over 20 000 years, human groups have used massacres and violent death is shaped by culturally specific motivations that are propose that massacres have a cultural logic of their own that is affected by social and historical dynamics. Hartley (2007, p. 238) shows that documenting forms of violence such as massacres through time is an important piece of understanding their persistence and use over time and space. Ultimately, the goal of bioarchaeology is to be able to say something about the meaning that cultures ascribe to the forms of violence that they use.

In order to establish that violent death has occurred, patterns of traumatic injuries, fractures, wounds, and cut marks are used to identify violence-related versus other causes of changes to skeletonized human remains, specifically those traumatic lesions occurring at or around the time of death. Termed perimortem lesions, these bony changes have the appearance of a vital reaction but lack any signs of healing. Vital (or antemortem) responses include as example hinge fracturing, which provides an indication of recently live organic components in the bone, thus allowing bone to bend before it breaks (Sauer 1998; Ubelaker and

Adams 1995). Other vital responses include osteogenic responses consisting of healing including initial callus formation. This implies that the trauma was survived and initially not lethal. However, lethal or perimortem injuries will have the appearance of antemortem fractures but lack any indications of healing and osteogenic response (Galloway et al. 2014). Because this definition for perimortem is descriptive, it is not limited to a specific time frame. Wounds may be described as perimortem if they occur weeks or even months after death if preservation of the organic components of bone is sufficient to allow for a vital response when the bone is altered. So, perimortem injuries may describe violent interaction that contributes to death, or it may be indicative of postmortem processing that occurs within the window where organic components are pronounced within the bone itself. Because of this, the nature of the bony injury is only one indicator for group-level violent death used in this chapter.

In addition to the identification of perimortem injury, the nature of the mortuary assemblage will be addressed as well. Different demographic signatures are expected for different types of group-level or collective violence including a wide range of culturally sanctioned "activities such as warfare, raiding, feuding, and ambushes (Durrant 2011, p. 429)" (Martin and Harrod 2015, p. 125). For massacres, as one example, often the entire population including both male and female adults as well as children and infants is represented in the mortuary assemblage (Hartley 2007; Harrod 2018a). But massacres can also be more demographically variable and raiding; warfare, captivity, and enslavement can be carried out on communities, or they can target subgroups within communities. For raiding, based on identified raiding assemblages, there is often an underrepresentation of young adults and adult males (e.g. Zimmerman 1997; Willey 1990; Wilkinson 1997). For assemblages resulting from warfare, there is often an abundance of young adult males (Chagnon 1988; Wrangham and Peterson 1996).

The context of the dead must also be examined, including the burial location. Burial locations near identified battlefields are more likely to be the result of warfare (e.g. Novak 2007), whereas massacre assemblages may be found within habitation sites (e.g. Alfsdotter et al. 2018). Differential post-mortem handling and processing of individuals from within such contexts may also be indicative of violent death. This is further explored below with respect to kretaphenous violence (witch destruction). In these cases, as well as with politically or ritually motivated killings that are socially sanctioned, there may be an identifiable pattern of taphonomic processing of the corpse (e.g. Walker 2008, 2009; Darling 1998). This patterning is important to the identification of violence carried out with specific motivations in mind.

5.2 Categories of group-level violent death

5.2.1 Bioarchaeology of Massacres

Bioarchaeology and forensic anthropology offer unique perspectives on studies of massacres, and this leads to the interpretation of human remains in a broader context. Massacres and other forms of large-scale violence have been documented in many different cultural contexts, ancient and contemporary. While the analysis is initially focused on the victims, moving the analysis to the broader political and cultural context necessitates using social theories about the nature of massacres. Dwyer and Ryan (2012, p. XV) define massacres as the "killing of one group of people by another group of people, regardless of whether the victims are armed or not, regardless of age or sex, race, religion and language, and regardless of political, cultural, racial, religious or economic motives for the killing". This is admittedly a broad and very inclusive working definition, but the breadth expressed here is important because too often massacres are seen as anomalies or a form of extreme deviance that is rare. In fact, massacres have been documented that are as old as 10 000 years (Erdal 2012; Lahr et al. 2016).

Another definition of massacres that has been useful in documenting extremely ancient cases is the one proposed by Alfsdotter et al. (2018, p. 428) where they state that massacres are "an act of intentional murder upon a mass of people who were not prepared for battle, with the killing being conducted by a group". Who is targeted and the overall demographics (composition of the victims by age and sex) show variability and nuance. Massacres have considerable time depth, and they show culturally specific variability in strategy and execution styles and have also been shown to be contextually contingent upon social, political, and ideological purposes in the societies in which they occur (Anderson and Martin 2018).

The following provides examples of violent deaths due to massacre events across different time periods and different cultures. As these case studies demonstrate, violent acts involved in massacres are preserved in the bioarchaeological record of the past and can serve to broaden the understanding about the origin, nature, and motivations of massacres in early groups. As anthropologists, bioarchaeologists have the tools and theoretical frameworks needed to go beyond simple descriptions of violent death into interpretations that illuminate motivation, planning, execution, and longer-term effects of massacre events.

5.3 Case studies illustrating integrative approaches to massacres in the past

5.3.1 Sandby borg Massacre (1500 BCE)

An overview of one team of researcher's methods provides a snapshot of how skeletal remains are analyzed. Alfsdotter et al. (2018) and Alfsdotter and Kjellström (2019, 2020) discuss evidence of a massacre that took place within the Sandbyborg ringfort (AD 400–550) on the island of Öland in modern southeast Sweden. Alfsdotter (2019, p. 433) notes that the remains exhibit a lack of defensive-related trauma, appear to have been killed with expedient lethal blows, and with no evidence of mutilation or trophy-taking, suggesting that the victims were taken by surprise and that the purpose of the attack was to kill an entire small village, including the animals.

Methodologically, in order to explore the particulars of the peri- and postmortem experiences and taphonomic processes affecting these remains, Alfsdotter and Kjellström (2020) present a taphonomic analysis of the massacred individuals using a combination of techniques including skeletal element preservation via zoning (Knüsel and Outram 2004), weathering stages (Behrensmeyer 1978), fracture analysis (Outram 2002), and archaeothanatology to determine the original depositional context of the massacred individuals. Also known as *anthropologie de terrain*, archaeothanatology is the in situ taphonomic analysis of a body that considers the postmortem manipulation and decomposition process of a corpse within different mortuary contexts (Alfsdotter and Kjellström 2020; Duday 2009, p. 267). Based on their analyses, Alfsdotter and Kjellström (2020) conclude that the spatial distribution, random positioning of the bodies, presence of rodent and carnivore gnawing, weathering, and the lack of evidence that the remains were manipulated from their primary depositional context by other humans at any point postmortem suggest the victims of this massacre were left exposed and unburied where they died and subsequently decomposed within the houses or streets. Furthermore, Alfsdotter (2019) points out that macrobotanical analyses, articulated and commingled skeletal remains of animals, and the overall archaeological context of the ringfort indicate that activity and habitation within the ringfort ceased after the massacre event with no evidence that it was resettled.

To understand how these remains were perceived by those who witnessed them and why these remains were left unburied, Alfsdotter (2019) integrates the osteological (Alfsdotter et al. 2018) and taphonomic analyses (Alfsdotter and Kjellström 2020) of these individuals with a theoretical framework that juxtaposes the final disposition of the bodies of the victims to contemporary normative mortuary practices and their postmortem treatment to contemporary Scandinavian Iron Age social responses and ideologies surrounding death and dying and contextualizes them within a discussion of the postmortem agency of human remains. By framing the lack of burial of the victims of the Sandby borg ringfort massacre as a deliberate and aggressive social tactic, Alfsdotter (2019, p. 438) proposes that the victims' bodies themselves were a source of political power for the perpetrators, which they used to manipulate the social and spatial memory of survivors and witnesses, and to redraw the social and territorial landscape. In this way, Alfsdotter (2019) and Kjellström (2020) present a theoretically rich case study that highlights the social and ideological implications inherently linked to the postmortem treatment of victims of violence and the tangible agency that dead bodies exert over the living, which arguably can have longer-lasting repercussions and significance for living and descendant generations than the initial act of violence itself.

5.3.2 Potočani, Croatia (6200 BCE)

Novak et al. (2021) combined bioarchaeological analyses with genome-wide DNA analyses to extrapolate the relationships and identities of 38 out of the 41 victims of a 6200-year-old massacre recovered from an Eneolithic (Copper Age) mass burial in Potočani, Croatia. The bioarchaeological analyses of the individuals recovered from the Potočani mass burial revealed the burial sample is equally represented by adult males and females and subadults from a wide range of age groups. At least 13 (6 subadults, 3 adult males, and 4 adult females) individuals exhibit perimortem cranial traumas to the back and side of the head, which were inflicted by different weapons and likely by numerous attackers. The archaeological context suggests that the collective groups were all interred in a single depositional event.

The paleogenomic DNA analyses revealed that the majority of the victims were not members of a closely related family group but likely represented a large farming community of several diverse lineages and that they were members of a homogenous population and therefore unlikely immigrants to the region. These results, Novak et al. (2021) conclude, indicate that the Potočani mass burial represents an indiscriminate massacre of an unrelated whole or part of a community and provides further evidence that large-scale massacres were a significant and important social process in pre-state societies. Novak et al.'s (2021) study is a good example of the necessity of a multidisciplinary approach to identify and interpret violence in the past and the utility of paleogenomic data in reconstructing the context of massacres and the identities of the victims.

These examples demonstrate new resources and ways of interpreting trauma and violence in increasingly nuanced ways. While skeletal trauma is evidence of warfare and massacres, the case studies above highlight other lines of evidence that provide more nuanced and compelling explanations for the data. Interpreting the reasons for skeletal trauma must take into consideration the cultural and environmental aspects while incorporating ethnographic analogy to enhance each study.

5.3.3 Spanish Civil War (1936–1939)

Contextualized trauma analysis and DNA analyses also play a significant role in the identification and recognition of human rights atrocities and genocides from historical and modern temporal contexts for medico-legal purposes. Owens (2021) details the 2017 exhumation and analysis of Timoteo Mendieta Alcalá and 27 other individuals who were executed and buried in a cemetery in Guadalajara Castilla La Mancha between July and November 1939, during the Spanish Civil War (1936–1939) and reign of fascist dictator Francisco Franco. The authors combine DNA identification, bioarchaeological analyses, and archaeological analysis of the material possessions included in the burial context to identify and interpret the executed individuals' lives, lived experiences of imprisonment, and subsequent executions. The bioarchaeological analyses of 24 burials in the primary grave revealed the victims exhibited gunshot trauma consistent with firing squads and execution-style wounds to the cranium as well as perimortem blunt and sharp force trauma.

The authors also found that 20.8% of the individuals exhibited healing antemortem trauma suggestive of extensive assault and torture in the period leading up to their executions (Owens 2021, p. 3). The bioarchaeological data presented by Owens (2021) reveal *unrecorded* and historically silenced dimensions of the Spanish fascist regime between 1936 and 1939, which contributes to extant research on global atrocities and speaks to the true human cost of the Spanish Civil War that historical and political narratives silenced through the 1977 Pact of Forgetting and other sociopolitical revisionist narratives of the period.

These case studies illustrate the ways that modern bioarchaeology documents the existence of massacre victims and also the ways that the cultural context is reconstructed so that the interpretations provide understanding the culturally specific ways that massacres were used. Understanding the social meaning behind massacres in any period begins with identifying who the victims were (e.g. age, sex, and place of origin), their relatedness to one another, and their genetic relatedness and relationships to the broader regional population. While bioarchaeological analyses can reveal some of these nuances, the more recent incorporation of paleogenomic analyses has greatly enhanced researchers' abilities to identify the subtle genetic relationships between the victims of massacres from mass grave contexts that taphonomy and commingling may obscure from. For instance, knowing if the massacred population is represented by a single sex versus both sexes, or a single genetically related family group versus a whole community, can significantly alter interpretations why and how massacres in the past took place.

5.3.4 Kratophanous violence and ritualized death

5.3.4.1 Ritualized death

Here, we also use a case study approach to illustrate ritualized and kratophanous violence (witch destruction). The focus of this is on ritualized destruction of the body in prehistoric contexts in the southwestern portion of the United States, identified in the literature as extreme processing (EP). This terminology was first introduced by Kuckelman et al. (2000). This pattern of body processing and deposition should be viewed as politically and/or religiously motivated violence.

Within the US Southwest, the discovery and analysis of assemblages with EP have occurred since the 1970s and show a wide variety of taphonomic indicators, including high degrees of fragmentation and commingling, burning, and evidence of tool marks and blunt force trauma. These disarticulated and fragmented assemblages show different demographic patterns from what would be expected from warfare in that they tend to reflect more of a living demography of a population, consisting of both males and females and individuals of all ages. All individuals show similar patterns of processing, inconsistent with an assemblage subject to raiding for females or warfare activities (Osterholtz 2018a). This demographic leveling of the assemblages suggests a different use of this pattern of violence. Individuals are broken down into fragments and mixed together in the depositions, a process that is formulaic and repetitive. Through examination of the elements, it is possible to reconstruct the systematic disassembly of the human body. Assemblages range in size from a few individuals to dozens of individuals, potentially representing clans or family groups singled out for this processing.

The identification of the assemblage at Sacred Ridge at around AD 810 throws causal explanations such as cannibalism or violence due to climate change or resource depletion into debate (Osterholtz 2018b; Potter and Chuipka 2010). Sacred Ridge contained two pit structures: one that may have acted as a processing center and the other that acted as the primary depositional space. The remains of at least 33 individuals of both sexes and all age categories were identified. All show significant amounts of perimortem fracturing, commingling, fragmentation, and burning (Stodder et al. 2010; Stodder and Osterholtz 2010; Osterholtz 2012, 2014, 2018a). Stratigraphically, this appears to be a single event and no materials postdate the creation of this assemblage.

In looking at EP assemblages, there are alternative hypotheses in addition to that of cannibalism. Raiding and warfare (explored elsewhere in this chapter in greater detail), politically motivated massacre (also explored elsewhere in this chapter), and witch execution or kratophanous violence can also be examined as potential causes. All of these would present different demographic signatures as well as present different rates for specific acts such as scalping, disarticulation, and processing methods. At its heart, this is a discussion about taphonomic processes as much as signs of direct trauma such as cranial depression fractures and postcranial trauma.

Instead of an approach predicated on a single explanation for violence within the Southwest, different types of violent interaction should be understood as serving different social functions. EP presents as qualitatively different than warfare and may be better understood if examined through a performative and poetic lens (e.g. Whitehead 2004a; Osterholtz and Martin 2017; Osterholtz 2020; Martin and Osterholtz 2020; Kuckelman 2020). This approach seeks to contextualize this pattern of violence, focused on the type and amount of body processing, how and when this processing occurred, and how it may have been viewed by both the participants and the witnesses to it. In this way, we can see EP events as a reflection of social change and a mechanism to restore balance (Martin and Osterholtz 2020; Palkovich 2012).

5.3.5 Kratophanous violence or witch execution

If EP events can be seen as society-level leveling mechanisms designed to bring communities back into a state of harmony or balance, then witch executions in the prehistoric southwest may be seen as smaller-scale mechanisms designed to remove an element that is pushing the community out of balance. The execution of witches has been identified ethnographically, with early researchers such as Parsons identifying the killing of witches (Parsons 1927, 1939). Witches are tied to origin stories as well as integral to understanding relationships between humans and the supernatural. They exist alongside humans but are not supernatural themselves. They are, in effect, the *other* living among the community, causing illness and death. The body of the witch becomes an object that becomes the focus of ritual destruction. Walker (1998) essentially views these bodies as ritually charged artifacts that need to have a special discard pathway as they are ritually charged in ways dangerous to community. Using Eliade's concept of kratophany, Walker describes violence directed toward witches as kratophanous, as this violence is intended to mitigate "darker and fearful aspects of sacred power" (Walker 1998, p. 264). He defines kratophanous behaviors as "activities or interactions that ritually redirect or end the life histories of people, portable artifacts, or architecture in order to contest their use within an ongoing ritual tradition" (Walker 1998, p. 265).

Punishment of witches could be an attempt to help right the course of the community toward balance. "..., the persecution and killing of witches was a way to ritually dispose of individuals, families and communities who were practicing sorcery and bringing droughts, illness and misfortune" (Martin and Harrod 2020, p. 308). Punishment could mean a variety of things, from fines to ostracism to physical torture and depending on the actions the witch had performed and the social position of the accused and the community from which they come (Darling 1999). Darling (1999, p. 737) sees the punishment of witches as a regulatory mechanism to decrease intracommunity tension by "redirecting 'violent' or potentially inappropriate actions in defined ways," noting that "ritual killing of witches effectively approximates an act of sacrifice in its attempt to reaffirm socioreligious norms of behavior and to protect the community through purification and destruction of evil". This interpretation draws on performative and ritual notions inherent within Whitehead's poetics model. Whitehead (2004a, 2005a, 2007) argued that ritual violence conducted in a performative format reinforced social structures and community identity. Following this line of argument, the punishment and execution of witches have tremendous power to reinforce social order, especially when conducted by religious specialists, and act both to destroy the negative elements within society while affirming group identity and to bring the community back into balance. This act "emphasizes the sacredness of the event" (Darling 1999, p. 738).

Archaeologically, both Darling (1999) and Walker (1998) discuss expected contexts for the identification of kratophanous depositions. Typically, these depositions are found either in pit structures believed to be dwellings or in ritual structures such as kivas. While processing may occur in other locations, depositions in these locations are common. These may appear either as secondary deposits (with increased commingling and incomplete representation of all expected skeletal elements) or as primary deposits with whole limbs in articulation. It is expected that these remains will be mixed in with structural fill or refuse as well as broken objects.

Walker (1998) examines differential disposal patterns of processed bodies as potential kratophanous violence at numerous sites within the Southwest. He asks the question "When is a Prehistoric Pueblo Witch?" (Walker 1998, p. 277), a specific phrasing designed to examine context over specific taphonomic indicators [such as those identified by Turner and others (e.g. Turner II et al. 1993; Turner II and Turner 1999; Turner II and Turner 1992; Turner II and Morris 1970; White 1992; Nickens 1975)to identify cannibalism]. He notes numerous incidences of intentional structural burning as closing rituals, ritual abandonment, and the presence of ritually important artifacts in association with processed individuals as possible indicators for witch depositions. At the site of Homol'ovi II, dating to between AD 1330 and 1400, numerous potential examples of kratophanous violence can be found. Structure 706, a kiva, contained the remains of three individuals (one adult female, an adolescent male, and a child) within a pile of boulders covered by an adobe cap. The left femur of the adolescent was severed above the knee perimortem, and the lower portion of the limb was not recovered with the body. All artifacts found in this structure were broken and deposited above the adobe cap. Structure 704 contained an individual lying on the structure's bench with the head protruding into the ventilator shaft. Hand and foot bones exhibited signs of burning; the excavators posited that the individual may have been alive when the structure was set on fire as the head was found within the ventilator shaft. Two projectile points were recovered from the fill surrounding the abdominal cavity (Walker 1998). The individual in

Structure 704 closely mirrors ethnographic accounts of witches being shot and then subjected to burning (Darling 1998), though in this case, the burning also acted as a ritual closing mechanism for the kiva in which it occurred.

5.4 Differentiating between kratophanous violence and ritualized death

Taphonomic indicators are similar between these two types of depositions, with high degrees of fragmentation, commingling, and signs of disarticulation and dismemberment. Also, both types of assemblages may be found in dwellings or in ritualized structures such as kivas. We argue here that this may simply be a matter of scale, with individuals or small numbers of individuals who transgress normative processes identified as witches and disposed of along highly ritualized lines. "The persecution and execution of witches was a way of ritually disposing of individuals, extended family, or even whole communities that were seen as transgressors" (Martin and Harrod 2020, p. 311). When this is no longer sufficient to rebalance the community, grander actions may necessitate a larger scale of violence, leading to the destruction of whole lineages or communities. Essentially, these are similar patterns, but differ in scale. In larger assemblages, such as that at Sacred Ridge, a larger group was targeted, and this necessitated the ritual closing of the entire site (it was not inhabited again by Puebloan groups). In these larger scale assemblages, which can be termed massacres, larger political ends may have been served than by the destruction of individual witches as evident in the smaller assemblages at Homol'ovi or the smaller sites surrounding Sacred Ridge. The scale sets them apart, but the underlying goals of returning to balance may be motivating factors for the violent acts themselves.

5.4.1 Captives and the enslaved

Bioarchaeological and archaeological signatures of captivity are evident in demographic composition of the sites (Kohler and Kramer Turner 2006; Cameron and Martin 2012), mortuary patterns of the burials (Martin and Akins 2001), and the bones of the individuals themselves (Harrod and Martin 2014; Martin and Harrod 2015). In most societies, women and children are more often targeted as potential captives; this is especially true when commercial and industrial activities are excluded, and one reality that this group faces more often than men is sexual assault. Based on the International Labour Organization (ILO) report of the individuals that are part of a system of forced sexual exploitation, women and girls make up at least 99% of the 4.8 million people identified as sex slaves (International Labour Organization 2017, p. 39).

The importance of highlighting who was the most likely to be impacted by slavery in the world today is that it can provide some insights into how it might have worked in the past, less politically complex societies (Patterson 1982). For example, researchers have noted that there is a higher risk for women and children in these societies to be targeted and selected as captives (see, for example, Cameron 2016; Barr 2005; Tung 2012; Wilkinson 1997; Martin 1997; Maschner and Reedy-Maschner 2007). In prior work by the authors, we have found ethnographic (Harrod et al. 2012) and bioarchaeological (Harrod 2018b; Martin 2008) evidence to support that women and children were the preferred target of captive-taking in small-scale societies. Industrialization and globalization presents a very different picture (Blakey et al. 2000; Rankin-Hill et al. 2000). In contemporary systems of forced labor, the International Labour Organization (ILO) compared males and females and found that "male victims were more likely to be subjected to threats against family, withheld wages, confinement, denial of food and sleep, and threats of legal action. In contrast, female victims of forced labour suffered higher rates of sexual violence and were more likely to have their passports withheld" (International Labour Organization 2017, p. 35). Looking specifically at women and girls together, the ILO report indicates that they account for over seventy percent of all the individuals identified in a system of modern slavery (International Labour Organization 2017, p. 10, 22). The pattern here indicates that while violence related to captives and slave labor can, and does, affect all genders, it is women who are generally targeted and sexual violence is often a component. These same patterns of unequal sex distribution are what we look for in archaeological contexts.

Female individuals are not only at greater risk but also often held captive in different spaces than the males. Forced labor includes a wide range of activities, but females are primarily involved in household work and the service industry, while males engage in commercial agricultural, construction, fishing industries, mining, and manufacturing work (ILO 2017, p. 32). The people often forced into these systems of inequality are not taken as captives during raids but exploited as a consequence of involuntary migration within their homeland and to new countries. According to the ILO, internal migration exceeds external migration in the percentage of people in debt bondage (International Labour Organization 2017, pp. 37–38). In the Southwest United States, the pattern of taking captive women from the region where similar cultural groups inhabited seems to hold in the past (Harrod 2018b; Harrod et al. 2017; Kohler and Kramer Turner 2006).

Forced marriage is described as any type of union that the individual has not consented to, which can include parents selling or trading their children, raiding and capture during conflict, or even entry into a foreign nation (International Labour Organization 2017, p. 43). Over 80% of the individuals in forced marriage arrangement were women and girls, and 96% of the children who entered into these unions were female (International Labour Organization 2017, pp. 44–45). Discussing the rights of women to choose their marriage arrangements in European society, John Stuart Mill (1869, pp. 53–54) suggest that the practice of father's selling their daughters or men forcibly capturing women was common. He also discussed how subjugation of wives was a problem in terms of inheriting property and suffering sexual abuse (Mill 1869, pp. 56–57). "...however brutal a tyrant she may unfortunately be chained to—though she may know that he hates her, though it may be his daily pleasure to torture her, and though she may feel it impossible not to loathe him—he can claim from her and enforce the lowest degradation of a human being, that of being made the instrument of an animal function contrary to her inclinations" (Mill 1869, p. 57). One major finding of this research was that regardless of the type of modern slavery, females, both women and young girls, are at risk of sexual assault and threats of actual physical violence (International Labour Organization, 2017, p. 36, Figure 10). The reality is that the capture of women in systems of raiding often leads to a type of "forced marriage" arrangement in the past as well. Retelling the account of the oral tradition among the Hopi of the destruction of Awat'ovi pueblo, Ekkhart Malotki mentions how the warriors from the Mishongnovi and Walpi pueblos had taken "...some of the more attractive ones and were returning home" while the people of Oraibi were busy destroying the last of Awat'ovi (Malotki 2002, pp. 187–188).

The reality, however, is that often women and children seized in raids and taken as captives and slaves did not always live long lives. Harrod and Martin (2015) cite Elisabeth Tooker (1962, p. 31), who provides accounts of the Huron in Eastern North America practicing the taking of women as replacements for lost loved ones. However, genetic work by Tung and Knudson (2008, 2011) found that occasionally women and children were killed and their bodies were used to create trophies. For example, in the story about the destruction of Awat'ovi, Malotki describes how many of the women and children were killed. When the Oraibis caught up with the other two groups who had taken the captives, they fought over the women and could not come to an agreement, so they decided to murder them so it was fair to each group. Malotki (2002, p. 188) provides the following quote attributed to an unidentified Oraibi individual, "In that case no one shall have them. Let's get rid of them. If we kill them all, nobody can have them." According to his account, they did kill most of the women and older girls but stated that they spared women who knew the "...art of rain-making", others "...who were versed in certain skills", and the children (Malotki 2002, p. 188), suggesting potential as laborers, knowledge carriers, marriage partners, and concubines but still highlighting that the women and children could be victims of lethal violence.

5.4.2 Group-level conflict: raiding and warfare

Here we will discuss both intra- and inter-group conflicts in the form of raiding or warfare. Martin and Harrod (2015) highlight the tendency for people to use the terms war, warfare, and raiding interchangeably. However, the motivations behind and the scale of these different behaviors are not equivocal. "One way to roughly differentiate hunter-gatherer 'feuding' from 'raiding' or 'warfare' would be simply to count with carefully kept scores based on one-at-a-time killings as feuds, while larger attacks with more generalized revenge these can run along the continuum from raiding to warfare – with warfare being seen as conflicts between whole local groups with at least one of the groups fully mobilized to attack" (Boehm 2013, p. 323). In many cases, the motivation for raiding may not be the same as warfare. Warfare might lead to the destruction of a community or lineage like at Sacred Ridge, while raiding feeds into a system of captive-taking. Ben Raffield et al. (2017) have suggested that the reason behind the raids by Viking people during the AD 700s was linked to an increase in social stratification that involved polygyny, which reduced the number of eligible women for low-status men to marry. Raiding in this case provided a means of obtaining new wives. In contrast, intragroup -level warfare can be seen as a mechanism for conflict resolution with a large distinction from intergroup -level conflict, namely, the goal of the conflict. In intragroup warfare, the goal may be non-lethal interaction with the purpose of relieving scalar stress or resolving conflict.

When we think of warfare, it is easy to immediately visualize modern, state-level warfare conducted by standing armies. But this is unlikely to have been the case for much of human history and prehistory (Gat 2006). Ceremonial or ritual warfare is complex and may be difficult to identify archaeologically. The documentary "Dead Birds" examines ritual fighting and ceremonial warfare among the Dani of West New Guinea. This type of ritual fighting places violent interaction in a socially acceptable frame, primarily consisting of nonlethal interactions. This mode of nonlethal or ceremonial warfare was likely common in the past as a mechanism for settling disputes as well as negotiating and gaining status. However, the documentary also shows a stealthy raid that is lethal for one boy in the community, which highlights the complex interplay between raiding and warfare in small-scale societies. How can these nuances be captured by the skeletal remains?

Bioarchaeological examples have been advanced by Lambert and Walker in their work with prehistoric Indigenous groups in California (see, for example, Lambert 1997; Walker 1989). Walker (1989) examined remains from the Santa Barbara Channel area and noted that for males, healed cranial depression fractures tend to occur on the left side of the frontal and on the cranial vault. He suggests that this pattern represents ritualized population-level fighting designed to injure but not kill and that this might have been a way to resolve conflict in areas of geographical circumscription. Older adult males have similar rates of trauma to younger adult males, suggesting that the pattern of ritualized violence was most common in young and middle adult males and that it was not necessary to continue the fighting once status was attained (Lambert 1997; Walker 1997). Ethnographic and bioarchaeological reconstructions of ceremonial or ritual warfare tend to have a focus on its non-lethal nature (Walker 2001; Martin et al. 2012a; Burbank 1994, 1999; Abbink 1999; Chacon et al. 2007). The goal of this type of warfare is to cause injury, including bleeding and bruises, but not necessarily death. In terms of demography that would be expected from this type of interaction, it should reflect those who engage in this type of behavior. For prehistoric California, this pattern of trauma holds for adult males as well as some nonadults (sex is not estimated in this age group) over the age of approximately 10 years (Walker 1997). If we assume that those in the nonadult category that exhibit this same pattern were males, then we can reconstruct that status-gaining and negotiation began for males around 10 years of age. This pattern of violence is also going to be reflected in antemortem trauma, as the goal of such violence is not death but injury. Perimortem injury may be present, but as this is not the goal, it is likely to be rare and difficult to interpret.

Intergroup warfare is more associated with lethal violence. It can also be seen as an example of cooperative behavior. Kim and Kissel (2018) argue that cooperative behavior is key to our evolutionary past, and one manifestation of cooperative behavior may be group-level intergroup conflict or warfare. Motivations for intergroup warfare can include competition over resources and/or political reorganization; oscillations in the amount of warfare reflect differing social factors when viewed in a historical lens (Arkush and Tung 2013). Warfare in the past was likely much more complex and likely not limited to adolescent and adult males as combatants (Tiesler and Cucina 2012; Harrod and Stone 2018, Scherer 2021).

5.5 Conclusions

The goal of this chapter was to highlight various elements of group-level violent death, examining factors such as context, demography, and interpretation of traumatic lesions. In many ways, starting with the bones (as proxy for the dead bodies) provides a close inspection of the processes of causing death through violent means. In this sense, bones are truth-tellers. From the types of violent death discussed here, it is clear that group-level violence: (i) should not be seen as a monolithic concept, but must instead be examined contextually; (ii) has different forms that illustrate different elements of lived experience; and (iii) has the power to serve important social functions, from mediating scalar stress to restoring balance within society to concrete gains in land, resources, or captives that can be added to the victors' population. As Martin et al. (2013, pp. 74–75) note, studying violence "requires researchers to understand the transformative powers of its use in social relations and cultural practice. To accomplish this, researchers must understand that they are not simply studying a punctuated event but rather a transformative process within a historical trajectory." There is no single mechanism with which to examine group-level violent death; instead violent death must be viewed within the historical and cultural context in which it occurs. Whitehead (2004a, 2004b, 2005a, 2007) shows that violence is both degenerative and regenerative, destructive and constructive. Violent death both severs social ties and reinforces the mechanisms by which social ties can be reformed and negotiated.

Through the types of violent death and interaction discussed in this chapter, we have shown that different types of violent death have different social functions and arise from different needs. As Whitehead (2001, p. 837) notes, "Violent performance discursively amplifies and extends the cultural force of violent acts so that violent acts themselves can generate a shared idiom of meaning for violent death that enfold both killer and killed. As a result of this the way in which persons are killed or mutilated is not arbitrary, haphazard or simply a function of perceived instrumentality." This quote captures the nuance and variability that is afforded through the analysis of skeletal remains for signs of violent death. Because violence across cultures is so variable, the nuance and culturally specific manner of using violence must be preserved in the analysis. Too many earlier broad studies on the origins and evolution of violence have obliterated the variability and focused on broad trends over time, collapsing widely diverse and dissimilar case studies into unserviceable categories that reflect modern notions of violence. Bioarchaeology offers a nonreductionist approach to violent death through case studies where the analysis moves from individual bodies and bones, to the death assemblage and victim demographic and profile, to the post mortem treatment of the violently killed, and on to the complex cultural and historical context that these deaths are found.

References

Abbink, J.G. (1999). Violence, ritual, and reproduction: culture and context in Surma dueling. *Ethnology* **3**(3): 227–242.

Alfsdotter, C. (2019). Social implications of unburied corpses from intergroup conflicts: postmortem agency following the Sandby borg massacre. *Cambridge Archaeological Journal* **29**(3): 427–442.

Alfsdotter, C. and Kjellström, A. (2019). The Sandby Borg massacre: interpersonal violence and the demography of the dead. *European Journal of Archaeology* **22**(2): 210–231.

Alfsdotter, C. and Kjellström, A. (2020). A taphonomic interpretation of the postmortem fate of the victims following the massacre at Sandby borg. Sweden. *Bioarchaeology International* **3**(4): 262–282.

Alfsdotter, C., Papmehl-Dufay, L., and Victor, H. (2018). A moment frozen in time: evidence of a late fifth-century massacre at Sandby borg. *Antiquity* **92**(362): 421–436.

Anderson, C.P. and Martin, D.L. (2018). Introduction. In: *Massacres: Bioarchaeology and Forenic Anthropology Approaches* (eds. C.P. Anderson and D.L. Martin), 1–11. Gainesville: University of Florida Press.

Arkush, E. and Tung, T. (2013). Patterns of war in the Andes fromt he Archaic to the Late Horizon: insights from settlement patterns and cranial trauma. *Journal of Archaeological Research* **21**: 66–81.

Barr, J. (2005). From captives to slaves: commodifying Indian women in the borderlands. *The Journal of American History* **92**(1): 19–46.

Baustian, K.M., Harrod, R.P., Osterholtz, A.J., and Martin, D.L. (2012). Battered and abused: analysis of trauma at Grasshopper Pueblo (AD 1275-1400). *International Journal of Paleopathology* **2**(2-3): 102–111.

Behrensmeyer, A.K. (1978). Taphonomic and ecological information from bone weathering. *Paleobiology* **4**: 150–162.

Blakey, M.L., Mack, M.E., Medford, E.G., Wilson, S.D., et al. (2000). Political economy of mortality of enslaved africans. *American Journal of Physical Anthropology* Supplemental **30**: 108.

Boehm, C. (2013). The biocultural evolution of conflict resolution between groups. In: *War, Peace, and Human Nature: The Convergence of Evolutionary and Cultural Views* (ed. D.P. Fry), 315–340. Oxford: Oxford University Press.

Burbank, V.K. (1994). *Fighting Women: Anger and Aggression in Aboriginal Australia*. Vol. Book, Whole. Berkeley: University of California Press.

Burbank, V.K. (1999). Fight! Fight! men, women, and interpersonal aggression in an Australian Aboriginal Community. In: To Have and To Hit: Cultural Perspectives on Wife Beating (eds. D. Ayers Counts, J.K. Brown, and J. Campbell), 43–52. Champaign: University of Illinois Press.

Cameron, C.M. (2016). *Captives: How Stolen People Changed the World*. Lincoln and London: University of Nebraska Press.

Cameron, C.M. and Martin, D.L. (2012). Archaeological and bioarchaeological perspectives on captivity and slavery. *Anthropology News* **53**(7): 4–5.

Chacon, R.J., Chacon, Y., and Guandinango, A. (2007). The Inti Raymi Festival among the Cotacachi and Otavalo of Highland Ecuador. In: *Latin American Indigenous Warfare and Ritual Violence* (eds. R.J. Chacon and R.G. Mendoza), 116–141. Tucson: University of Arizona Press.

Chagnon, N.A. (1988). Life histories, blood revenge, and warfare in a tribal population. *Science* **239**(4843): 985–992. doi: 10.1126/science.239.4843.985. http://www.sciencemag.org/content/239/4843/985.abstract.

Darling, A.J. (1998). Mass inhumation and the execution of witches in the American Southwest. *American Anthropologist, New Series* **100**(3): 732–752.

Darling, A.J. (1999). Review of man corn: Cannibalism and violence in the prehistoric American Southwest by Christy G. Turner, II and Jacqueline A Turner. *Latin American Antiquity* **10**(4): 441–442.

Duday, H. (2009). The Archaeology of the Dead: Lectures in Archaeothanatology, translated by. In: Studies in Funerary Archaeology (eds. A.M. Cipriani and J. Pearce), Vol. 3. Oxford: Oxford Books.

Durrant, R. (2011). Collective violence: an evolutionary perspective. *Aggression and Violent Behavior* **16**: 428–436.

Dwyer, P.G. and Ryan, L. (2012). Introduction: the massacre and history. In: Theatres of Violence: Massacres, Mass Killings and Atrocity Throughout History (eds. P.G. Dwyer and L. Ryan). New York: Berghahn Books.

Erdal, Ö.D. (2012). A possible Massacre at early bronze age Titriş Höyük Anatolia. *International Journal of Osteoarchaeology* **22**(1): 1–21.

Galloway, A., Zephro, L., and Wedel, V.L. (2014). Diagnostic criteria for the determination of timing and fracture mechanism. In: *Broken Bones: Anthropological Analysis of Blunt Force Trauma* (eds. V.L. Wedel and A. Galloway), 47–58. Springfield: Charles C. Thomas.

Gat, A. (2006). *War in Human Civilization*. Vol. Book, Whole. Oxford: Oxford University Press.

Harrod, R.P. (2018a). Conclusion: What bioarchaeology and forensic anthropology reveal about massacres. In: *Massacres: Bioarchaeology and Forenic Anthropology Approaches* (eds. C.P. Anderson and D.L. Martin), 184–194. Gainesville: University of Florida Press.

Harrod, R.P. (2018b). Subjugated in the San Juan basin: identifying captives in the American Southwest. *Kiva* **84**(4): 480–497.

Harrod, R.P. and Martin, D.L. (2014). Signatures of captivity and subordination on Skeletonized human remains: a bioarchaeological case study from the ancient Southwest. In: *Bioarchaeological and Forensic Perspectives on Violence: How Violent Death is Interpreted from Skeletal Remains* (eds. D.L. Martin and C.P. Anderson), 103–119. Cambridge: Cambridge University Press.

Harrod, R.P. and Martin, D.L. (2015). Bioarchaeological case studies of slavery, captivity, and other forms of exploitation. In: The Archaeology of Slavery: A Comparative Approach to Captivity and Coercion (ed. L.W. Marshall). Center for Archaeological Investigations, Occasional Paper No. 41., 41–63. Carbondale: Southern Illinois University.

Harrod, R.P. and Stone, P.K. (2018). Mother, laborer, captive, and leader: reassessing the various roles that females held among the Ancestral Pueblo in the American Southwest. In: *Bioarchaeological Analyses and Bodies: New Ways of Knowing Anatomical and Archaeological Skeletal Collections* (ed. P.K. Stone), 191–212. New York: Springer.

Harrod, R.P., Liénard, P., and Martin, D.L. (2012a). Deciphering violence: the potential of modern ethnography to aid in the interpretation of archaeological populations. In: *The Bioarchaeology of Violence* (eds. D.L. Martin, R.P. Harrod, and V.R. Pérez), 63–80. Gainesville: University of Florida Press.

Harrod, R.P., Martin, D.L., and Pérez, V.R. (2012b). Conclusion: Implications and future directions. In: *The Bioarchaeology of Violence* (eds. D.L. Martin, R.P. Harrod, and V.R. Pérez), 276–280. Gainesville: University of Florida Press.

Harrod, R.P., Thompson, J.L., and Martin, D.L. (2013). Hard labor and hostile encounters: what human remains reveal about institutional violence and Chinese immigrants living in Carlin, Nevada (1885–1923). *Historical Archaeology* **46**(4): 85–111.

Harrod, R.P., Martin, D.L., and Fields, M. (2017). Across a Spectrum of Inequality: Hierarchy, health, and culturally sanctioned violence in the precontact U.S. Southwest. In: Bones of Complexity: Bioarchaeological Case Studies of Social Organization and Skeletal Biology (ed. M.N. Cohen), 363–387. Gainesville: University Press of Florida.

Hartley, R.J. (2007). To Massacre: a perspective on demographic competition. *Anthropological Quarterly* **80**(1): 237–251.
International Labour Organization (2017). *Global Estimates of Modern Slavery: Forced labour and forced marriage*. Geneva: International Labour Organization (ILO).
Kim, N.C. and Kissel, M. (2018). *Emergent Warfare in our Evolutionary Past*. New York: Routledge.
Klusemann, S. (2012). Massacres as process: a micro-sociological theory of internal patterns of mass atrocities. *European Journal of Criminology* **9**(5): 468–480.
Knüsel, C.J. and Outram, A.K. (2004). Fragmentation: the Zonation method applied to fragmented human remains from archaeological and forensic contexts. *Environmental Archaeology* **9**(1): 85–98.
Kohler, T.A. and Kramer Turner, K. (2006). Raiding for women in the pre-hispanic northern Pueblo Southwest? *Current Anthropology* **47**(6): 1035–1045.
Kuckelman, K.A. (2020). Ritual modification in the context of social unrest among ancestral Pueblo peoples of the Northern San Juan. In: *The Poetics of Processing: Memory Formation, Cosmology, and the Handling of the Dead* (ed. A.J. Osterholtz), 66–84. Boulder, CO: University Press of Colorado.
Kuckelman, K.A., Lightfoot, R.R., and Martin, D.L. (2000). Changing patterns of violence in the Northern San Juan region. *Kiva* **66**(1): 147–165.
Lahr, M., Rivera, F., Power, R.K., Mounier, A., et al. (2016). Inter-group violence among early Holocene Hunter-Gatherers of West Turkana, Kenya. Nature **529**(7586): 394–398.
Lambert, P.M. (1997). Patterns of violence in prehistoric hunter-gatherer societies of Coastal Southern California. In: *Troubled Times: Violence and Warfare in the Past* (ed. D.L. Martin), 77–109. Amsterdam: Gordon and Breach.
Malotki, E. (eds.) (2002). *Hopi Tales of Destruction. Narrated by Michael Lomatuway'ma, Lorena Lomatuway'ma and Sidney Namingha*. Lincoln and London: University of Nebraska Press.
Martin, D.L. (1997). Violence against women in the La Plata River Valley (A.D. 1000–1300). In: Troubled Times: Violence and Warfare in the Past (eds. D.L. Martin and D.W. Frayer), 45–75. Amsterdam: Gordon and Breach.
Martin, D.L. (2008). Ripped flesh and torn souls: evidence for slavery in the prehistoric Southwest, AD 800-1500. In: *Invisible Citizens: Captives and Their Consequences* (ed. C.M. Cameron), 159–180. Salt Lake City: The University of Utah Press.
Martin, D.L. and Akins, N.J. (2001). Unequal treatment in life as in death: trauma and mortuary behavior at La Plata (AD 1000–1300). In: *Ancient Burial Practices in the American Southwest: Archaeology, Physical Anthropology, and Native American Perspectives* (eds. D.R. Mitchell and J.L. Brunson-Hadley), 223–248. Albuquerque: University of New Mexico Press.
Martin, D.L. and Frayer, D.W. (1997). Introduction. In: *Troubled Times: Violence and Warfare in the Past* (eds. D.L. Martin and D.W. Frayer), xiii–xxi. Amsterdam: Gordon and Breach.
Martin, D.L. and Harrod, R.P. (2012). Body parts and parts of bodies: traces of violence in past cultures. *International Journal of Paleopathology* **2**(2–3): 49–52.
Martin, D.L. and Harrod, R.P. (2015). Bioarchaeological contributions to the study of violence. *Yearbook of Physical Anthropology* **156**(S59): 116–145.
Martin, D.L. and Harrod, R.P. (2020). The climate change-witch execution connection: living in environmental uncertainties on the Colorado Plateau (AD 800–1350). In: The Routledge Handbook of the Bioarchaeology of Climate and Environmental Change (ed. G.R. Schug), 301–315. London: Routledge.

Martin, D.L. and Osterholtz, A.J. (2012). A bioarchaeology of captivity, slavery, bondage, and torture. New directions in bioarchaeology, special forum. The SAA Archaeological Record **12**(3): 32–34.

Martin, D.L. and Osterholtz, A.J. (2020). The Poetics of Corpse Fragmentation and Processing in the Ancient Southwest. In: *The Poetics of Processing: Memory Formation, Cosmology, and the Handling of the Dead* (ed. A.J. Osterholtz), 85–102. Boulder, CO: University Press of Colorado.

Martin, D.L., Harrod, R.P., and Fields, M. (2010). Beaten down and worked to the bone: bioarchaeological investigations of women and violence in the ancient Southwest. *Landscapes of Violence* **1**(1), Article 3.

Martin, D.L., Harrod, R.P., and Pérez, V.R. (2012a). *The Bioarchaeology of Violence*, Vol. Book. Gainesville: University Press of Florida.

Martin, D.L., Harrod, R.P., and Pérez, V.R. (2012b). Introduction: bioarchaeology and the study of violence. In: *The Bioarchaeology of Violence* (eds. D.L. Martin, R.P. Harrod, and V.R. Pérez), 1–10. Gainesville: University of Florida Press.

Martin, D.L., Harrod, R.P., and Pérez, V.R. (2013). *Bioarchaeology: An Integrated Approach to Working with Human Remains*. Vol. Book, Whole. New York: Springer.

Maschner, H.D.G. and Reedy-Maschner, K.L. (2007). Heads, women, and the baubles of prestige: trophies of war in the arctic and subarctic. In: *The Taking and Displaying of Human Body Parts as Trophies by Amerindians* (eds. R.J. Chacon and D.H. Dye), 32–44. New York: Springer Science and Business Media.

Mill, J.S. (1869). *The Subjection of Women*. Longmans. London: Green, Reader, and Dyer.

Nickens, P.R. (1975). Prehistoric Cannibalism in the Mancos Canyon, Southwestern Colorado. Kiva **40**(4): 283–293.

Novak, S.A. (2007). Battle-related trauma. In: *Blood Red Roses: The Archaeology of a Mass Grave from the Battle of Towton AD 1461* (eds. V. Fiorato, A. Boylston, and C. Knüsel), 90–102. Oxford: Oxbow Books.

Novak, M., Olalde, I., Ringbauer, H., Rohland, N., et al. (2021). Genome-wide analysis of nearly all the victims of a 6200 year old massacre. *PLoS One* **16**(3): e0247332.

Osterholtz, A.J. (2012). The social role of hobbling and torture: violence in the prehistoric Southwest. *International Journal of Paleopathology* **2**(2–3): 148–155.

Osterholtz, A.J. (2014). Patterned processing as performative violence at sacred ridge. Paper presented at the 79th Annual Meeting of the Society for American Archaeology, Austin.

Osterholtz, A.J. (2018a). Each one the same: performance, demography, and violence at sacred ridge. In: *Massacres: Bioarcheaology and Forensic Anthropology Approaches* (eds. C.P. Anderson and D.L. Martin), 82–93. Gainesville: University of Florida Press.

Osterholtz, A.J. (2018b). Interpreting and reinterpreting sacred ridge: placing extreme processing in a larger context. *Kiva* **84**(4): 461–479.

Osterholtz, A.J. (2020). Introduction: processing and poetics, examining the model. In: *The Poetics of Processing: Memory Formation, Cosmology, and the Handling of the Dead* (ed. A.J. Osterholtz), 3–14. Boulder, CO: University Press of Colorado.

Osterholtz, A.J. and Martin, D.L. (2017). The poetics of annihilation: on the presence of women and children at massacre sites in the ancient Southwest. In: *Bioarchaeology of Women and Children in Times of War: Case Studies from the Americas* (eds. D.L. Martin and C. Tegtmeyer), 111–128. New York: Springer.

Outram, A.K. (2002). Bone fracture and within-bone nutrients: an experimentally based method for investigating levels of marrow extraction. In: *Consuming Passions and Patterns of Consumption* (eds. P. Miracle and N. Milner), 51–64. Cambridge: McDonald Institute for Archaeological Research.

Owens, L.S. (2021). Timoteo Mendieta Alcalá and the Pact of Forgetting: trauma analysis of execution victims from a Spanish Civil War mass burial site at Guadalajara, Castilla la Mancha. *Forensic Science International: Synergy* **3**, Article 100156.

Palkovich, A.M. (2012). Community violence and everyday life: death at Arroyo Hondo. In: *The Bioarchaeology of Violence* (eds. D.L. Martin and R.P. Harrod). Gainesville: University Press of Florida.

Parsons, E.W.C. (1927). Witchcraft among the Pueblos: Indian or Spanish? *Man* **27**: 106–112.

Parsons, E.W.C. (1939). *Pueblo Indian Religion*, Vol. 1 & 2. Vol. Book, Whole. Chicago: University of Chicago.

Patterson, O. (1982). *Slavery and Social Death*. Vol. Book, Whole. Cambridge: Harvard University Press.

Pérez-Flórez, A.M. and Harrod, R.P. (2021). Más de dos décadas de investigación: el estudio de la violencia directa a partir del registro bioarqueológico. *Cuicuilco Revista de Ciencias Anthropológicas* **80**: 295–323.

Potter, J. and Chuipka, J.P. (2010). Perimortem mutilation of human remains in an early village in the American Southwest: A case for ethnic violence. *Journal of Anthropological Archaeology* **29**(4): 507–523.

Raffield, B., Price, N., and Collard, M. (2017). Male-biased operational sex ratios and the Viking phenomenon: an evolutionary anthropological perspective on Late Iron Age Scandinavian raiding. *Evolution and Human Behavior* **38**(3): 315–324.

Rankin-Hill, L.M., Blakey, M.L., Carrington, S.H.H., and Howson, J.E. (2000). Political economy of fertility and population growth among enslaved Africans in Colonial New York. *American Journal of Physical Anthropology* **111**(S30): 259.

Sauer, N.J. (1998). The timing of injuries and manner of death: distinguishing among antemortem, perimortem, and postmortem trauma. In: *Forensic Osteology: Advances in the Identification of Human Remains* (ed. K.J. Reichs), 2 e, 321–332. Springfield: Charles C. Thomas.

Scherer, A.K. (2021). Recent research on the archaeology of war and violence. *Annual Review of Anthroopology* **50**: 403–421.

Seidel, A.C. and Fulginiti, L.C. (2014). The first cut is the deepest: looking for patterns in cases of human dismemberment. In: *Bioarchaeological and Forensic Perspectives on Violence: How Violent Death is Interpreted from Skeletal Remains* (eds. D.L. Martin and C.P. Anderson), 63–82. Cambridge: Cambridge University Press.

Stodder, A.L.W. and Osterholtz, A.J. (2010). Analysis of the processed human remains from the sacred ridge site: methods and data collection protocol. In: *Animas-La Plata Project: XV-Bioarchaeology* (eds. E.M. Perry, A.L.W. Stodder, and C.A. Bollong), 243–278. Pheonix: SWCA Environmental Consultants.

Stodder, A.L.W., Osterholtz, A.J., Mowrer, K., and Chuipka, J.P. (2010). Processed human remains from the sacred ridge site: context, taphonomy, interpretation. In: Animas-La Plata Project: Bioarchaeology. SWCA Anthropological Research Papers No. 10 (eds. E.M. Perry, A.L.W. Stodder, and C.A. Bollong), Vol. XV, 279–415. Phoenix: SWCA Environmental Consultants.

Tiesler, V. and Cucina, A. (2012). Where are the warriors? Cranial trauma patterns and confict among the ancient Maya. In: *The Bioarchaeology of Violence* (eds. D.L. Martin and R.P. Harrod). Gainesville: University Press of Florida.

Tooker, E. (1962). *An Ethnography of the Huron Indians, 1615-1649*. Vol. Book, Whole. Bureau of American Ethnology. Bulletin, No. 190. Washington, DC: Smithsonian Institution Press.

Tung, T.A. (2012). Violence against women: differential treatment of local and foreign females in the heartland of the Wari Empire, Peru. In: *The Bioarchaeology of Violence* (eds. D.L. Martin, R.P. Harrod, and V. Pérez), 180–198. Gainesville: University of Florida Press.

Tung, T.A. and Knudson, K.J. (2008). Social identities and geographical origins of wari trophy heads from Conchopata Peru. *Current Anthropology* **49**(5): 915–925.

Tung, T.A. and Knudson, K.J. (2011). Identifying locals, migrants, and captives in the wari heartland: a bioarchaeological and biogeochemical study of human remains from Conchopata Peru. *Journal of Anthropological Archaeology* **30**(3): 247–261.

Turner, C.G. II and Morris, N. (1970). A massacre at Hopi. American Antiquity **35**(3): 320–331.

Turner, C.G. II and Turner, J.A. (1992). The first claim for cannibalism in the Southwest: Walter Hough's 1901 discovery at Canyon Butte Ruin 3, Northeastern Arizona. *American Antiquity* **57**(4): 661–682.

Turner, C.G. II and Turner, J.A. (1999). *Man Corn: Cannibalism and Violence in the Prehistoric American Southwest*. Salt Lake City: University of Utah Press.

Turner, C.G. II, Turner, J.A., and Green, R.C. (1993). Taphonomic analysis of Anasazi skeletal remains from Largo-Gallina sites in Northwestern New Mexico. *Journal of Anthropological Research* **49**(2): 83–110.

Ubelaker, D.H. and Adams, B.J. (1995). Differentiation of perimortem and postmortem trauma using taphonomic Indicators. *Journal of Forensic Sciences* **40**(3): 509–512.

Walker, P.L. (1989). Cranial injuries as evidence of violence in prehistoric Southern California. *American Journal of Physical Anthropology* **80**(3): 313–323.

Walker, P.L. (1997). Wife beating, boxing, and broken noses: skeletal evidence for the cultural patterning of violence. In: *Troubled Times: Violence and Warfare in the Past* (eds. D.L. Martin and D.W. Frayer), 145–180. Amsterdam: Gordon and Breach.

Walker, W.H. (1998). Where are the witches of prehistory? *Journal of Archaeological Method and Theory* **5**(3): 245–308.

Walker, P.L. (2001). A bioarchaeological perspective on the history of violence. *Annual Review of Anthropology* **30**: 573–596.

Walker, W.H. (2008). Witches, practice, and the context of Pueblo Cannibalism. In: *Social Violence in the Prehispanic American Southwest* (eds. D.L. Nichols and P.L. Crown), 143–183. Tucson: University of Arizona Press.

Walker, W.H. (2009). Warfare and the practice of supernatural agents. In: *Warfare in Cultural Context: Practice, Agency, and the Archaeology of Violence* (eds. A.E. Nielsen and W.H. Walker), 109–138. Tucson: University of Arizona Press.

White, T.D. (1992). *Prehistoric Cannibalism at Mancos 5MTUMR-2346*. Princeton: Princeton University Press.

Whitehead, N.L. (2001). A history of research on warfare in anthropology - Reply to Keith Otterbein. *American Anthropologist* **102**(4): 834–836.

Whitehead, N.L. (2004a). Introduction: cultures, conflicts, and the poetics of violent practice. In: *Violence* (ed. N.L. Whitehead), 3–24. Santa Fe: School of American Research Press.

Whitehead, N.L. (2004b). On the poetics of violence. In: *Violence* (ed. N.L. Whitehead), 55–78. Santa Fe: SAR Press.

Whitehead, N.L. (2005a). War and violence as cultural expression. *Anthropology News* **46**(5): 23–26. doi: 10.1525/an.2005.46.5.23.1.

Whitehead, N.L. (2007). Violence and the cultural order. *Daedalus* **136**(1): 40–50. doi: 10.2307/20028088. http://www.jstor.org/stable/20028088.

Wilkinson, R.G. (1997). Violence against women: raiding and abduction in prehistoric Michigan. In: *Troubled Times: Violence and Warfare in the Past* (eds. D.L. Martin and D.W. Frayer), 21–44. Amsterdam: Gordon and Breach.

Willey, P.S. (1990). *Prehistoric Warfare on the Great Plains: Skeletal Analysis of the Crow Creek Massacre Victims*. Vol. Book, Whole: Garland Publishing, New York.

Wrangham, R.W. and Peterson, D. (1996). *Demonic Males: Apes and the Origins of Human Violence*. Vol. Book, Whole. Boston: Houghton Mifflin Company.

Zimmerman, L.J. (1997). The Crow Creek massacre: archaeology and prehistoric Plains warfare in contemporary contexts. In: *Material Harm: Archaeological Studies of War and Violence* (ed. J. Carman), 75–94. Glasgow: Cruithne Press.

CHAPTER 6

Destruction, mass violence, and human remains: Dealing with dead bodies as a "total social phenomenon"

Élisabeth Anstett

UMR 7268 ADES anthropologie bio-culturelle, droit, éthique et santé, Faculté des sciences médicales et paramédicales, Aix-Marseille Université, Marseille, France

> In these *total* social phenomena, as we propose to call them, all kinds of institutions find simultaneous expression: religious, legal, moral, and economic. In addition, the phenomena have their aesthetic aspect and they reveal morphological types (Mauss 1966, p. 1).

6.1 Introduction

One rather surprising feature of the research carried out within the human and social sciences on the subject of mass killings is that, for a long time, it either side-lined or indeed completely ignored the question of the treatment of corpses. Yet this observation is perhaps not quite so surprising when one considers the extent to which the material reality of death has always been, and still remains, a distinctly uncomfortable subject for societies and researchers alike.

The fate of corpses in situations of mass violence has thus only become the subject of scientific interest rather late in the day, driven on the one hand by the advent of the "Forensic Turn" and, on the other, by the development of transitional justice, which has increasingly come to consider the humanitarian treatment of human remains and the dignified reburial of victims as an essential tool of resilience in societies scarred by extreme violence. It was only in the early 2000s that the pioneering work of social anthropologists, Sanford (2003) in Guatemala and Ferrándiz (2006) in Spain, began to concentrate specifically on corpses, human remains, and the ways in which they are used. For the first time,

Anthropology of Violent Death: Theoretical Foundations for Forensic Humanitarian Action, First Edition.
Edited by Roberto C. Parra and Douglas H. Ubelaker.

researchers began to take an interest in the – very real – skeletons hidden away, sometimes for decades, in the closest symbolic or otherwise – of many contemporary societies.

What is revealed in particular by the advent of the Forensic Turn (understood from an anthropological point of view as being the moment when communities became sufficiently invested in the search for their dead to consider disinterring their remains; Anstett and Dreyfus 2015) and, alongside it, the recent emergence of the field of humanitarian forensics, is the continuing importance of mortal remains as a focus of societal interest. For the fact is that, in spite of the fear, anguish, and disgust elicited by corpses, the material and ritual handling – in both a figurative and a literal sense – of the bodies of the dead is a process that few societies are ready to abandon. In numerous contexts, a powerful sense of indignation is thus felt when such remains are absent. In this respect, the pressing need to locate the dead in order to bring them back as far as possible into normal social structures constitutes a moral imperative, the mechanisms of which are in many respects yet to be fully understood.

Yet even though we do not entirely understand the material and symbolic motivations behind this imperative need, social anthropologists working with groups scarred by the experience of mass killing have observed an identical refusal to accept the absence, or the disappearance of mortal remains, an absence that is often likened to a theft, a despoliation, a basic deprivation, and as such is felt to be unbearable. Whether working in Spain on the exhumations carried out in Francoist mass-graves (Renshaw 2011), in Bosnia on the secondary and tertiary burials from the genocides and crimes against humanity committed during the wars in the former Yugoslavia (Wagner 2008), in Argentina on the reappearance of remains of the "disappeared" victims of the military junta (Panizo 2016), in Peru on the treatment of mass graves from the country's internal conflict (Robin Azevedo 2021), in Zimbabwe on the mass burials scattered across the forests of Matabeleland (Eppel 2014), in Uganda on the process of moving the graves of war victims (Jahn and Wilhelm-Solomon 2015), in Cambodia on the ritual treatment of the traces of massacres carried out by the Khmer Rouge (Guillou 2016), or in Vietnam on the mediation efforts put in place to make peace with the ghosts of soldiers who died in battle (Sorrentino 2016), there is a high degree of consensus among the accounts provided by social anthropologists of the problems posed either by the absence of the dead, or by the fact that their remains had been treated with insufficient care.

The recurrent nature of these forms of social resistance, along with their sheer scale and variety, has thus led us to consider the idea that the treatment of corpses might constitute a total social phenomenon, in the Maussian sense of the term among (Mauss, 1978 [1950], 1966), the analysis of which promises to reveal the mechanisms essential to the functioning of every society, along with the logics on the basis of which the latter are both maintained under normal circumstances and rebuilt in times of crisis. How, then, can the human and social sciences, and above all social and cultural anthropology, document the treatment of human remains in these contexts of mass violence and destruction? And what fresh insights are they able to offer us?

6.2 Understanding the forms taken by the Forensic Turn, and its effects

From the early 2000s onwards, the human and social sciences have worked to gain an understanding of the vast phenomenon of the search for the dead, and of the different objectives that this search and the exhumations carried out as part of it may seek to achieve. Attention has thus been focused not only on the forms taken by these disinterments and their symbolic and social effects, but also on the preconditions necessary for them to be carried out at all.

The very existence of these situations of absence is due in the first instance to deliberate practices, which aim to render the human remains in question invisible or inaccessible. In this respect, the various ways in which corpses are treated by the perpetrators themselves constitute a preliminary step in the process by which the dead can return, and they subsequently define many aspects of this process. Numerous studies have thus sought to gain a close understanding of the *modus operandi* employed by these criminals, aiming, in particular, to elucidate the logic of destruction underpinning their actions, building on the work of Alexander Hinton in his pioneering article "Why Did You Kill?" published almost a quarter of a century ago (Hinton 1998). Feeding steadily into the emerging field of Perpetrator Studies, these studies all show how the actual killing of victims is only one stage in a complex process of destruction, which can also be seen at work in the funerary treatment of their remains (see the Chapter 7 by Roberto C. Parra, Digna M Vigo-Corea and Pierre Perich in the present volume).

Our own analysis of these various funerary treatments (Anstett 2018) has shown that they all involve the combinatory articulation of a regime of appropriation of human remains (polarized between holding onto the corpse and disposing of it) and a regime of visibility (polarized between displaying the corpse and concealing it). Four different types of treatment may thus be distinguished: display, disposal, concealment, and destruction.

At one of the poles of the "visibility" spectrum are to be found those practices of display that seek to underline, or even (quite literally) showcase the reality of the appropriation of corpses by the perpetrators. Emblematic as they are of the trophyization of the enemy's corpse, the forms and symbolic aspects of which have been brilliantly analyzed by the British anthropologist Simon Harrison in his *Dark Trophies* (Harrison 2012), these funerary treatments rely on the staging of a set of power relations that may possess multiple political dimensions, as the research carried out by Onek Adyanga on the treatment of human remains from the Luwero War in Uganda (Adyanga 2015) has shown. At a later stage, such remains will therefore be correspondingly easier to locate, given that they will often not have left the public space in the meantime.

By contrast, at the opposite pole of the visibility spectrum are to be found practices of camouflage and concealment, and even of total physical destruction by mechanical or chemical means (the Nazi crematoria being the absolutely archetypal example of this), reminding us that relations of power and domination also govern the material appropriation of people's bodies, and not just of their possessions.[1] These practices of concealment have an extremely direct and sometimes very long-lasting impact on the process of searching for, exhuming, identifying, and reburying victims.

Between these two poles are to be found practices involving the disposal, or more precisely the discarding of corpses, which stem directly from a principle of disqualification applied to the groups and individuals who are the target of the violence in question. Victims of genocides and crimes against humanity are systematically denied their status as individuals and indeed their basic quality as human beings, finding themselves denigrated and frequently likened to worthless objects, vermin, and even excrement. Following such massacres, these "remains of things," as the killers see the corpses of their victims, and themselves suffer further denigration. Their mortal remains are thus treated not merely *like* but literally *as* rubbish.

Indeed, despite being totally lifeless, these corpses give rise to the same level of hatred among perpetrators as the latter showed in their brutal determination to destroy their living victims. In this second (but by no means secondary) stage of the crime, an analysis of the treatment of these remains reveal that they are often considered by the perpetrators as mere waste, and are therefore subject to practices of physical expulsions, such as being thrown onto rubbish dumps.[2] In contexts of mass violence, corpses and human remains become nothing more than worthless objects, and are consequently treated as waste matter.

The work of Rémi Korman, for example, has shown how in the case of the genocide committed against the Tutsis in Rwanda, the killers frequently disposed of their victims in latrines (Korman 2014) and we know that, during the Holocaust, the ashes from the cremation ovens at Auschwitz II were disposed of on rubbish dumps situated within the discharge zone of the camp's sewers.[3] Quite logically, then, it is in such waste disposal zones that the search for victims' remains should subsequently be carried out.

The physical treatment of the remains of victims of mass violence – insofar as this process constitutes a total social phenomenon – thus reveals the moral economies and value systems underpinning the practices of disqualification and annihilation of the individuals and groups targeted by this violence, as well as determining whether or not it will possible to find these remains, and which practical methods will need to be employed from among the huge range of techniques available.

Other research carried out within the human and social sciences has thus sought to understand the phenomenon of the search for and disinterment of the dead by focusing more particularly on the various forms taken by the Forensic Turn. The numerous studies carried out in Europe, Latin America, Africa, and Asia into large-scale practices of exhumation over the last fifteen years have been able to shed light not only on the great variety of actors involved, as can be seen, for example, in the comparative study carried out on exhumations in Spain, Poland, and Bosnia by Ferrándiz and Hristova (2019), but also the heterogeneity – indeed in some cases the incompatibility – of their respective agendas, as has been revealed by the research conducted by Ernesto Schwartz-Marin and Arely Cruz-Santiago in Mexico (Schwartz-Marin and Cruz-Santiago 2016a), as well as the enduring influence of local cultural and religious specificities, to which the standardized practices and scenarios of transitional justice often have difficulty in adapting. The research carried out by the social anthropologist Dorothée Delacroix in Peru has thus revealed how the meaning attached by local populations to the methods employed in the material treatment of the human remains exhumed (taking and storing samples, conducting physical and chemical analyses), can sometimes awaken very ancient notions of death and dead bodies, which stand in radical opposition to the judicial and hygiene-centered approaches promoted by forensic experts, whether local or international (Delacroix 2021).

These studies also reveal the variety of logistical and technical resources mobilized for this task, and in particular, the increasingly prominent role played by the tools and methods of physical anthropology and biology, as the use of DNA sequencing has become widespread. These two disciplines have in this way contributed to the birth of a new area of expert knowledge and an entirely new discipline – forensic anthropology, – which has quickly become internationalized and professionalized, as the French political scientist Selim Smaoui has shown in the case of Spain (Smaoui 2015). This field of knowledge has contributed *de facto* to the growing prevalence of a biological reading of identity that raises its own set of questions, particularly insofar as it may be involved in making certain victims invisible (such as individuals targeted for being transgender, for example) as the research carried out by Adriana Díaz del Castillo, María Fernanda Olarte Sierra, and Tania Pérez-Bustos in Colombia (Díaz del Castillo et al. 2012) has shown. However, these forms of knowledge are also now being appropriated by communities on the ground, as the social anthropologists Ernesto Schwartz-Marin and Arely Cruz-Santiago have shown in their work on Colombia and Mexico (Schwartz-Marin and Cruz-Santiago 2016b).

Studies examining the forms taken by the Forensic Turn also shed light on the particular issues underpinning the search for remains on the one hand, and their identification on the other. The question of the way in which these remains can contribute – or not – to rebuilding a social body left damaged by destructive violence, along with the question of whether it is possible or indeed necessary to identify remains individually, has been explored in particular in the context of the Balkans by the anthropologists Jugo and Wastell (2015), following up on earlier research by Petrovic-Steger (2009). There is general agreement among anthropologists examining this issue that, together with the mistreatment inflicted on corpses by perpetrators, the invasive methods associated with forensic investigations can themselves endanger a society's ability to rebuild itself.

The analysis of these features of the Forensic Turn, thus allows us to understand how the societal issues underpinning the treatment of human remains relate directly to a fundamental principle of perpetuation within societies. The fact is that this principle has difficulty coping with the disappearance of specific links in the generational chain, just as it sometimes has great trouble dealing with the uncertainty and doubt surrounding the identification of some of these same links. For logic of family and lineage, and representations of the diachronic reproduction of a social group more generally, presuppose an unbroken link between the generations. This idea of a necessary link is sometimes hard to reconcile with the fragmentation and scattering of remains, or indeed their complete disappearance. The analysis of vernacular representations of the principle of the transmission of hereditary characteristics, and of the different regimes of truth constructed by societies around these representations, thus opens up some interesting avenues for research into these societies' logics of perpetuation, as the work conducted by the social anthropologist Dorothée Delacroix on DNA and the symbolic adoption of bodies recovered from mass graves in Peru and Spain has shown (Delacroix and Noûs 2020).

By studying the consequences of the Forensic Turn, then, the human and social sciences have sought to understand both the phenomenon of mass exhumations and the impact of the reappearance of the dead after a lengthy absence on the societies, which either actively bring about this return or have it forced upon them.

The initial effects of these exhumations are also visible in the legal field. The question of the legal status assigned to human remains (neither "things" nor "persons": Dziuban 2017b; Lopez Mazz and Anstett 2022) is still unresolved and looks set to remain so, so great is the tension that it creates between conflicting representations of the human person. However, the question of what can or should now be done with human remains has given rise to a growing number of regulatory measures. Those – such as the NAGPRA in the United States and the Human Tissue Act in the United Kingdom – which were initially meant to provide a regulatory framework for the collection, storage, and study of human biological material, have increasingly facilitated the restitution (or "relocation" as the return of bodies is sometimes euphemistically described) of human remains resulting from practices of predation which are often linked to contexts of mass violence; as a result of this, as the work of Mountain (2017) has shown, many museum institutions are now having to confront significant ethical and scientific challenges. In another legal area, the question of the right to obtain the truth regarding the fate of victims of mass crimes – a question currently being studied closely by the *Right to Truth, Truth through Rights* research program led by Professor Sévane Garibian at the University of Geneva – has increasingly focused on the question of the dignified treatment of these victims' remains, given that as yet no precisely defined legal framework exists to govern this treatment (Garibian et al. 2020). The related question of the protection of mass graves themselves is also starting to be considered (Klinkner 2017).

The study of the practices surrounding the return of human remains to society (Dreyfus and Anstett 2016) shows that, in addition to its legal implications, this phenomenon also has consequences in the cultural and religious domain, in particular owing to the tension that it creates around issues linked to the funerary and patrimonial spheres. For the sudden appearance of fragmented bodies, of anonymous bodies, or indeed the continuing absence of certain individuals' remains inevitably obliges societies affected by episodes of extreme violence to revise the grammar and lexicon of their traditional religious habits. For the latter suffers a drop in efficacy when faced with completely unprecedented realities and scenarios linked to the reappearance of corpses and human remains in large quantities. Surprisingly, however, the religious sphere in general, and in particular the impact on funerary rituals of having to deal with fragmented, absent, or supernumerary corpses, along with the ritual reconfigurations made necessary by the collective – as opposed to individual – character of such funeral ceremonies, which are also greatly delayed, have only very recently begun to be studied by social anthropologists.[4] By contrast, the strictly patrimonial – as opposed to funerary – treatment of these human remains (through their incorporation within memorials or museums) quickly became a focus of attention. Research in this area has concentrated in particular on the consequences of lasting spatial inscriptions of the materiality of death (giving rise to the phenomenon of dark tourism; see Olson and Korstanje 2020) and the impact of these on the memory and identities of various social groups affected by mass violence, as well as examining the conflicts of appropriation which often arise with the building of memorials, as may be seen from the historian Jean-Marc Dreyfus' study of the patrimonialization of the Bergen-Belsen concentration camp (Dreyfus 2006).

Many practices that aim to bring back the bodies of the dead or oversee their return thus shine a light on power relations. As a result, the resurfacing of bones is never a neutral process. The different forms taken by this return, its potential orchestration or staging, and its timing, are all governed by objectives that are essentially political in nature, and not just cultural or religious, as has been convincingly demonstrated by the anthropologist Joost Fontein's work in Zimbabwe (Fontein 2010). The material treatment of the corpse – insofar as the latter necessarily remains bound by power relations – thus allows light to be shed on the specific forms of biopolitical logic that underpin the functioning of societies, as the political scientist and philosopher Yehonatan Alsheh reminds us (Alsheh 2014). Following on from the foundational work of Mbembe (2006) on the notion of "necro-politics," the research carried out by the political scientist Finn Steputtat, along with studies coordinated by the anthropologists Ferrándiz and Robben (2015), have thus contributed to the emergence of an entirely new field of research centered on questions linked to the governance and governability of dead bodies. The principle that state institutions, whether national or national, should necessarily have a predominant role in the governance of human remains is now starting to be challenged, to the extent that initiatives aiming to enable simple citizens to conduct exhumations and oversee DNA identifications – or even carry these out fully by themselves – are beginning to emerge, paving the way for the development of "citizen-led forensics," a phenomenon studied by the social anthropologist Arely Cruz-Santiago in Mexico, for example (Cruz-Santiago 2020).

6.3 Understanding the genealogy of professional practices of disinterment

In a second, more recent development, the human sciences have also begun to investigate the genealogy of practices surrounding the search for and disinterment of remains on a mass scale. It is to be noted that this latest stage in the research being conducted into extreme violence and its social effects has received crucial contributions from the disciplines of history and archaeology. Thanks to various studies focusing both on contexts of genocide and on contexts of armed conflict, we are now able to look back over the period preceding the late twentieth century in order to examine what became of corpses and what kinds of treatment they received in situations of mass violence prior to the development of the forensic sciences as we now understand them.

The genocides of the twentieth century, which, in the words of the anthropologist Alexander Hinton, have shaped the "dark side of modernity," constitute an area of study that is absolutely essential to our understanding of contemporary developments in the mortuary and funerary treatment of human remains in times of crisis.

The studies carried out on the Herero and Nama genocide in Namibia from 1904 onwards, and in particular, the conclusions of the Charité Human Remains Project led by Stoecker and Winkelmann (2018), have thus revealed that the trephination and theft of human remains, which accompanied the destruction of these indigenous communities – and also contributed to the vogue enjoyed by racialized physical anthropology at the time – left a lasting mark on these societies which were robbed of their dead. The work of the Namibian historian Vilho Shigwedha (Shigwedha 2018) has shown how, by making it impossible for funerals to be held, the confiscation of remains suspended the entire symbolic economy of grief for a long period and had a radical impact not just on individual families, but on the identity of whole communities.

The recent research carried out by forensic anthropologists (Ferllini and Croft 2009) on the mass graves of the Armenian genocide – perpetrated less than 20 years after the extermination of the Hereros and the Nama – confirms the work of historians who had already shed light on the various forms of mistreatment inflicted on the victims' remains, whether through their display or through their concealment and/or destruction by water, earth or fire (Kévorkian 2014). The historian Elyse Semerdjian has thus shown that this treatment gave rise to a unique form of memorial geography – in a very real sense, a necro-geography – by creating a specific and lasting identity-based relationship between the communities targeted by this violence and the sites where the destruction took place (Semerdjian 2018).

The research carried out in the search for human remains from the Holocaust, meanwhile, has shown how this process gradually evolved from the unauthorized digging of treasure-hunters (Dziuban 2020) and the small number of judicial exhumations carried out in the immediate postwar period (Finder 2015), through to the progressive rejection of any intrusive practices in accordance with the prescriptions of the Jewish faith, which now govern the practices of Holocaust archaeologists (Sturdy Colls 2012, 2017). These developments underline the extent to which human remains are still highly sensitive objects, meaning that exhumation sites are similarly sensitive places, subject to lasting cultural and religious considerations. Disinterring human remains thus implies a close engagement with the materiality of death which in turn raises a number of debates, regarding both the social uses of what is brought up from beneath the ground (Dziuban 2017a) and the problematically intrusive and invasive character of the act of exhumation itself. It should be remembered that many cultures consider disturbing the dead to be wrong, to the extent that some of them mount determined opposition to the very idea of disinterring human remains at all.

The case of the genocide in Cambodia has led researchers to focus on a context posing another set of technical, social, and political challenges. The predominant method of disposal employed during the crimes committed by the Khmer Rouge consisted quite simply of leaving victims' corpses in rice paddies or in roadside ditches while preventing neighboring rural communities from conducting funerals. Now totally decomposed, or partially entangled within subsequent plant growth, these human remains (or merely the memory of them) are honored by expiatory rites, whether *in situ* or remotely. In addition to these material difficulties hampering the search for human remains from the genocide, further problems are posed by the legacy of the Khmer Rouge regime, a legacy which still exerts great influence over many aspects of the functioning of Cambodian society today, and weighs heavily on the judicial process. The research carried out by the social anthropologists Guillou (2012) and Bennett (2018), and the forensic anthropologist Fleischman (2016) on the treatment of human remains from the Khmer Rouge period is unanimous in emphasizing just how hard it is to make the small number of exhumations and forensic analyses carried out long after the fact comprehensible to local communities, who tend to prioritize funerary expectations over judicial ones. Studies on the genocides of the twentieth century, then, serve to underline the enduring power of cultural and political questions not just to shape the search for and exhumation of human remains, but even to govern the entire process of their funerary treatment.

Other recent studies have shed light on the specific context of the two world wars, and of contemporary armed conflicts more widely, and – as we now know – the determining role of these in creating an environment where the knowledge and techniques which would later form the basis of the forensic sciences were first developed and consolidated.

The research carried out by the anthropologist Adrien Douchet and the historians Taline Garibian and Benoît Poget (Douchet et al. 2021) on the protocols for handling the remains of French soldiers who died on the battlefield in the early years of the Great War, for example, along with that conducted by the historian Romain Fathi on the activity of the Australian Grave Detachment in the same period (Fathi 2018), shows how the treatment of corpses and human remains on the battlefield was governed in the first instance by hygienic and moral objectives, which led the belligerents to conduct various medical and technological experiments, including attempts to accelerate the cremation of bodies. The historian Béatrix Pau, meanwhile, has shown how the funerary handling of such remains, however fragmentary and hard to identify these may be, can also be dictated by political objectives (conceived of in terms of maintaining social harmony and gaining support for new nationalist projects) in an immediate post-conflict context (Pau 2016).

Research into the treatment of human remains from the Second World War, in particular, that carried out by Mauriello (2017) on the practice of "forced confrontation" with corpses, and by the social anthropologist Sarah Wagner (Wagner 2019) on the work of the Defense POW/MIA Accounting Agency, has shown the extent to which the process of searching for and identifying the remains of combatants or civilian victims, along with practices of visibilization and invisibilization of corpses, are a response both to geopolitical and diplomatic priorities and to internal political demands, all of which seek to legitimize particular national postures and narratives. The psychological power of these factors was a strong motivating force behind the decision by the United States in 1941 to create a military institution dedicated to the search for and identification of the remains of soldiers killed in combat and exerted great influence over the consolidation of military forensic techniques both in the United States and in the Soviet Union in the very specific context of the documentation of the crimes perpetrated by the Nazis (Sorokina 2005). The subsequent management of military funerary spaces, and the exchanges of remains that often occur as part of their construction and ongoing maintenance, likewise reveal how human remains function as a backdrop (occasionally in a transactional, monetized context) against which the long-term relations between former warring parties play out, both in the case of conventional armed conflicts and of asymmetrical warfare. In this sense, exhumations and reburials represent potentially endless processes, insofar as they can always be restarted for reasons (linked to the value assigned to the remains or to the spaces of inhumation) that have come to be seen as priorities, despite having previously been considered unfeasible.

At a methodological and epistemological level, recent studies carried out on the treatment of human remains in the context of armed conflict can shed light on contemporary theatres of war as well as older conflicts (Coleman 2006). These studies remind us, lest we had forgotten, that groups in uniform are the biggest producers of corpses, and therefore also the first to have to decide on a position to take regarding how to deal with them. These studies, thus feed into a debate – already begun in other quarters – regarding the strategic and military use of scientific knowledge, which is now underway both in the domain of forensic anthropology, with the development of the emerging field of battlefield forensics (Wilson et al. 2019), and in the domain of conflict archaeology, where for almost fifteen years the crucial work carried out by the Argentine archeologist Alfredo González-Ruibal has investigated the relationship between archaeology and the wars and mass crimes of the past (González-Ruibal 2008; González-Ruibal and Moshenska 2014). Working as they do on the actual sites of wars, archaeologists are faced with many ethical dilemmas linked not only to the potential misuse of their research but also to the potential judicial significance of the artifacts they unearth, especially when several layers of extreme violence are superimposed on top of one another at a single site, as is the case for example in Syria or the Balkans.

6.4 The blind spots of a total social phenomenon of great complexity

In spite of the large volume of knowledge that has thus been accumulated regarding the treatment of human remains in contexts of mass violence, many blind spots still exist. In particular, we possess relatively little information regarding how large numbers of corpses have been treated in certain remote contexts (in terms of their separation from us in both time and space), and also regarding the various relationships (technical, social, cultural, judicial, religious) that have been established between societies and their corpses in the context of crises of mortality more generally.

We do know that, in addition to those episodes intentionally caused by humans (such as armed conflicts or practices of extermination), numerous crises of mortality of various types (natural disasters, epidemics) have left their mark on the history of humanity across all the continents. Archaeologists have revealed the existence of disaster burials and emergency funerary rites dating from epidemics, which ravaged the societies of the ancient world[5]. Yet the ways in which corpses are treated and the effects of this treatment on the resilience of the societies in question is a subject, which remains under-explored with respect both to the number of dead and the number of societies affected by such crises, even in purely demographic terms. However, in addition to isolated studies produced in response to individual episodes, such as Hurricane Katrina (Giroux 2006) or the 2010 earthquake in Haiti (Corbet 2011), there is now growing interest in the treatment of the dead as well as that of the living in the context of humanitarian crises. This can be seen in the creation of various academic research networks and permanent research structures, such as IRIDES (International Research Institute of Disaster Science), which focus on improving our understanding of situations of destruction.[6] An analysis of the way in which mortal remains are handled in times of crisis is indeed essential to gaining a full understanding of the reconstruction mechanisms at work within societies, as it provides insights into the risks involved in this process, whether these are material, hygienic or symbolic [the latter manifesting themselves, for example, through the presence of ghosts, zombies and other supernatural beings considered to be dangerous, as documented by Kwon (2017) in Vietnam and Corbet (2011) in Haiti]. It also helps build the argument in favor of making the voice of humanitarian forensics heard more loudly within initiatives, such as the World Bosaï Forum, created in Japan after the 2011 tsunami, which studies the effects of disasters with a view to preventing them in the future or at least reducing their impact.

Another area that still requires further examination – and recognition – is the specifically colonial nature of the production of large numbers of dead within contexts that either stem directly from the process of colonial conquest, or more indirectly – as is the case in particular with the asymmetric conflicts that typify wars of decolonization, or the propping-up of authoritarian regimes in Latin America in the second half of the twentieth century – ad the implications of this colonial aspect for the treatment of the corpses of victims. There is also a direct correlation between this question and that of the handling of human remains generated by this violence in today's postcolonial context, particularly within scientific institutions, such as universities (for instance, see Tony Platt's study of the osteological collections held by Berkeley; Platt 2011) or cultural institutions, such as museums (for instance, see the work by Ciraj Rassool on the multiple implications of the repatriation of human remains back to South African museums; Rassool 2015). And what of the ancient forms (which only archaeology can reveal) and the indigenous or precolonial versions (on which historians and archaeologists can shed light) of dealing with large quantities of human remains, and the status that was assigned to the latter? The question of the extent to which the objectivation of precolonial corpses and human remains – literally transformed into *objects* to study and collect through a process which, as we know, was the fruit of historical relations of domination – helps perpetuate an enduring pattern of "brutalism," in the sense applied to this term by the philosopher Achille Mbembe (Mbembe 2020), thus remains unresolved.

6.5 Conclusion

Overall, then, it is clear that in spite of the knowledge accrued so far, drawing the dividing line between mortuary practices and funerary practices remains a complex task. This is perhaps due to the fact that the "total" social phenomenon that is the handling of corpses – particularly in contexts of mass violence, where these are present in large numbers – simultaneously mobilizes a variety of registers (religious, legal, moral, and political) and multiple regimes of value, from the symbolic to the highly material or even monetary, and in so doing gives rise to a necro-economy. This necro-economy now fits into highly monetized and globalized circuits, which are stimulated by a market logic, itself driven by the practices involved in the search for and conservation of human bodies (supply) and in their patrimonialization (demand) that have been described in numerous studies cited here. And, while the search for and identification of corpses produced by mass violence and genocides has given rise to a market in forensic expertise, we have also witnessed the emergence – as a consequence of this first market – of a whole new economy based on thanatourism, along with a leisure economy involving the creation of permanent or temporary museum spaces, documentaries and film dramas, and indeed all forms of cultural production. In the final analysis, we have yet to understand fully how the moral economies born from the return of the dead to society now interact with the major economic and (geo-)political configurations on a global scale. This interaction occurs at a very concrete level when, for example, a museum curator needs to estimate the value (expressed in euros or dollars) of a skull or a humerus, a valuation of this kind being necessary to insure the object during transportation or if it is lent to another institution. What, then, is the value of this piece of bone? The study of this interaction between a symbolic necro-economy and a monetary necro-economy is, to my mind, becoming all the more crucial and urgent given the current context of steadily increasing scrutiny of the way in which human remains are used within cultural and scientific institutions.

Notes

1. See also the work of the French historian Karine Ramondy on the treatment of the remains of political dissidents murdered in central Africa in the late 1950s and early 1960s (Ramondy, 2020).
2. See the articles in the special issue of the journal *Human Remains and Violence* devoted to "Corpses in rubbish dumps," available in Open Access https://www.manchesteropenhive.com/view/journals/hrv/5/1/hrv.5.issue-1.xml
3. The ash removed from the four crematory ovens (numbered 2–5 on the map available on the website of the United States Holocaust Memorial Museum) was flushed away into the sewage treatment area (number 10 on the map): https://encyclopedia.ushmm.org/content/fr/map/auschwitz-ii-birkenau-camp-summer-1944
4. See the comparative research program "Europe/Amérique Latine Transfunéraire" launched in 2020: https://funeraire.hypotheses.org/
5. See in particular the impressive doctoral thesis produced by Catherine Rigeade, *Les sépultures de catastrophe: approche anthropologique des sites d'inhumations en relation avec des épidémies de peste, des massacres de population et des charniers militaires*. Thèse de doctorat, Université Aix-Marseille 2, 2006.
6. Such as the International Network of Disaster Studies and the Disaster-STS Network

References

Adyanga, O.C. (2015). A macabre exhibit: Ugandan President Museveni's public display of the Luwero Triangle War's human remains. *Advances in Historical Studies* **4**(5): 389–402.

Alsheh, Y. (2014). The biopolitics of corpses of mass violence and genocide. In: *Human Remains and Mass Violence: Methodological Approaches* (eds. J.-M. Dreyfus and E. Anstett), 12–43. Manchester, England: Manchester University Press.

Anstett, É. (2018). What is a mass grave? Toward an anthropology of human remains treatment in contemporary contexts of mass violence. In: *A Companion to the Anthropology of Death* (ed. A.C.G.M. Robben), 177–188: Wiley and Blackwell.
Anstett, É. and Dreyfus, J.-M. (eds.) (2015). *Human Remains and Identification: Mass Violence, Genocide and the 'Forensic Turn'*: Manchester University Press.
Bennett, C. (2018). Living with the dead in the killing fields of Cambodia. *Journal of Southeast Asian Studies* **49**(2): 184–203.
Bernard, P. (2017). The politics of the Luweero skulls: the making of memorial heritage and post-revolutionary state legitimacy over the Luweero mass graves in Uganda. *Journal of Eastern African Studies* **11**(1): 188–209.
Coleman, B.L. (2006). The dead of winter: how battlefield investigators, WWII Veterans, and Forensic Scientists Solved the Mystery of the Bulge's Lost Soldiers. *The Journal of Military History* **70**(3): 872–873.
Corbet, A. (2011). *Les morts et la mort à Haïti suite au séisme du 12 janvier 2010*. Paris: Grotius.
Cruz-Santiago, A. (2020). Lists, maps, and bones: the untold journeys of citizen-led forensics in Mexico. *Victims and Offenders* **15**(3): 350–369.
Delacroix, D. (2021). L'État cannibale. Rumeurs de trafic d'os exhumés au Pérou. *Cultures and Conflits* **121**(1): 73–97.
Delacroix, D. and Noûs, C. (2020). Politiques du doute et régimes de vérité à l' 'ère de l'os'. ADN et adoptions symboliques des corps récupérés dans les charniers au Pérou et en Espagne. *Ethnologie française* **50**(2): 327–344.
Díaz del Castillo, A., Olarte Sierra, M.F., and Pérez-Bustos, T. (2012). Testigos modestos y poblaciones invisibles en la cobertura de la genética humana en los medios de comunicación colombianos. *Interface-Comunicação, Saúde, Educação* **16**: 451–467.
Douchet, A., Garibian, T., and Pouget, B. (2021). Managing the remains of citizen soldiers: France and its war dead in 1914 and 1915. *Human Remains and Violence: An Interdisciplinary Journal* **7**(1): 37–51.
Dreyfus, J.-M. (2006). Conflit de mémoires autour du cimetière de Bergen-Belsen. *Vingtieme Siecle. Revue d'histoire* **2**: 73–87.
Dreyfus, J.-M. and Anstett, E. (eds.) (2016). *Human Remains in Society: Curation and Exhibition in the Aftermath of Genocide and Mass-violence*. Manchester: Manchester University Press.
Dziuban, Z. (eds.) (2017a). *Mapping the 'Forensic Turn': Engagements with Materialities of Mass Death in Holocaust Studies and Beyond*: New Academic Press.
Dziuban, Z. (2017b). Between subjectification and objectification: theorizing ashes. In: *Mapping the 'Forensic Turn': Engagements with Materialities of Mass Death in Holocaust Studies and Beyond* (ed. Z. Dziuban). VWI zur Holocaustforschung, Vol. 5, 261–288: New Academic Press.
Dziuban, Z. (2020). Atopic objects: the afterlives of gold teeth stolen from Holocaust dead. *Journal of Material Culture* **25**(4): 408–427.
Eppel, S. (2014). Bones in the forest in Matabeleland, Zimbabwe: exhumations as a tool for transformation. *International Journal of Transitional Justice* **8**(3): 404–425.
Fathi, R. (2018). We refused to work until we had better means for handling the bodies. discipline at the Australian graves detachment. *First World War Studies* **9**(1): 35–56.
Ferllini, R. and Croft, A.M. (2009). The case of an Armenian mass grave. *Journal of Human Rights* **8**(3): 229–244.
Ferrándiz, F. (2006). The return of Civil War ghosts: the ethnography of exhumations in contemporary Spain. *Anthropology Today* **22**(3): 7–12.

Ferrándiz, F. and Hristova, M. (2019). Mass grave exhumation sites as agonistic fora: a Comparative Study of Spain, Poland and Bosnia. In: *Repensar el pasado: La memoria (trans)cultural Europea* (eds. J. Vollmeyer and M.F. Bueno), 101–122. Madrid: Dykinson.
Ferrándiz, F. and Robben, A.C.G.M. (eds.) (2015). *Necropolitics: Mass Graves and Exhumations in the Age of Human Rights*. Philadelphia: University of Pennsylvania Press.
Finder, G.N. (2015). Final chapter. Portraying the exhumation and reburial of Polish Jewish Holocaust victims in the pages of yizkor books. In: *Human Remains and Identification: Mass Violence, Genocide, and the 'Forensic Turn'* (eds. E. Anstett and J.-M. Dreyfus), 34–58.
Fleischman, J.M. (2016). Working with the remains in Cambodia: skeletal analysis and human rights after atrocity. *Genocide Studies and Prevention: An International Journal* **10**(2): 10.
Fontein, J. (2010). Between tortured bodies and resurfacing bones: the politics of the dead in Zimbabwe. *Journal of Material Culture* **15**(4): 423–448.
Garibian, S., Tidball-Binz, M., Araguete Toribio, Z., Schnyder, A., et al. (2020). The development of guiding principles for the proper management of the dead in humanitarian emergencies and help in preventing their becoming missing persons: First Expert's Meeting. *International Review of the Red Cross* **101**(912): 1213–1229.
Giroux, H.A. (2006). Reading Hurricane Katrina: race, class, and the biopolitics of disposability. *College Literature* **33**(3): 171–196.
González-Ruibal, A. (2008). Time to destroy: an archaeology of supermodernity. *Current Anthropology* **49**(2): 247–279.
González-Ruibal, A. and Moshenska, G. (eds.) (2014). *Ethics and the Archaeology of Violence*: Springer.
Guillou, A.Y. (2012). An alternative memory of the Khmer Rouge genocide: the dead of the mass graves and the land guardian spirits [*neak ta*]. *South East Asia Research* **20**(2): 207–226.
Guillou, A.Y. (2016). Traces of destruction and the thread of continuity in post-genocide Cambodia. In: *Religion, Place and Modernity: Spatial Articulations in Southeast Asia and East Asia* (eds. M. Dickhardt and A. Lauser), 729–742: Brill.
Harrison, S. (2012). *Dark Trophies: Hunting and the Enemy Body in Modern War*: Berghahn Books.
Hinton, A.L. (1998). Why did you kill? The Cambodian genocide and the dark side of face and honor. *The Journal of Asian Studies* **57**(1): 93–122.
Hinton, A.L. (2002). I. The dark side of modernity: toward an anthropology of genocide. In: *Annihilating Difference*, 1–40: University of California Press.
Jahn, I.R. and Wilhelm-Solomon, M. (2015). 'Bones in the wrong soil': reburial, belonging, and disinterred cosmologies in post-conflict northern Uganda. *Critical African Studies* **7**(2): 182–201.
Jugo, A. and Wastell, S. (2015). Disassembling the pieces, reassembling the social: the forensic and political lives of secondary mass graves in Bosnia and Herzegovina. In: *Human Remains and Identification: Mass Violence, Genocide and the Forensic Turn* (eds. E. Anstett and J.-M. Dreyfus), 142–174. Manchester: Manchester University Press.
Kévorkian, R.H. (2014). Earth, fire, water: or how to make the Armenian corpses disappear. In: *Destruction and Human Remains: Disposal and Concealment in Genocide and Mass Violence* (eds. E. Anstett and J.-M. Dreyfus), 89–116. Manchester: Manchester University Press.

Klinkner, M. (2017). Towards mass-grave protection guidelines. *Human Remains and Violence: An Interdisciplinary Journal* **3**(1): 52–70.
Korman, R. (2014). The Tutsi body in the 1994 genocide: ideology, physical destruction, and memory. In: *Destruction and Human Remains: Disposal and Concealment in Genocide and Mass Violence* (eds. E. Anstett and J.-M. Dreyfus), 226–242. Manchester: Manchester University Press.
Kwon, H. (2017). Revolution in the Afterlife. *Religions* **8**(8): 146.
Lopez Mazz, J.Y. and Anstett, E. (2022). *Los restos óseos humanos. ¿Cosas o personas?* Montevideo: Banda Oriental.
Major, L. (2015). Unearthing, untangling and re-articulating genocide corpses in Rwanda: Déterrer, démêler et réarticuler les corps du génocide au Rwanda. *Critical African Studies* **7**(2): 164–181.
Mauriello, C.E. (2017). *Forced Confrontation: The Politics of Dead Bodies in Germany at the End of World War II*: Lexington Books.
Mauss, M. (1966). *The Gift: Forms and Functions of Exchange in Archaic Societies (translated by Ian Cunnison).* London: Cohen and West.
Mauss, M. (1978 [1950]). *Sociologie et anthropologie.* Paris: PUF.
Mbembe, A. (2006). Nécropolitique. *Raisons politiques* **1**: 29–60.
Mbembe, A. (2020). *Brutalisme.* Paris. France: La Découverte.
Mountain, R. (2017). The future of the past: reclassification of 'culturally unidentifiable' human remains under NAGPRA. *Arizona Anthropologist* **28**: 66–75.
Olson, D.H. and Korstanje, M.E. (eds.) (2020). *Dark Tourism and Pilgrimage.* Wallingford and Boston: CABI.
Panizo, L. (2016). Among bodies: reflections on ethnographic work and the repercussions of exhumations and identifications of the disappeared of the last military dictatorship in Argentina. *Human Remains and Violence: An Interdisciplinary Journal* **2**(2): 21–38.
Pau, B. (2016). *Le ballet des morts. État, armée, familles: S'occuper des corps de la Grande Guerre.* Paris: La Librairie Vuibert.
Petrovic-Steger, M. (2009). Anatomising conflict—accommodating human remains. In: *Social bodies* (eds. H. Lambert and M. McDonald), 47–76. New York: Berghahn.
Platt, T. (2011). *Grave Matters: Excavating California's Buried Past.* Berkeley, CA: Heyday.
Ramondy, K. (2020). *Leaders assassinés en Afrique Centrale (1958-1961): Entre construction nationale et régulation des relations internationales.* Paris: L'Harmattan.
Rassool, C. (2015). Re-storing the skeletons of empire: return, reburial and rehumanisation in Southern Africa. *Journal of Southern African Studies* **41**(3): 653–670.
Renshaw, L. (2011). *Exhuming Loss: Memory, Materiality and Mass Graves of the Spanish Civil War*: Routledge.
Robin Azevedo, V. (2021). From dignified burial to 'Terrorist Mausoleum': exhumations, moral panic and mourning policies in Peru. *Bulletin of Latin American Research* **40**(1): 21–39.
Sanford, V. (2003). *Buried Secrets: Truth and Human Rights in Guatemala*: Palgrave Macmillan.
Schwartz-Marin, E. and Cruz-Santiago, A. (2016a). Pure corpses, dangerous citizens: transgressing the boundaries between experts and mourners in the search for the disappeared in Mexico. *Social Research: An International Quarterly* **83**(2): 483–510.
Schwartz-Marin, E. and Cruz-Santiago, A. (2016b). Forensic civism: articulating science, DNA and kinship in contemporary Mexico and Colombia. *Human Remains and Violence: An Interdisciplinary Journal* **2**(1): 58–74.

Semerdjian, E. (2018). Bone memory: the necrogeography of the Armenian Genocide in Dayr al-Zur, Syria. *Human Remains and Violence: An Interdisciplinary Journal* **4**(1): 56–75.

Shigwedha, V.A. (2018). The homecoming of Ovaherero and Nama skulls. *Human Remains and Violence: An Interdisciplinary Journal* **4**(2): 67–89.

Smaoui, S. (2015). Fouiller. . . Militer. Penser la cause des 'disparus' du franquisme à l'aune des carrières d'archéologues et d'anthropologues. *Politix* **110**(2): 35–62.

Sorokina, M.A. (2005). People and procedures: toward a history of the investigation of Nazi Crimes in the USSR. *Kritika: Explorations in Russian and Eurasian History* **6**(4): 797–831.

Sorrentino, P. (2016). The 'Ghost Room': space, death and ritual in Vietnam. In: *Religion, Place and Modernity: Spatial Articulations in Southeast Asia and East Asia* (eds. M. Dickhardt and A. Lauser), 290–311: Brill.

Stoecker, H. and Winkelmann, A. (2018). Skulls and skeletons from Namibia in Berlin. *Human Remains and Violence: An Interdisciplinary Journal* **4**(2): 5–26.

Sturdy Colls, C. (2012). Holocaust archaeology: archaeological approaches to landscapes of Nazi genocide and persecution. *Journal of Conflict Archaeology* **7**(2): 70–104.

Sturdy Colls, C. (2017). The archaeology of cultural genocide: a forensic turn in holocaust studies? In: *Mapping the 'Forensic Turn': The Engagements with Materialities of Mass Death in Holocaust Studies and Beyond* (ed. Z. Dziuban). Vienne: New Academic Press.

Wagner, S. (2008). *To Know Where he Lies: DNA Technology and the Search for Srebrenica's Missing*. Berkeley: University of California Press.

Wagner, S. (2019). *What Remains: Bringing America's Missing Home from the Vietnam War*. Cambridge, MA: Harvard University Press.

Wilson, L.E., Gahan, M.E., Lennard, C., and Robertson, J. (2019). The black sheep of forensic science: military forensic and technical exploitation. *Australian Journal of Forensic Sciences* **51**(6): 636–648.

CHAPTER 7

Kill, kill again and destroy: when death is not enough

Roberto C. Parra[1,2*], Digna M. Vigo-Corea[3] and Pierre Perich[4]

[1]*Technical Assistance Team. United Nations Joint Human Rights Office (UNJHRO), MONUSCO, Democratic Republic of Congo*

[2]*Unité mixte de recherche d'Anthropologie bio-culturelle, Droit, Éthique & Santé (UMR 7268 - ÁDES), Aix Marseille University, Marseille, France*

[3]*Unidad Medico Legal II Ancash, Instituto de Medicina Legal y Ciencias Forenses, Ministerio Publico del Perú*

[4]*Forensic Department, Hôpital de la Timone, Aix Marseille University, Marseille, France*

**The views expressed herein are those of the author and do not necessarily reflect the views of the United Nations.*

7.1 Introduction

Humanity, in an act of absolute irreverence and vehemence in its violent actions, has gone far beyond the unimaginable. Violent death[1] by decision or decisions of other people has not only surpassed the human nature of killing but also exacerbated the kill again and demonstrated the fascination with excess (Sémelin 2007). Violence against the living and the dead, as well as an extreme and growing variety of sophisticated modes of body destruction, has been facilitating an enormous production of inert bodies and body parts (Parra et al. 2020; Anstett 2018). Fascination for the excess is reflected in the destruction with the clear objective of, somehow, provoking the social death[2] of the killed and killed again. *The* "brute stuff of violent death itself"[3] is a source of manifestations of such violent processes, which have been remarkably impacting the worldview of affected populations, due to the enormous multiplicity of meanings found embedded in human remains (Anstett and Dreyfus 2015; Verdery 1999; Sémelin 2007, Hinton 2002, 2005, 2016; among others). In addition, the places where bodies are finally deposited concentrate a set of meanings (Anstett 2018)

Anthropology of Violent Death: Theoretical Foundations for Forensic Humanitarian Action, First Edition. Edited by Roberto C. Parra and Douglas H. Ubelaker.

that in various situations become negative deathscapes[4] (Parra et al. 2022; Kwon 2006, 2008; Mueggler 2001).

Following Elizabeth Anstett (2018) concerning the treatment of human remains, she highlights that four different types of treatment by aggressors could be distinguished: display, disposal, concealment, and destruction. In all of them, violent death keeps executing and representing itself through a complex series of manipulations of signs and symbols (Whitehead 2004) from which it is possible to build, reconstruct, and interpret the meanings of the act. Anstett (see Chapter 6 in this volume) also emphasizes that the treatment of human remains articulates a regime of appropriation (polarized between retaining the corpse and disposing of it) and a regime of visibility (polarized between exhibiting the corpse and hiding it). All this is reflected in a "plot" of meanings that involves the participation of the victims, the witnesses (collectivities), and the perpetrator (Whitehead 2004; Riches 1986 pp. 19–86). This complex interaction is closely related to the social control that the perpetrators (aggressors) have motivated over the witnesses and victims by subjugating their victims through pain and suffering. These interactions have a changing dynamic where perpetrators can at some point become victims and witnesses become either perpetrators or victims. The change of roles contains an impressive load of volitional attitudes that can be reflected in human remains and show the ferocity of such actions. To understand these bloody episodes, the panorama must be observed in an integral way, where the dynamics that lead to the performance of lethal violence must be recognized mainly in their cultural motivations (Whitehead 2004, 2005, 2007). In most cases, the perpetrators are motivated to legitimize violent actions by denying the human condition of the victims, dehumanizing them (Whitehead 2004; Smith 2011, 2014, 2016, 2020, 2021; Vaes et al. 2021; Haslam 2019; Haslam et al. 2008, 2011; Haslam and Loughnan 2014; Taylor 1999; Hinton 2005, 2016; among others). Nevertheless, there are other positions that do not necessarily give credence to it (Over 2021).

The human remains of the victims, on the one hand, can be perceived as filthy, useless, culturally contaminated, and even dangerous objects, which must be disposed of as garbage or excrement. In contrast to this perception, bodies can also be an important source of symbolic energy that the owner or possessor (perpetrator) can dispose of to make them visible for various interests, among them, with the intention of facilitating social control. The exercise of the practice of power is revealed by disposing of people's lives and, above all, in the mechanisms to transform the body into a source of communication; in other words, in the way of killing again and destroying it and how it will be perceived by society through the ritualization of violence that stigmatizes but empowers the event at the same time. On the other hand, the intentionality of causing pain and all the actions of destruction tears down not only the body but also its identity and memory, thus deconstructing its essence as a human being as well as damaging the cultural order and the social fabric. Violent death will always be closely linked to a matter of degree, intensity, and culturally competent motivations, which constructs such vehement actions as violent and also destructive (Whitehead 2004).

7.2 Dehumanizing

Perpetrators of exacerbated or cruel violent deaths often perceive or categorize their victims as lacking any essential human characteristic. They are even seen as an object of disparagement (Taylor 1999; Sémelin 2007; Hinton 2005, 2016; Smith 2011, 2014, 2016, 2020, 2021). All this becomes from the fact of not simply guaranteeing death, but of making it effective and functional, under the perception of rejection and deserving, of the cultural valorization of death and the type of death they should receive. Christopher Taylor (1999), for the case of Rwanda, proposed an anthropological interpretation to understand massacres, which considered that the anatomy of the enemy was inextricably articulated to the anatomy of an animal, particularly with oxen, so that the sectioning of the Achilles tendon was frequent. The animalization of the human reflected a Rwandan symbol of the body that was related to the worldview where the main characteristic of this was mobilization. Therefore, an immobilized body due to the sectioning of the Achilles tendon was a clogged, useless body, and it constituted a danger to itself and to the society, so it was ready to be sacrificed. Other anthropological approaches that emphasize dehumanizing processes have offered new perspectives for the analysis of massacres as proposed by Alexander Hinton (2005, 2016) for the particular scenario of Cambodia.

In ***On Inhumanity: Dehumanization and How to Resist It***, Smith (2020) argues that "given the looming threat of catastrophic climate change, and the devastating social consequences that are sure to follow in its wake, a descent into the worst sort of barbarism is overwhelmingly likely before the century is out." For him, the scenario of violence is ready to continue dehumanizing each other and building arguments to facilitate and justify mass atrocity. Hobsbawm (2008) in "War, Peace and Hegemony at the Beginning of the Twenty-First Century" also argued that humans are living in a period of history that has accelerated to a "dizzying pace" and advances at a speed that endangers our species. If the future is one in which human beings will have to compete more and more with each other for resources, in response to the progressive worsening of the effects of global warming and climate change, then we have to consider "what to do and what to avoid."[5] These times include the rise of authoritarian policies around the world and of hate crimes against minority groups, the brutal advances of crimes for the control of drug trafficking areas, illegal exploitation of natural resources and other power struggles that lead to mass deaths, as well as the crisis of migrants and refugees who are also exposed to discrimination and hate. Dehumanization is the appropriate fuel that motivates such behaviors, making it a brutal tool to cause pain, suffering, and destruction.

Smith also warns against falling into the grave error of directing the same way of thinking that implies dehumanization toward those who dehumanize others, in other words dehumanizing dehumanizers:

> *Describing other human beings as monsters is an obstacle to seriously addressing the problem. It doesn't matter how repugnant or destructive their beliefs and actions are. Monsters are fictional, but dehumanizers are real, and they are mostly ordinary people like you and me (Smith* 2020, *p. 20).*

Harriet Over (2021), in clear opposition to these dehumanizing positions, published a paper entitled "Seven Challenges for the Dehumanitation Hypothesis," where, among other statements, she points out that the type of argument associated with "dehumanization" is not absolutely negative because being non-human is not always susceptible to being attacked, for example, pets; "dehumanizers" often see them even as humans, like Adolf Hitler, who adored his dog, and that certain acts of "dehumanization," such as torture and humiliation, in fact, only make sense if they think of their victims as humans. Soon, Over's criticisms were harshly replicated (Smith 2021; Vaes et al. 2021; Giner-Sorolla et al. 2021) considering that Over's critique does not in any way destroy the existing evidence on dehumanization, and on the contrary, they push to be clearer and test the coherence of his arguments (Giner-Sorolla et al. 2021).

On his part, Smith stressed that considering what dehumanizers talk about and act, it seems to indicate that if they think of their victims as humans, it is much less satisfactory to achieve their goals. However, Smith accepts that the "dehumanizers" might still think that their victims are human, but at the same time, they are also thinking that their victims are not human at all. Smith writes that the dehumanization of the other removes inhibitions to act extremely: "Our inhibition against killing other human beings gets switched on automatically when we recognize another person as a human being. And when this mechanism gets overridden, dampened down, or switched off entirely—whether by dehumanization or some other process—this clears the way for viciously destructive moral fury." Although if we understand violence as a discursive practice, dehumanization is an indispensable aspect that must be interpreted from cultural forms. Whitehead (2007) argues that we should pay more attention to the schemes that generate culturally appropriate behavior as well as to the historically constituted matrix of symbolic and ideational forms on which cultural representations, expressions, and performances are based (Whitehead 2007). The aggressors may not really stop thinking completely that those they are massacring have not ceased to be human; on the contrary, they are humans who at the same time have assumed a contaminated and dirty subhuman posture by which they must be eliminated. If a human being is eventually perceived as a cockroach, as in the case of the Rwandan Genocide, that human being must be exterminated to avoid polluting the spaces where humans live and thus prevent them from mixing with each other (Taylor 1999, 2004). Hinton (2005) also reported that the victim's body during the events in Cambodia was no longer a human being due to its contamination by dirty entities, so the bodies had to be disposed of.

Anstett (Chapter 6, in this volume) has highlighted that the "victims of genocides and crimes against humanity are systematically denied their status as individuals and indeed their basic quality as human beings, finding themselves denigrated and frequently likened to worthless objects, vermin and even excrement. Following such massacres, these 'remains of things', as the killers see the corpses of their victims, themselves suffer further denigration. Their mortal remains are thus treated not merely like but literally as rubbish." Even if, despite all the humiliation, an attempt is made to offer a dignified treatment to the body or body parts, identification is achieved, and their identity is restored, it will not always be possible to compensate for the degradation he suffered as a human being and a member of society because the dead continue to maintain their damaged agency, linked to the bad death. When the inert body is destroyed with cruelty, there is an intention to be denied, to force it to cease to be who it is in order to become what the aggressor wants it to become: a complex mechanism for transmitting information that encourages a state of vulnerability. Dehumanization is a functional way for this task, hidden in several cases, but made invisible due to the fact that it is often minimized. However, when it becomes notorious, the lethal ferocity of its results is inevitable. As Smith emphasizes, the latter is even more important because we all have the potential to develop a dehumanizing mindset toward other people, a mindset that cannot be effectively addressed unless we recognize it as human beings and as a society.

Finally, Over (2021) concludes by acknowledging the central meaning of the discussion of the theory of dehumanization by pointing out the following:

> It may be that the dehumanization hypothesis, or some variants of it, can withstand the challenges I outlined in my original article and in this response. It may be that we do not need to reject the dehumanization hypothesis, but rather to refine it (as Smith and Giner-Sorolla et al. suggest in their commentaries). Whatever the case, the field will benefit from further theoretical clarification and empirical data as we continue to address our shared goal of reducing the terrible, real-world consequences of intergroup bias.

In *On Inhumanity*, Smith (2020) takes us to graphic descriptions of the excesses that can stem from dehumanization. One of the author's most striking examples is the documented massacre of black population in the United States between

1877 and 1950. Smith points to the cases of victims who were forced to eat their own amputated genitalia; in another case, a woman's unborn baby was cut from her womb and trampled to death. As he explains, racist lynching were not just extrajudicial executions but also involved torture and body mutilation, often while the victim was still alive. The cut body parts were displayed or kept as souvenirs. Some victims were even burned alive, which is why white people occasionally referred to these abuses as "barbecues." Rather than being understood as heinous and inhumane spectacles, massacres were often considered public holiday events. In her work *"Matar, rematar y contramatar,"* Maria Victoria Uribe (1990) describes various behaviors and actions of mutilation through the dismemberment of people during the eighties in the Colombia of paramilitarism. Her narratives have also shown that one of the mechanisms that led to moving the perpetrators toward these levels of "carnage" has been to deny the category of human to the victims and to even represent them as objects and trophies. Like Uribe's (1990) narrative, hundreds of examples have been reported in the published literature that demonstrate that slaughter is only one stage on the road to destruction (Sémelin 2007; Anstett, Chapter 6 of this volume).

7.3 When death is not enough

7.3.1 Violent death in a Democratic Republic of Congo (DRC) context

Violent death in the special cultural context of DRC has been studied very little. DRC is a social scene with an impressive cultural richness, at both a multiethnic and multilingual level, as well as the harshness of its basic needs that are increasingly a breeding ground for diseases and for the escalation of conflicts and physical violence. In this particular scenario with a long history of violence of all kinds (Van Reybrouck 2015), cultural expressions have been deeply constructed and internalized as violence occurred. The violence that this country has experienced, and still continues to experience, has been gradually transformed, blending it with the customs and beliefs, and has also become a part of the worldview through the production of symbols that can be notoriously perceived when making decisions to kill and kill again people. Between 2016 and 2017, the Kasai region, an area that had remained quiet without violent events of magnitude, was the scene of the Kamuina Nsapu rebellion, which became one of the main humanitarian crisis zones of the contemporary world.[6] For the Kamuina Nsapu, the magical-religious cultural conception was fundamental to their combat actions, which helped them to attack, defend and resist, and attack again. The Kamuina Nsapu introduced notions and perceptions that adjusted or manipulated the cultural essence of the population to strengthen the magical world of animism, fetishes, and violence without limits.[7] In the context of Kasai, the events after the beginning of the Kamuina Nsapu phenomenon can be summarized in three phases, according to the level of escalation of violence:

First phase: From April to August 2016, the escalation of violence in the territory of Dibaya (Kasai Central) begins. The disagreement and refusal of the DRC government to recognize the customary Kamuina Nsapu chief Jean-Prince Mpandi, culturally acclaimed, led to the request of a so-called "political-customary" armed movement of the same name, which opposed the status quo materialized in the presence of institutions that were associated with state authority, such as the Congolese National Police (PNC), the Armed Forces of the Democratic Republic of Congo (FARDC), public servers, and other elements in political positions. The militia recruited many minors in and around Dibaya, attacking state symbols and beheading people associated with the state, such as police, military, members of the electoral commission, and so on. Public property, for example, offices and police stations, was vandalized and looted. The private property of individuals also met the same fate. Often, other civil buildings such as schools, churches, and health centers were also not spared. The influence of ritual beliefs linked to customary traditions on the recruitment and actions of the militia cannot be underestimated, since many elements, including children, were initiated into the "baptism rituals" in the so-called *Tshiotas* (Extended Families in the Tshiluba language), who were believed to have supernatural powers that made them, for example, immune to gunfire, capable of carrying invincible mystical fetish weapons manufactured with pieces of wood and painted red, or, in the case of girls, capable of stopping bullets with their skirts. However, state repression was brutal and characterized by an "asymmetric war," in which national forces armed with assault rifles and rocket launchers mostly fought children and youth armed with wooden sticks, spears, machetes, and hunting rifles at best. On August 12, 2016, Jean-Prince Npandi was killed in the village of Kamuina Nsapu, which led to the exacerbation of hostilities.[8]

Second phase: From September to December 2016, despite the brutal repression, the Kamuina Nsapu movement became popular among the Luba-speaking communities (like the *Tshiluba*, here called lubaphones) from the majority group of Luba people, and they continued to fight the state authority, reaching the city of Kananga, the capital of Kasai Central, and other areas in the provinces of Kasai Oriental and Kasai, with significant activity on the Kananga-Tshikapa road axis. In areas that fell under militia control, not only was state authority repressed but also local customary chiefs were forced to declare themselves allies with the movement otherwise be beheaded, and minors were largely recruited to plan upcoming attacks. As mentioned before, the repression by the state was very harsh. For example, in the city of Kananga, after the airport area was attacked by the militia and retaken by the military, follow-up operations by militia elements were carried out "door to door" and were marked by testimonies of serious human rights violations, with allegations of looting, summary executions, enforced disappearances, and gang rapes. In the village of Mzanza Lomba, a video recorded by the army in December 2016 showed FARDC elements firing indiscriminately at people, including minors and young women, allegedly linked. Then, it would be known that those young women could be serving as human shields who had the magical powers to stop the bullets.[9]

Third phase: from January to July 2017, violence reached a peak level and there was an ethnic dimension in hostilities. In places under militia control, the *Tshiotas* were used as initiation centers for newly recruited members and also as parallel courtrooms, where informal accusations of robbery, rape, and witchcraft would be tried and often punished with death. In the city of Luebo, a highly emblematic case of sexual assault in public was committed, in the middle of a central square after a woman was accused of treason by the militia and forced to have sex in public with her stepson. After that, both were beheaded. All aspects of daily life were controlled by the militia, including access to and use of mobile phones, for instance. The recovery of these areas by government forces was marked by acts of extreme violence, including the indiscriminate use of force against civilians, looting, sexual violence, enforced disappearances, and summary executions. As the militia advanced westward, it expanded into areas inhabited by ethnic groups other than the Luba, such as the Chokwe and the Pende, who did not speak *Tshiluba* as a first language and did not identify with the political-customary elements that led to the emergence of the militia. In response to hostilities toward non-lubaphone populations, other armed groups were soon organized as self-defense militias, some allegedly receiving government support, such as the *Bana Mura*. Over time, populations opposed to the militia's arrival progressively associated lubaphone populations with the Kamuina Nsapu militia, and the Bana Mura armed groups started to direct acts of extreme violence specifically against those who, for example, did not speak *Chokwe* or *Pende*, including summary executions, forced displacement, sexual violence, and other inhumane treatment. The UN received complaints about the abduction of women and children who were taken to farms and used as forced laborers and sex slaves. On the other hand, Kamuina Nsapu's violent actions also intensified with attacks on civilians who were not lubaphones. A significant part of the population in these areas became internally displaced person (IDP), trying to escape from violence toward other provinces or Angola.

7.3.2 The power of symbols, beliefs, and violent death in Kasai

An interesting report from July 2018, by *Congo Research Group* of the *Center on International Cooperation New York University,* presented the testimonies of two people from Kananga, who mentioned that the girls were also recruited to perform subordinate tasks for the male combatants, basically to be spouses. They also reported that other women who were young were put on the front line, as they were able to stop the bullets. The specially selected women were virgins, who while menstruating had especially that power. We agree with the Congo Research Group report when it highlights that "both versions reflect a cultural understanding of purity and pollution, in which the militia groups sought to mobilize the girls' potency either through the 'purity' of their virginity, or through their temporary state of 'pollution' while menstruating" (2018, p. 12). Douglas (2002) [1966] argues that each culture perceives the world through a system of categories of purity that define the natural order by assigning things a proper place or considering them as an anomaly, dirty, impure, and threatening, "matter out of place." During 2019 and 2021, we frequently visited the territory of Nganza, near the city of Kananga, where we managed to verify such testimonies. Numerous women who had been sexually assaulted and forced to join the militia commented that several dozen young women from Nganza participated as shields in the front line, due to their powers during menstruation, but when they died, their bodies were not to be touched and were left out in the open because of the dirt of their condition.

The population as a whole, including especially the children who were recruited by the militia, was convinced that their rituals were powerful and contained magical elements that prevented them from dying in combat. According to them, the same thing happened when a fighter fell into action; they did not use the word "death" because they did not die—they only became another type of a more powerful force capable of defeating anyone. The Kamuina Nsapu understood that it was not a death as such, but rather the incorporation of greater powers to continue fighting, and only the most powerful reached that privilege. There were even children who assumed the representation of combatants who had fallen in combat but who managed to "revive" or "settle" inside the body of those children after a ceremony in the *Tshiota*. The children drank the blood of the enemies who were captured and then beheaded in their presence, becoming powerful fighters or assuming a new identity capable of destroying the enemy. These children and young people always wore a red bow around their heads, the symbol of which identified them as powerful warriors of the militia. When the Kamuina Nsapu executed someone, usually in public, they often beheaded the prisoner and subsequently dismembered him. In addition to that, only the heads were displayed in the *Tshiota*, as a symbol of power; the other body parts were thrown away as garbage or burned, but they were never buried. Blood was the magical vehicle that transported the new force to another body through concoction, but it was possible only if the new possessor of that force beheaded the prisoner and then ingested the blood directly from the hemorrhage. According to the interpretation of the Kamuina Nsapu, the strength and anima of the fallen combatant entered the body of the enemy and was deposited in his blood, so it was absolutely important to take prisoners and behead them in life to facilitate the hemorrhage.

Currently, if you ask in the rural population and in larger cities like Kananga as well, from elderlies to children, they are convinced that Kamuina Nsapu had special powers that made them powerful and feared. Even during 2021, several people interviewed maintained the speech affirming that, in the special scenario of Kasai, diseases such as Ebola and COVID-19 never entered the area due to the particular powers of the traditional chiefs, who are in charge of driving away these evil forces from the region. People felt firmly protected by the magical power during the quarantine that humanity lived through. In the region of the great Kasai, life continued magically healthy. This widespread belief in the powers of Kamuina Nsapu and the fear it aroused among the Kasai population may partly explain how an almost unarmed militia, with sticks, arrows, and red cords surrounding its head as a symbol of magical power, composed largely of children and teenagers, was able to withstand for more than a year the offensives of a regular army of fire-armed and well-trained state fighters. Most of those members of the army and PNC were part of the Tshiluba-speaking cultural group that fought other Tshiluba but with a supernatural force of almost invincible magical adversaries. Nonetheless, as it is known, a very well-armed platoon of 40 PNC members who came from Kinshasa (where they speak another language, Lingala) by the Tschikapa–Kananga route, was captured in the village named Dambu Mukanga by Kamuina Nsapu fighters. According to the mission of the PNC platoon, they had to support the security of the city of Kananga. However, 40 members of that platoon were beheaded and finished off as the militia styled; before that, the members of the platoon were publicly humiliated and called pigs, that is, they were perceived as less than human, so they had to die as such. As expected, the militiamen seized the ammunition and weapons carried by this platoon. One of the survivors of this massacre whom we had the opportunity to interview was sure that they had an impressive power—when they wanted to defend themselves, their weapons never worked. In addition, several of them felt fear of the power they had, so they were taken into captivity for a long time. Apparently, the power of Kamuina Nsapu had transcended cultural boundaries where it was thought that they did not die but obtained more power and returned to take revenge in the midst of brutal actions of kill again and destruction.

In other DRC regions, this same situation was observed in 2021, mainly in Northern Kibu, where members of a rebel militia, who committed abuses against the population, were captured by the civilian population itself and subsequently dehumanized as if they were goats; therefore, they had to follow the same path as a goat. After the death of these rebels, they were roasted in the middle of the main square as part of a kind of symbolic festival so that an armed group never again enters their territory to abuse its population. The captive body of a rebel was devoured by members of the population as part of the festival.

7.3.2.1 Symbolic significance of mass graves

The United Nations Joint Human Rights Office (UNJHRO) has reported, for the specific context of Kasai, about 150 sites containing human remains, which are popularly known as mass graves. In the context of Kasai, the graves and the places where human remains were deposited have a harmful symbolic meaning, which may become culturally dangerous. From our conception, humanitarian reasons would explain the importance of recovering these bodies to be delivered to their families in ceremonies that can contribute to dignify the memory of the deceased and also facilitate the mourning of the relatives. However, in this particular scenario of violence, and in others in DRC such as North and South Kivu, these places containing human remains are highly complex to manage, especially when violent deaths occur. Parra et al. (2020), on this subject, mentioned that:

> "In the Kasai culture of the Democratic Republic of Congo, burials are an essential part of life as well, and if the dead are not properly buried and accompanied in their new journey, their spirit can haunt the living. As for the opening of mass graves, for the Kasai cultural context would mean the production of a living dead whose power would be considered absolute, a kind of invincible zombie." (Parra et al. 2020, p. 84)

In Nganza, during our forensic work for the reconnaissance prior to any forensic intervention of mass graves, we have received testimonies that various local chiefs have been working to relieve those places of danger through the use of ritual ceremonies. Nevertheless, those places continue to be forbidden places where the evil charge continues, and they should not be "opened" because many people are buried there, even villagers who were powerful fighters of Kamuina Nsapu. *"They should not leave there,"* has been a remarkable testimony of a local. Population of the area is convinced that by opening these places, their *"spirits will reincarnate in the children and new battles will begin because those spirits are already confused."* For them, the only way to open those places is to drive away the children during the process. *"It is important to keep the children away to avoid risks of danger."* On the other hand, they at all times did not conceive the reason why the authorities and the forensics wanted to open those places if everything was quiet and it was not necessary to disturb those beings.

When humanitarian reasons were surveyed in order to explain that in those places, there could be several relatives of them who would be missing, the villagers explained to us that their relatives were not missing, because they knew where they were. In addition, they did not need to remove them from these contaminated places. Conversely, they mentioned that their relatives had been reincarnated into another child because they themselves had seen not only that reincarnation but also how their relatives had become more powerful in the Tshiota. So, the dead buried in those places were no longer their relatives; they were just evil beings who should not leave there. Villagers claimed that their relatives had returned home after the fighting and are now dissolved in concoctions they had ingested themselves. For them, it was not possible for their relatives to be buried there; their relatives were with them, and they were part of them. Apparently, the dimension of death in this cultural context would be behaving independently of the materiality of the body, and its prominence would be much more relevant to process suffering. For them, the body was out of place; it was no longer the body of a relative because of the form and violent circumstances. The representation of the good death can be intrinsic and takes place in the ingrained grieving process through the rituals with which they assimilate the transformation of presence–absence. We have noticed that the dignity and memory of the deceased have nothing to do with the usual forensic processes and the so-called dignified handover of the body.

The loss of a member in contexts of violence, such as the one exposed, has evolutionary meanings that condense mechanisms of reorganization and continuity of the social order, which is altered with forensic interventions; even if they are humanitarian from our own vision, for them, the humanitarian meaning may mean leaving things as they are. In this regard, it is doubtful whether the symbolic power that surrounds violent death and the processes of individual and collective mourning are negotiable to fulfill legal effects—a complex scenario that forensic work faces, even from its humanitarian aspect.

A particularly interesting case took place in Tshisuku when the authorities decided to exhume bodies for legal reasons, mainly to document deaths and forms of violence. The villagers of Tshisuku strongly requested the authorities that the mass graves be immediately covered and the bodies taken away from Tshisuku. They mentioned that traditional chiefs would work to minimize the problem that forensics had caused through a series of local rituals. They also mentioned that those who were in that place were not people but beings who were looking to return in order to cause trouble instead. Moreover, authorities and forensics had been influenced by these beings to achieve what they wanted, that is, to be released from those places. Nonetheless, these bodies had to return to Tshisuku, where the villagers themselves would lock them in a mausoleum specially built according to the treatment that was customary for the good death.

Therefore, those beings would be under control. The confinement of these beings was carried out in a public ceremony, where the whole township and local and national authorities attended the event as a cultural way to practice and make visible transitional justice. Other social contexts in DRC have shown similar reactions regarding the meaning of what are popularly called mass graves. Similar reports are exposed for other African contexts, such as those reported for a region of Uganda by Redeker-Hepner et al. 2018; Redeker-Hepner and Steadman (Chapter 16, in this volume).

7.4 Dismembering/mutilating: the perspective from culture

The behavior of the mutilator can vary depending on his interests and the way in which he understands social and cultural life, and he can do it when the person is still alive or when they are already dead; indeed, the latter may not matter to him. In the published literature, there is consensus on the type of behavior that causes dismemberment, classifications, patterns, forensic implications, differences, and approach methodology for the analysis of dismemberment (Konopka et al. 2007, 2016; Dogan et al. 2010; Rajs et al. 1998; Puschel and Koops 1987; Ehrlich et al. 2000; Mellor 2016; Ross et al. 2019; Black et al. 2017; Persaud and Häkkänen-Nyholm 2012; Hakkanen-Nyholm et al. 2009; among others). Usually, we can find behaviors that explain these actions and define the functional sense of dismemberment/mutilation, which even have a complex combination between themselves. A brief description based on the literature previously mentioned has been elaborated, including some notes from our own practical experience with the intention of locating the violent expressions found in the Kasai scenario.

(1) The dismemberer tries to prevent his victim's body from being found. Usually, this occurs after a murder, where the perpetrator tries to get rid of the body to prevent him from being dragged. For that purpose, he proceeds to dismember the body with the intention of facilitating the transport of the remains and dispersing them in different areas as a way to hide the corpse. He attempts, in this way, to eliminate all evidence, and if it fails to prevent the finding, at least the murderer tries to avoid or hinder the victim from being identified through various mechanisms that involve, but are not limited to, mutilation of the fingers, disfigurement of the face, and so on. This first behavior is not new; in fact, it is the most common in various societies (Black et al. 2017; Ross et al. 2019) and can be labeled as the classic conception that causes the dismemberment of someone. It is usually known as *defensive mutilation*.

(2) When there is impulsivity due to the anger of the perpetrator caused by some situation, where the perpetrator does not seem enough to have killed the victim and requires to kill again, including overkiller (destroy it). This process, which is classified as *aggressive mutilation*, can even initiate before killing. This action is gradually intensified until the perpetrator satisfies his anger.

(3) *Communicational mutilation*, focused on generating two-way messages, causes terror among enemies or in society as a whole and sends messages of offense to the memory of the executed, killing him slowly, viciously, and with the greatest suffering to make clear there is no mercy at all. It is a way of symbolizing power through clear messages to opponents, demonstrating a complete disregard for their life or total abhorrence against them. Practices like this have been frequently reported in Latin America (Ross et al. 2019), mainly in countries that are part of the northern Central American triangle, in addition to Costa Rica, Panama, and Mexico; and in South America, in countries such as Brazil, Colombia, Ecuador, and Venezuela.

(4) The act of killing motivated by a state of basically sexual indignation, which provokes rewarding feelings to the perpetrator when killing and killing again, due to the revenge for having been humiliated. These actions tend to look at visible areas such as the victim's face and intimate areas such as their genitalia. It is also linked to lustful and sadistic behavior, since there is need to carry out sexual activities that infringe pain or the desire for killing to complement sexual pleasure. Beyond these conditions, *offensive mutilation* can be initiated on a living person, who may be aware or unaware of the acts that take place on his or her body, and may continue after the victim has died and include actions of cannibalism too.

(5) Mutilation is linked to compulsive desires to relate sexually with a corpse (necromaniac impulse), either before or after organ mutilation (*necromaniac mutilation*). The body parts thus mutilated could be used as a trophy or fetish. Such cases are rare but have been reported (Ehrlich et al. 2000).

In our particular scenario of dismemberment/mutilation, it seems that our observed cases would not be located in any of these classifications that include but are not limited to the fact that the perpetrators do not intend to try to hinder or completely avoid the identification of the body; they do not require to facilitate the transport and disposition of the body with the intention of eliminating the evidence, and there is no need for a demonstration of complete disregard for human life or total abhorrence for the victim. However, it seems that these practices would approach the framework of mutilating actions as vehicles of communication, although in these particular cases, the intention of sending messages of terror from direct messages to the enemy or society as a whole is not precisely the main motivation. Rather, it seems to be a kind of mutilation that contains a strong burden linked to the local belief system that configures the dismemberment/mutilation that holds a complex practical functionality from the cultural worldview. Ross et al. (2019) in their work *"The pattern of Violence and Aggression,"* included cultural considerations as a way of understanding the reasons for dismemberment/mutilation. The authors even were encouraged to offer the hypothesis that dismemberment patterns can also vary between cultures. Salfati and Park (2007) also considered culture as a source of explanation for the cases they observed. Labuschange (2004) completed a detailed review of cultural motivations as the main way to dismember/mutilate within a belief system in the South African context. Parra et al. (2020) showed a pattern of mutilation in a Colombian setting, which was closely associated with animism, witchcraft, and sorcery.

Mutilation, which we call cultural, implies a strong symbolic charge that has its origin in the conception of the energy of the body and its fluids, as a transporter of meanings of power, linked to a system of beliefs that include, but are not limited to, magic, witchcraft, and sorcery, and its performance can be linked to animism. Parra et al. (2020) described a scenario of dismemberment/mutilation among Afro-descendant societies of the Columbian Pacific coast, mainly in the port of Buenaventura, where these practices were connected to cultural conceptions. Nevertheless, it is necessary to make clear that the trigger of a violent death in that particular context has its origins in the power dispute over drug trafficking and intersects with communicational mutilation.

Usually, the perpetrators of these crimes subject their victims to dismemberment while still alive, with the intention of provoking a severe hemorrhage, since they believe that ripping the body apart facilitates the release of the spirit through exsanguination—the spirit leaves the body with the blood. In this way, the perpetrator avoids possible persecution by the deceased's soul and also blocks any possibility of a spell that could be practiced by the deceased person's family to find them. The soul, after leaving the body through the hemorrhage, loses its course in the world of the living without any chance of locating its executioner. In order to achieve the perpetrator's goal, the parts of a single body must be buried together in a specific place, still carrying its belongings (Parra et al. 2020, p. 81).

As observed in the great Kasai and probably in other African regions, what Parra et al. (2020) observed regarding dismembering a living person to facilitate bleeding and the exit of the spirit has similarities with the facts of Buenaventura, because in both cases blood has a fundamental role as a vehicle of power. While for Kasai, the blood must be drunk to acquire magical powers that lead to adopting new energies, for the special place of Buenaventura, the blood contains a type of spiritual energy that must come out and disappear in order that the body does not manage to get up and look for its aggressor; otherwise, the person or persons involved in the death will be reprimanded and suffer severe punishments that may result in their own death. Though, in both cases, dismemberment/mutilation must happen in life since it fulfills an important function: to facilitate hemorrhage and, with it, its cultural functionality.

Other examples of cultural mutilation have been reported in African contexts (Steyn and Brits 2019; Labuschange 2004). Steyn and Brits (2019) showed that in South Africa, cultural beliefs and the action of dismembering/mutilating had been combined for the trade of Muti, a powerful medicinal potion that is regarded as the essence of life. For the Muti to be effective, human parts must be removed when the person is still alive (Labuschange 2004). Labuschange (2004) stressed that the mutilation that takes place in a Muti murder, which may include dismemberment or beheading, is not done with the intention of delaying identification, nor provoked by an outburst of rage. Since the murder is carefully planned and a victim is selected, neither any sexual activity nor fantasy is involved in the mutilation. Finally, in a Muti murder, body parts must be removed while the victim is alive, thus excluding necromaniac mutilation.

If we compare the events mentioned here, related to current life, with those facts reported for ancestral times, we will find similarities regarding their cultural motivations, mainly as an internalizing mechanism with the supernatural to end the existence of something living or the functional destruction of something inanimate (Schwartz 2012). These could be one of the most ancient motivations from the culture of dismemberment/mutilation together with communicational mutilation. For example, ritual violence in the ancestral Andes (Klaus and Toyne 2016; Verano 2013; Verano and Phillips 2016; Verano and Toyne 2011; among others) highlighted archaeological discoveries concerning mutilations in the North coast of Peru. These discoveries have been combined with ethnohistorical and iconographic information to prove such practices involving human executions, ritual killing, and sacrifices. These violent actions have been contrasted with a diversity of characteristics including, but not limited to, the demographic profile of the victims, the contexts in which the victims were found, the presence or absence of associated offerings, and the manner in which the individuals were sacrificed and/or executed. The diversity of the cases evidenced range from executed prisoners to companions sacrificed in honor of the dead dignitaries or their deities.

Verano (2014), for the particular case of Moche, argues that the means to kill the captives was slaughter, with the intention of producing massive bleeding that led to recovering the blood of the victim. Likewise, the strictly practical action was not enough, since it seemed that the repetitive cuts found would suggest the performative action of cutting the throat. In the same way, it has been reported for captives in Punta Lobos (Verano and Phillips 2016; Verano and

Toyne 2011). In fact, Verano and Phillips (2016) have argued that in Moche and Chimu societies, the execution of prisoners was a persistent and pervasive practice. Associated with these actions, beheading has also been one of the repeated practices in various scenarios of Peru (Verano 2018; Tung 2016), mainly as a form of trophy among the Wari (Tung 2016). Several other societies have also used beheading as a way to symbolically express certain meanings such as protecting power, sacred forces, personification, and prestige, including social identity (Tiesler and Lozada 2018). In the archaeological context in the Moche valley itself, more than a hundred children are reportedly sacrificed with evidence of cuts in the thorax, which would be suggesting the intention of accessing the heart to be removed as an offering (Prieto et al. 2019).

In more recent events related to cultural mutilation, Whitehead (2002) examines the complex cultural practice of Kanaimà in the interior of Guyana, which borders Venezuela and Brazil. The conception of Kanaimà, in a wide cultural scenario of the area, describes specific methods of mutilation, murder, and ingestion of liquids from the decomposing corpse that are called *maba*. Whitehead describes the latter as follows *"It consists of the juices produced through the putrefaction of a dead victim's body that has been mutilated anally to permit the introduction of various magical substances that catalyze that putrefaction and add vital elements to the maba"* (Whitehead (2004, p. 71)). The cultural conception of Kanaimà is dual. On the one hand, it depicts evil spirits not only as a particular way of a murderous protective spirit but also as a relationship between the human and the natural forces that describe the native commitment to Kanaimà and its contribution to life forms as a *"cultural proclivity."* Whitehead (2004, p. 46) highlights that this practice of cultural mutilation is about *"an authentic and legitimate form of cultural expression."*

7.4.1 How to understand Kasai's violent events

On the topic of the events in Kasai and the actions of dismemberment/mutilation, these could be explained from the perspective of understanding patterns of meanings and their expressive forms (Whitehead 2004). Like Taylor (2004), we follow what Aijmer (2000, p. 2) has called the *"symbological approach,"* which involves three different but at the same time juxtaposed levels of analysis. There is a first level that brings together the imaginary and the importance of symbols. A second level that involves the discursive containing a strong load of intentions, including but not limited to, performative acts, statements, disagreement, and ideological aspects. Finally, the ethological level that includes the materiality of the facts, that is, *"brute stuff of violent death itself,"* in addition to the psychic representation of its image, its meaning, and its implications (Aijmer 2000, 2001). At this level, the treatment of the body as a transmitter of meanings assumes relevance. It becomes the culturally communicative bridge between the previous levels. In this regard, Whitehead (2001, p. 831) argues that:

> Violent performance discursively amplifies and extends the cultural force of violent acts so that violent acts themselves can generate a shared idiom of meaning for violent death that enfold both killer and killed. As a result of this the way in which persons are killed or mutilated is not arbitrary, haphazard or simply a function of perceived instrumentality.

The need to consume blood, in the particular case of Kasai, among the Kamuina Nsapu, has a meaning that embodies the desire of the imaginary to strengthen itself and put aside its fears in order to continue fighting while these events are being performatively shaped by ideological statements that drive to move forward—a way to instrumentalize power where the body and its fluids are used as vehicles to perform violence. In this case, beheading, dismembering/mutilating, looking for young menstruating virgins to avoid being harmed, and labeling women as dirty during this period become such a symbolic vehicle that results in destroying the enemy. Hinton (2004), in his analysis of the consumption of human livers during the Cambodian genocide, argues that these practices bring together meanings of belonging and difference, solidarity, and power. Based on Turner's (1967) meanings of polarization, Hinton (2004) argues that:

> "Turner ́s conception of embodied symbols provides us with one way of explaining how ideological discourse come to have motivating force in the violent encounter, as they resonate ontologically with felt 'sensory', qualities of given symbols, particularly the symbolic being under assault. In particular, it suggests a further 'grammatical rule' of the vernacular of violence: violence has a mimetic structure, as victims serve as highly symbolic icons reflecting back the subjectify of the perpetrator. This 'mimetics of difference' is a one constructs and image of the self as one manufactures the subjectivity of symbolic 'other'." (2004, p. 180)

The subjectivity to which he refers is the precise moment in which the dehumanization of the victim is given way. As mentioned before, the process of dehumanization is the perfect way to initiate an escalation of suitable and appropriate meanings that contribute to degrading the victim. In the particular case of Kasai, the decapitated and dismembered/mutilated victims were conceived as pigs and goats, but they contained the incarnate power of humans, which after facilitating the hemorrhage, the strength of them whom could be acquired by drinking their blood.

7.5 Conclusions

As humans, a difficult obstacle to overcome is to cease our own system of values and beliefs in order to try to understand various situations, which involve the knowledge of certain bloody episodes such as the dismemberment/mutilation of people. Normally, we understand these events as dehumanizing, appalling, and horrendous, which in fact, are some of the most shocking ways to observe the death of someone, or their kill again, which even leads to their destruction as a human being. However, there is a content of intrinsic meanings that make these types of manifestations a way to explore as far as we are capable of acting, although it seems that we have no limits. Certainly, other ways of violence, such as those shown in this writing, contribute to our conception of life, as unimaginable forms from our own conception, but which can explain to us that culture and its manifestations of violent death are only the repercussions solidly rooted in the world of imagination and symbolism, which we use to perform violence and magnify it for various reasons. We agree with Ortersholtz et al. (Chapter 5 in this volume) who emphasize that *"There is no single mechanism with which to examine group-level violent death, instead violent death must be viewed within the historical and cultural context in which it occurs."* These manifestations are so complex that they require the general approach of anthropology to understand these forms of violence, which can *"… illuminates the social processes of our own times and may show us, if we are ready to listen to its teachings, what to do and what to avoid"* (Boas 1928, p. 11). These teachings will help us to explain the effervescence and vehemence of violence, which has a critical humanitarian impact, as we know. All these episodes of violent deaths demand new reflections so that humanitarian action will be carried out in a suitable and culturally appropriate manner. To achieve this purpose, Parra et al. 2020, p. 79 have highlighted that *"in many ways, social sciences and forensic sciences need to unite to face such humanitarian challenges"*. However, as we have noted, what is considered for certain human groups as a humanitarian need, for other human groups, it does not necessarily have the same meaning (Fassin 2012). Moreover, other types of understandings are required that for now are escaping our notion.

Notes

1. We refer here to violent death within the framework of the concept of mass violence as highlighted by Anstett and Dreyfus (2015).
2. In the sense described by Parra et al. (2020).
3. Expression adapted from Engelke (2019), originally coined as "brute stuff of death yourself."
4. Concept that focuses on the relationships between space/place and death, which are imbued with special meaning and associations (Maddrell and Sidaway 2010; Olds et al. 2005).
5. In words of Boas (1928, p. 11), who argued to principles of century past "that a clear understanding of the principles of anthropology illuminates the social processes of our own times and may show us, if we are ready to listen to its teachings, what to do and what to avoid."
6. UN Human Rights Council (2018), "Rapport de l'Equipe d'experts internationaux sur la situation au Kasaï," June 6, 2018.

7. For further information, see "Setting Fire to Your Own House: Crisis in Kasai, the Manipulation of Customary Power and the Instrumentalization of Disorder, Congo Research Group of the Center on International Cooperation New York University Jul, 2018."
8. UN Human Rights Council (2018), "Rapport of l'Equipe d'experts internationaux sur la situation au Kasaï," June 6, 2018.
9. For further information, see "Setting Fire to Your Own House: Crisis in Kasaï, the Manipulation of Customary Power and the Instrumentalization of Disorder, Congo Research Group of the Center on International Cooperation New York University Jul, 2018".

References

Aijmer, G. (2000). Introduction: the idiom of violence in imagery and discourse. In: *Meaning of Violence: A cross Cultural Perspective* (eds. G. Aijmer and J. Abbik), R1–R9. NY: Rutledge.

Aijmer, G. (2001). The symbological project. *Cultural Dynamic* **13**(1): 66–91.

Anstett, E. (2018). What is a mass grave? Toward an anthropology of human remains treatment in contemporary context of mass violence. In: *A Companion to the Anthropology of Death* (ed. A.C.G.M. Robben), 177–188. Chichester: John Wiley and Sons, Inc.

Anstett, É. and Dreyfus, J.-M. (2015). Introduction. Corpses and mass violence: an inventory of the unthinkable. In: *Human Remains and Mass Violence: Methodological Approaches* (eds. J.-M. Dreyfus and É. Anstett), 1–11: Manchester University Press.

Black, S., Rutty, G., Hainsworth, S., and Thomson, G. (2017). Appendix II. In: *Criminal Dismemberment Forensic and Investigative Analysis* (eds. S. Black, G. Rutty, S. Hainsworth, and G. Thomson), 200–202. Boca Raton: CRC Press.

Boas, F. (1928). *Anthropology and Modern Life*. New York: W. W. Norton & Company.

Dogan, K.H., Demirci, S., Deniz, I., and Erkol, Z. (2010). Decapitation and dismemberment of the corpse: a matricide case. *Journal of Forensic Science* **55**(2): 542–545.

Douglas, M. (2002 [1966]). *Purity and Danger: An Analysis of Concepts of Pollution and Taboo*. London and New York: Routledge.

Ehrlich, E., Rothschild, M.A., Pluisch, F., and Schneider, V. (2000). An extreme case of necrophilia. *Legal Medicine* **2**(4): 224–226.

Engelke, M. (2019). The anthropology of death revisited. *Annual Review of Anthropology* **48**(1): 29–44.

Fassin, D. (2012). *Humanitarian Reason. A Moral History of the Present*. Berkeley: University of California Press.

Giner-Sorolla, R., Burgmer, P., and Demir, N. (2021). Commentary on Over (2021) Well-taken points about dehumanization, but exaggeration of challenges. *Perspectives on Psychological Science* **16**: 24–27. doi: 10.1177/1745691620953788.

Hakkanen-Nyholm, H., Weizmann-Henelius, G., Salenius, S., Lindberg, N., et al. (2009). Homicides with mutilation of the victim's body. *Journal of Forensic Sciences* **54**(4): 933–937.

Haslam, N. (2019). The many roles of dehumanization in genocide. In: *Confronting Humanity at its Worst: Social Psychological Perspectives on Genocide* (ed. L.S. Newman), 199–139. Oxford: Oxford University Press.

Haslam, N. and Loughnan, S. (2014). Dehumanization and infra-humanization. *Annual Review of Psychology* **65**: 399–423.

Haslam, N., Kashima, Y., Loughnan, S., Shi, J., et al. (2008). Subhuman, inhuman, and superhuman: contrasting humans and nonhumans in three cultures. *Social Cognition* **26**: 248–258.

Haslam, N., Loughnan, S., and Sun, P. (2011). Beastly: what makes animal metaphors offensive? *Journal of Language and Social Psychology* **30**: 311–325. doi: 10.1177/0261927X 11407168.

Hinton, A.L. (2002). The dark side of modernity: toward an anthropology of genocide. In: *Annihilating Difference*, 1–40: University of California Press.

Hinton, A.L. (2004). The poetics of genocidal practice: violence under the khmer rouge. In: *Violence* (ed. N.L. Whitehead), 157–184. Santa Fe: SAR Press.

Hinton, A.L. (2005). Why did you kill? The Cambodian genocide and the dark side of face and honor. *The Journal of Asian Studies* **57**(1): 93–122.

Hinton, A.L. (2016). *Man or Monster? The Trial of a Khmer Rouge Torturer*. Durham: Duke University Press.

Hobsbawm, E. (2008). War, peace and hegemony at the beginning of the twenty-first century. In: *War, Peace and Hegemony in a Globalized World: The changing balance of power in the twenty-first century* (ed. C. Chari), 15–24. Oxon: Routledge.

Klaus, H.D. and Toyne, J.M. (eds.) (2016). *Ritual Violence in Ancient Andes. Reconstructing Sacrifice on the North Coast of Peru*. Austin: University of Texas Press.

Konopka, T., Strona, M., Bolechala, F., and Kunz, J. (2007). Corpse dismemberment in the material collected by the department of forensic medicine, Cracow, Poland. *Legal Medicine* **9**(1): 1–13.

Konopka, T., Bolechała, F., Strona, M., and Kopacz, P. (2016). Homicides with corpse dismemberment in the material collected by the Department of Forensic Medicine, Krakow Poland. *ArchiwumMedycynySadowej I Kryminologii* **66**(4): 220–234.

Kwon, H. (2006). *After the Massacre: Commemoration and Consolation in Ha My and My Lai*. Berkeley: University of California Pres.

Kwon, H. (2008). *Ghosts of War in Vietnam*. Cambridge: Cambridge University Press.

Labuschange, G. (2004). Features and investigative implications of muti murder in South Africa. *Journal of Investigative Psychology and Offender Profiling* **1**: 191–206.

Maddrell, A. and Sidaway, J.D. (2010). *Deathscapes: Spaces for Death, Dying, Mourning, and Remembrance*. Farnham: Ashgate Publishing Limited.

Mellor, L. (2016). Mincing words: refining the language and interpretation of mutilation. In: *Understanding Necrophilia: A Global Multidisciplinary Perspective* (eds. L. Mellor, A. Aggrawal, and E.W. Hickey), 25–39. San Diego: Cognella.

Mueggler, E. (2001). *The Age of Wild Ghosts: Memory, Violence, and Place in Southwest China*. Berkeley: University of California Press.

Olds, K., Sidaway, J.D., and Sparke, M. (2005). White death. *Environment and Planning D: Society and Space* **23**(4): 475–479.

Over, H. (2021). Seven challenges for the dehumanization hypothesis. *Perspectives on Psychological Science* **16**: 3–13. doi: 10.1177/1745691620902133.

Parra, R.C., Anstett, E., Perich, P., and Buikstra, J.E. (2020). Unidentified deceased persons: social life, social death, and humanitarian action. In: *Forensic Science and Humanitarian Action: Interacting with the Dead and the Living* (eds. R.C. Parra, S.C. Zapico, and D.H. Ubelaker), 1 e, 79–99. Hoboken, NJ: John Wiley & Sons.

Parra, R.C., Vigo-Corea, D.M., Palma, M.R., Condori, L.A., et al. (2022). Anthropology as a humanitarian action in Peru: violent death and deathscapes out of place. *Human Organization* **81**(2): 180–181.

Persaud, R. and Häkkänen-Nyholm H. (2012) The psychology of corpse dismemberment. The motivation behind the most grotesque crimes. The Blog. Huffington Post. http://www.huffingtonpost.co.uk/dr-raj-persaud/the-psychology-of-corpse-dismemberment_b_1577919.html (accessed May 01, 2022).

Prieto, G., Verano, J.W., Goepfert, N., Kennett, D., et al. (2019). A mass sacrifice of children and camelids at the Huanchaquito-Las Llamas site, Moche Valley Peru. *PLoS ONE* **14**(3): e0211691.

Puschel, K. and Koops, E. (1987). Dismemberment and mutilation (2). *Archives fur Kriminologie* **180**: 88–100.

Rajs, J., Lundstrom, M., Broberg, M., Lidberg, L., et al. (1998). Criminal mutilation of the human body in Sweden – a thirty year medico-legal and forensic psychiatric study. *Journal of Forensic Sciences* **43**(3): 563–580.

Redeker-Hepner, T., Wolfe Steadman, D., and Hannebrink, J.R. (2018). Sowing the Dead: Massacres and the Missing in Northern Uganda. In: *Massacres: Bioarchaeological and Forensic Anthropology Approaches* (eds. C. Anderson and D. Martin), 136–154. Gainesville: University of Florida Press.

Riches, D. (eds.) (1986). *The Anthropology of Violence*. Oxford: Blackwell.

Ross, A.H., Humphries, A., and Cunha, E. (2019). The pattern of violence and aggression. In: *Dismemberments: Perspectives in Forensic Anthropology and Legal Medicine* (eds. A.H. Ross and E. Cunha), 183–194: Academic Press.

Salfati, C.G. and Park, J. (2007). An analysis of Korean homicide crime-scene actions. *Journal of Interpersonal Violence* **22**(11): 1448–1470.

Schwartz, G.M. (2012). Archaelogy and sacrifice. In: *Sacred Killing: The Archeaology of Sacrifice in the Ancient Near East* (eds. A.M. Porter and G.M. Schwartz), 1–32: Eisenbrauuns.

Sémelin, J. (2007). *Purify and Destroy: The Political Uses of Massacre and Genocide*. New York: Columbia University Press.

Smith, D.L. (2011). *Less than Human: Why we Demean, Enslave, and Exterminate Others*. New York: Macmillan.

Smith, D.L. (2014). Dehumanization, essentialism, and moral psychology. *Philosophy Compass* **9**: 814–824.

Smith, D.L. (2016). Paradoxes of dehumanisation. *Social Theory and Practice* **42**: 416–443. doi: 10.5840/soctheo rpract201642222.

Smith, D.L. (2020). *On Inhumanity: Dehumanization and How to Resist It*. Oxford: Oxford University Press.

Smith, D.L. (2021). Challenge 8: a response to over (2021). *Perspectives on Psychological Science* **16**: 22–23.

Steyn, M. and Brits, D. (2019). Dismemberment in South Africa: case studies. In: *Dismemberments: Perspectives in Forensic Anthropology and Legal Medicine* (eds. A.H. Ross and E. Cunha), 183–194: Academic Press.

Taylor, C.C. (1999). *Sacrifice as Terror: The Rwandan Genocide of 1994*. Oxford: Berg Press.

Taylor, C.C. (2004). Dealy images: king sacrifice, President Habyarimana, and the iconography of pregenocidal Rwandan. In: *Violence* (ed. N.L. Whitehead), 79–106. Santa Fe: SAR Press.

Tiesler, V. and Lozada, M.C. (eds.) (2018). *Social Skins of the Head: Body Beliefs and Ritual in Ancient Mesoamerica and Andes*: University of New Mexico Press.

Tung, T.A. (2016). Practicing and performing sacrifice. In: *Ritual Violence in Ancient Andes. Reconstructing Sacrifice on the North Coast of Peru* (eds. H.D. Klaus and J.M. Toyne), 361–370. Austin: University of Texas Press.

Turner, V. (1967). *The Forest of Symbols: Aspects of Ndembu Ritual*. Ithaca: Cornell University.

UN Human Rights Council (2018) Rapport de l'Equipe d'experts internationaux sur la situation au Kasaï," June 6.

Uribe, M.V. (1990) Matar, rematar y contramatar. Las masacres en el Tolima 1948–1964. Controversia. CINEP, Bogotá.

Vaes, J., Paladino, M.P., and Haslam, N. (2021). Seven clarifications on the psychology of dehumanization. *Perspectives on Psychological Science* **16**: 28–32. doi: 10.1177/1745691620953767.

Van Reybrouck, D. (2015). *Congo: The Epic History of a People*: Ecco press.

Verano, J.W. (2013). Many faces of death: warfare, human sacrifice, and mortuary practices of the elite in late pre-Hispanic northern Peru. In: *The Routledge Handbook of the Bioarchaeology of Human Conflict* (eds. C. Knüsel and M.J. Smith), 355–370. London and New York: Routledge Press.

Verano, J.W. (2014). Warfare and captive sacrifice in the moche culture: the battle continues. In: *Embattled Bodies, Embattled Places: War in Pre-Columbian Mesoamerica and the Andes* (eds. A. Scherer and J.W. Verano), 283–310. Washington, DC: Dumbarton Oaks Pre-Columbian Symposia and Colloquia.

Verano, J.W. (2018). Afterlives of the decapitated in ancient Peru. In: *Social Skins of the Head: Body Beliefs and Ritual in Ancient Mesoamerica and the Andes* (eds. V. Tiesler and M.C. Lozada), 175–185: University of New Mexico Press Albuquerque.

Verano, J.W. and Phillips, S.S. (2016). The killing of captives on the north coast of Peru in Pre-Hispanic Times: Iconographic and Bioarchaelogical evidence. In: *Ritual Violence in Ancient Andes. Reconstructing Sacrifice on the North Coast of Peru* (eds. H.D. Klaus and J.M. Toyne), 244–265. Austin: University of Texas Press.

Verano, J.W. and Toyne, J.M. (2011). Estudio bioantropológico de los restos humanos del Sector II, Punta Lobos, valle de Huarmey. In: Arqueologia de la costa de Ancash. ANDES 8: Boletín del Centro de Estudios Precolombinos de la Universidad de Varsovia (ed. M. Giersz), 421–446. Varsovia/Lima: l'Institut français d'études andines.

Verdery, K. (1999). *The Political Lives of Dead Bodies: Reburial and Post Socialist Change*. New York: Columbia University Press.

Whitehead, N.L. (2001). A history of research on warfare in anthropology – reply to Keith Otterbein. *American Anthropologist* **102**(4): 834–836.

Whitehead, N.L. (2002). *Dark Shamans: Kanaimà and the Poetics of Violent Death*. Durham: Duke University Press.

Whitehead, N.L. (2004). On the poetics of violence. In: *Violence* (ed. N.L. Whitehead), 55–78. Santa Fe: SAR Press.

Whitehead, N.L. (2005). War and violence as cultural expression. *Anthropology News* **46**(5): 23–26.

Whitehead, N.L. (2007). Violence and the cultural order. *Daedalus* **136**(1): 40–50.

CHAPTER 8

Mourning violent deaths and disappearances

Antonius C. G. M. Robben
Department of Anthropology, Utrecht University, Utrecht, The Netherlands

8.1 Introduction

The Universal Declaration of Human Rights was born from the slaughter of the Second World War, but where are the dead who inspired the world's nations to call for an international bill of rights? The rights of the dead are missing from the declaration, and so are those of the bereaved. Forensic humanitarianism has tried to fill this gap by restoring the human worth and dignity of the dead and relieve the sorrow of the bereaved (Cordner and Tidball-Binz 2017; Ubelaker et al., 2019).[1]

Unlike forensic exhumations, which are primarily carried out to gather legal evidence to convict perpetrators, humanitarian exhumations aim to clarify the fate of the dead and the disappeared. Positive identifications and the recovery of human remains enable the bereaved to bury their dead and allow them to work through their loss. The painful past is put to rest, and the bereaved can make a new beginning through a mourning process that ends in closure; at least, this is commonly assumed. In this chapter, I will show that this understanding is based on four misconceptions that may hinder the ways people come to terms with the violent death or disappearance of loved ones.

First, disappearances do not inhibit mourning because facing the difficult reality of a missing relative or friend is already a process of mourning. Second, people construct meaningful lives despite the uncertainty of whether their missing loved ones are dead or alive. Third, if a death is confirmed and the body has received the proper funerary treatment, then closure is not the inevitable outcome of mourning because bereaved individuals may maintain ongoing

Anthropology of Violent Death: Theoretical Foundations for Forensic Humanitarian Action, First Edition.
Edited by Roberto C. Parra and Douglas H. Ubelaker.

relationships with the dead. Finally, personal mourning should not be confounded with social and national mourning.

I shall begin with a discussion of the mourning of dead and missing soldiers of the First World War to explain the differences and tensions between personal, social, and national mourning. The postwar monopolization of national mourning by the state provoked protests from civil society and marginalized the personal mourning of the bereaved. Throughout the twentieth century, states have directed the national memory of the dead and missing, and some even took possession of the corpses for political ends. This politics of national mourning violates the rights of the dead and the bereaved.

In the next section, I examine why people care for the dead and search for the missing. Forensic humanitarianism defines its mission as helping people to mourn their losses but narrowly interprets mourning as a process aimed at closure so that the mourners can get on with their lives, and nations are freed from the burdens of the past. Using illustrations from post-authoritarian Argentina, I will show that this emphasis on care is important for humanitarian assistance but is insufficient as an explanation for people's care for the dead and the missing. Care is a surface manifestation of an enduring attachment and trust among human beings, including forensic experts, which originates in the home. Care enacts a relationship between the dead, the disappeared, and the living rooted in their social attachment and trust and often continues after the mortuary rituals have been performed.

The final section demonstrates that mourning, at whichever level of social complexity, is directed at primary and secondary losses. Mourning is not exclusively focused on the dead and disappeared but also on having a meaningful life without the presence of the loved persons. Mourning is about people, groups, societies, and states finding a sense of existence in the wake of massive violence. I shall conclude that forensic humanitarian work should be sensitive to the potential conflicts between personal, social, and national mourning and that more attention should be paid to the relationship between the dead, the disappeared, and the living, which may end in closure but may just as well give continuous new meaning to life, death, and history.

8.2 The conflictive mourning of the dead and missing after the First World War

The soldiers who died or went missing during the First World War were regarded as martyrs, irrespective of the country for which they fell. The postwar creation of what George Mosse has called the Myth of the War Experience increased their martyrdom. The misery of trench warfare made way for the national commemoration of a holy war fought by brave men. "The memory of the war was refashioned into a sacred experience which provided the nation with a new depth of religious feeling, putting at its disposal ever-present saints and martyrs, places of worship, and a heritage to emulate" (Mosse 1990, p. 7). Fallen British soldiers were resembled to Christ who was purified by his suffering and also sacrificed his life for humankind, and like Christ on Easter, the soldiers would rise from the grave on Resurrection Day. The military cemeteries were therefore hallowed places. However, they lacked the symbolic power of national shrines. For this reason, tombs of the unknown soldier were erected in 1920 in France and Great Britain that could unite people's personal sentiments. These tombs intended "to glorify the nation and the greatness of killing and dying in war" (Zambernardi 2020, p. 10).

Still, for all the worship and honor bestowed on the dead, there were many bereaved relatives who had never visited their deceased loved ones at some foreign graveyard or had been unable to bury them because the bodies had fragmented or were missing. National shrines acknowledged all war casualties, allowing relatives to mourn the dead and the missing collectively. Winter (1995) is right when he writes that the war memorials and annual commemorative ceremonies of the First World War gave collective meaning to the human losses and created a community of mourners consoled by their common fate. His conclusion that this collective mourning was instrumental in making people cope with their individual bereavement is, however, based on an unfortunate conflation of personal, social, and national mourning.

National mourning is orchestrated by the state. The state defines who, what, and how the dead and missing will be mourned and remembered. Monuments, memorial plaques, and commemorations are public forms of national mourning, but there are also less visible forms such as reparation payments, pensions, and the consignment of art works. The state may pursue policies of national reconciliation to end domestic and international animosities that may undermine the smooth functioning of economy and society.

These official measures may be contested by social groups whose interests are underrepresented or whose dead and missing are ignored in the state's national mourning. Social mourning is a group process of mourners who have a similar social attachment to the dead because of a shared marker, such as ethnicity, religion, political conviction, regiment, unit, city, and region. Their public initiatives might be at odds with the national mourning politics. For example, the grief of Australian mothers who lost their sons was officially acknowledged immediately after the First World War, but the bereaved women were increasingly marginalized from public commemorations as time passed because only fallen soldiers were honored for their sacrifice to the nation (Damousi 1999a). Another example of the tensions between social and national mourning is the differential treatment of soldiers who died during and after the war. Australian servicemen who returned home wounded and then died were not considered to be war deaths, and their wives were not regarded as war widows. Both were excluded from the national commemorations of the First World War. Widows of the post-war dead did, however, receive recognition from community organizations of veterans and war widows who acknowledged their grief and provided support when needed. It would take till 1928 when the postwar dead were officially acknowledged by having their names added to Roll of Honour of the Australian War Memorial in Canberra (Larsson 2009).

The historian Jay Winter has suggested that national and social mourning can overlay personal mourning. He infers that people achieved closure after the First World War by displacing their grief on national shrines and finding consolation in official commemorative acts. Winter defines mourning as a process "of separating from the dead and beginning to live again" and writes that this "process of separation from the dead, of forgetting as much as remembering" is the central thesis of his much-cited book (Winter 1995, pp. 115, 224). Unfortunately, he confuses personal, social, and national mourning and uses an outdated conceptualization of personal mourning.

Personal mourning concerns the combination of an individual's grief and the cultural ways of coping with bereavement. However, the term "bereavement denotes the social status of having lost someone, which may be a deceased or missing person; "Grief is a response to bereavement. It is how the survivor feels. It is also how the survivor thinks, eats, sleeps, and makes it through the day. . .. Mourning refers to the culturally patterned expressions of the bereaved person's thoughts and feelings" (Kastenbaum 1977, pp. 242–244). The bereaved person wages an inner struggle about how to relate to the dead or missing loved person. One person's coping with loss may differ greatly from the sense of loss experienced by a relative or friend who mourns the same dead person.

Several studies have shown that national mourning concealed rather than resolved personal mourning after the First World War. For more than a decade, British families visited military cemeteries in Belgium and France because the national memorials and commemorations didn't satisfy their emotional needs (Jalland 2010). In Italy, commemorative pamphlets were printed for distribution among family, comrades, and friends. The small booklets contained obituaries, eulogies, and letters from officers and comrades who had witnessed the soldier's death. These pamphlets were substitutes of the mortuary rituals that bereaved families had been unable to perform and indicated that people didn't trust their dead to the state's politics of national mourning (Janz 2009). In Germany, war widows didn't wear the customary mourning garments in order to express their loyalty to the state and approval of the human sacrifices made to the nation. Privately, however, the emotions might break through their publicly cultivated stoicism (Siebrecht 2014). In Australia, similar feelings of maternal sacrifice and stoicism were replaced by public protests against the state that increasingly ignored their enduring grief, while the proud Australian fathers who had imbued their sons with a sense of patriotism and manliness, and had encouraged them to enlist, bitterly mourned their deaths in private (Damousi 1999b).

The state's dominance over people's personal mourning after the First World War is relevant to forensic humanitarian action. Forensic teams must be aware of state authorities that try to employ human remains for political ends, as happened in Chile, Spain, and Cambodia. Chilean relatives were asked to bury the victims of Pinochet's military regime in a memorial at the General Cemetery in Santiago for the sake of national reconciliation (Robben 2015). The Spanish dictator Franco ordered the exhumation of tens of thousands of corpses of Nationalist and Republican soldiers that had died during the Civil War and interred them in the Valley of the Fallen memorial without obtaining permission from the relatives (Ferrándiz 2019). The Cambodian government erected communal memorials containing the skeletal remains of the victims of the Cambodian genocide against the wishes of relatives who wanted a Buddhist cremation (Kidron 2020).

The uproar about the treatment of human remains in countries as culturally diverse as Chile, Cambodia, and Spain suggests that the dead hold human rights because, as Moon (2014, p. 59) has pointed out: "they can be seen to be rights holders insofar as the living behave as if they have obligations towards the dead, treat them as if they have rights, and confer rights upon them in practice". Adam Rosenblatt is hesitant about conferring human rights on the dead and the missing but nevertheless concludes perceptively that withholding care is a violation of their rights. "The care that relatives and mourners offer a dead body, whether it takes the form of washing, cremation, viewing, or any other practice, cannot be carried out when the body is in a mass grave" (Rosenblatt 2015, p. 165). By extension, not only the dead have human rights but also the bereaved have the human right to mourn the dead, as I have argued elsewhere (Robben 2012).

Why is mortuary care so important for the living and the dead? The historian Laqueur (2015, pp. 5–10) has argued that people have a need to acknowledge the dead as deceased members of a community and humanize them through funerary rituals that differentiate them from animals as cultural beings. Laqueur builds on the seminal work of anthropologist Robert Hertz, who stated that a person's death is both a biological and a cultural fact that entails moral and social obligations from the living. "The body of the deceased is not regarded like the carcass of some animal: specific care must be given to it and a correct burial; not merely for reasons of hygiene but out of moral obligation" (Hertz 2018, p. 19). Rosenblatt (2015, p. 189) also gives central importance to care by arguing that forensic exhumations allow relatives to care for the dead: "The violence visited upon the dead bodies in a mass grave was an attempt to place them beyond the reach of care. . .. Among the most important tasks of the forensic expert who exhumes bodies and objects . . . are the unearthing of these networks of affective connection and the expansion of opportunities for care".

These are important and sensitive observations based on historical and empirical analyses. Yet, people are not born with care. Care is a manifestation of deeper lying social attachments nurtured in early childhood and extended later in life to others, including the dead and the disappeared. This nuance is important. If the ethics of forensic humanitarian action is defined solely in terms of providing care, then the cultural variation in the ways to satisfy the human rights of the dead, the disappeared, and the bereaved is ignored and may even be suppressed. What is proper humanitarian care can only be determined after understanding people's social attachments and how these bonds influence their mourning of the dead and the disappeared.

8.3 Enduring bonds of the living, the dead, and the disappeared in Argentina

Forensic humanitarianism aims to restore the human dignity of the victims of political violence and provide emotional relief and closure to the bereaved by exhuming and identifying their remains. "For the families of the missing, the combination of lack of news and uncertainty about the fate of their loved ones amounts to unbearable suffering. The unresolved grief often remains active as long as 'closure' is not possible" (Tidball-Binz 2013, p. 341).[2] This understanding owes much to Freud.

Sigmund Freud argued that mourning requires grief work to overcome the initial disbelief of death. The bereaved fantasize that the loved ones have not died – they had seen them in good health only days ago or had talked to them on the phone just recently – but reality will prove them wrong. They must face the truth and slowly loosen the personal bond with the deceased. Bereaved persons may even contemplate suicide to join the deceased in their fate, but they will most often choose life over death and "sever [the] attachment to the object [i.e. the deceased] that has been abolished" (Freud 1955, p. 255). Influential theorists interpreted Freud as saying that severing the relationship between the deceased and the bereaved is essential to have a meaningful life again. Psychotherapists concentrated their counseling therefore on the acceptance of loss and untying the emotional relationship with the deceased and whatever reminded of them (Silverman and Klass 1996, pp. 7–14; Stroebe and Schut 1999, pp. 197–201; Valentine 2006, p. 60).

The disappearance of a loved person complicates the mourning process. The loss is hoped to be temporary, and the ongoing uncertainty confirms the denial of death. Argentine parents who didn't find their disappeared sons and daughters in hospitals and morgues assumed that they were still in the hands of the military dictatorship. The belief that the disappeared were dead would be emotionally unacceptable because that would imply ending the search and mentally killing their loved ones.

The unsure fate of the disappeared caused different forms of mourning. Many relatives suffered from impaired mourning because they didn't want to accept that the person was dead. Others displayed anticipatory grief or chronic anxiety. They prepared themselves for the worst to come or felt unmoored from life because of the ongoing uncertainty. Feeling powerless, many searching relatives suffered from multiple psychological and psychosomatic problems such as depression, insomnia, and loss of appetite (Kordon et al. 1988). Still others assumed from the start that the disappeared were dead. This was the price of waging a revolution.

Increasingly more relatives resigned themselves to the inevitable during the first years of democracy when numerous anonymous graves were discovered, but a number of them still had difficulty coping with the loss. Argentine psychotherapists argued that the absence of a physical proof of death hindered the grief work: "one doesn't know what it is that one has to accept, and what the nature of the loss is. This has a destructuring effect on the psyche, and is confusing for the person who has to accompany this process of working-through. It is worth remembering that the presence of a corpse is an important element that helps a person to escape denial mechanisms when trying to work through a death" (Edelman and Kordon 1995, p. 107). This Freudian interpretation of the mourning process proved to be crucial in convincing an influential group of searching mothers to reject forensic exhumations.

In line with Freud's grief work hypothesis, the psychologists who assisted the Mothers of the Plaza de Mayo explained that the exhumation, identification, and reburial of the skeletal remains of the disappeared would provide emotional closure and dissolve their political drive to denounce the disappearances and the regime's perpetrators. The organization's president, Hebe de Bonafini, accused the Argentine government in 1984 of a scheme to undermine their activism by setting grief work in motion through exhumations and financial compensations: "What are you going to protest about when you accept the exhumations and the indemnification? In no way whatsoever do I want a dead body. What I want is the murderer!" (Diago 1988, p. 157). The group around Hebe de Bonafini began to interrupt forensic exhumations and demanded that the Argentine government made haste with prosecuting and convicting the perpetrators. Their resistance to the forensic exhumations was based on the belief that mourning would make the searching relatives leave the past behind: "Convert the mothers of the disappeared into the mothers of the dead. And so close the problem of the disappeared" (del Rosario de Cerruti 1984, p. 2). She was wrong on both counts. Relatives who buried the remains of their exhumed loved ones didn't stop their political engagement but continued to protest the impunity of the Argentine military and police, and personal mourning didn't sever the relationship with the dead. The reason is that many people maintain an enduring bond with the dead, even though some may wish and succeed in achieving closure.

Psychological studies have shown "that the bereaved remain involved and connected to the deceased, and that the bereaved actively construct an inner representation of the deceased that is part of the normal grieving process" (Silverman and Klass 1996, p. 16). This inner representation reproduces a continuing bond that should not be diagnosed as pathological. Also, the sociologist Tony Walter has emphasized that mourners integrate the dead in their lives. "The purpose of grief is not to move on without those who have died, but to find a secure place for them" (Walter 1996, p. 20). People may cut their ties to the dead, but they may equally refashion the relationship, remembering them daily and maintaining inner conversations with the dead. Finally, the anthropology of death has shown that people in many societies forge enduring spiritual relations with their ancestors, including those who died violent deaths (e.g. Kwon 2006; Nelson 2008).

The violent death and disappearance of loved persons is painful to the relatives and friends because of their social attachment. Bowlby (1997, p. 371) defined attachment as follows: "To say of a child that he is attached to, or has an attachment to, someone means that he is strongly disposed to seek proximity to and contact with a specific figure and to do so in certain situations, notably when he is frightened, tired or ill". With the exception of neglectful homes and abusive parents, attachment creates in caregivers the disposition to cherish children and protect them from danger. They try to be near them as much and closely as possible and put the children's safety above that of their own (Weiss 1993, pp. 274–275). This protective urge is illustrated by the following case of an Argentine mother and son who were abducted together.

On April 15, 1976, five armed men forced their way into the house of Iris Etelvina Pereyra de Avellaneda in search of her husband, but he succeeded to escape. In response, the assault team abducted her and their 14-year-old son, Floreal. They were beaten and taken into the street. Iris related in 1985 at an Argentine court how she had clung to her son when they were hooded. "We had our hands free and instinctively I searched for those of my son but I didn't find them. I then raised my voice asking for him, and the police commissioner answered unwillingly: 'I'll bring him right now.' And, in fact, they put us together in the same vehicle. They put us in the back seat. My son squeezed my right hand as if to give me courage" (Pichel 1985, p. 2). Iris was tortured about her husband's hiding place and then granted three wishes before she was going to be executed. "I asked him about my son, and he answered that I shouldn't ask anymore because 'We already tore your son to pieces'" (Pichel 1985, p. 3). After being released in July 1978, Iris learned that her son, Floreal, had washed ashore in Uruguay in May 1976. According to the autopsy report, he had died from impalement (Almirón 1999, p. 194; Feitlowitz 1998, p. 208).

Attachment differs cross-culturally. The mother–baby relationship is hegemonic in Western societies but not necessarily elsewhere. Cultures differ in terms of the meaning, importance, and closeness of the maternal bond. Small children may be raised by multiple caregivers who play different roles in the child's life. Biological mothers and fathers may maintain a greater social and physical distance than other caregivers. Caregivers and children may also communicate in more nonverbal ways and develop other notions of safety and independence than in the Western middle-class families on which John Bowlby based his attachment theory (Keller 2014; Quinn and Mageo 2013).

Attachment creates trust in the child, as the psychologist Erik Erikson explained: "The infant's first social achievement . . . is his willingness to let the mother out of sight without undue anxiety or rage, because she has become an inner certainty as well as an outer predictability" (Erikson 1963, p. 247). The infant is confident that the mother will return. This trust will also develop the mother's trust toward her child. The mutual trust continues into adulthood. Furthermore, the trust nurtured among family members will extend during childhood and adolescence to friends and other members of society. Trust gives them a fundamental sense of security, which allows them to engage in new relationships and feel at ease outside the home (Giddens 1991, pp. 39–40). This mature trust means that people suspend the doubt that relationships may go awry, that they may be betrayed and taken advantage of by others (Möllering 2006, pp. 109–111; Robben 2018, pp. 15–16). This leap of faith is based on each other's past behavior and future expectations. Frequent social interaction tests the mutual trust and calibrates the relationship.

Like attachment, trust and trusting relationships vary cross-culturally (Broch-Due and Ystanes 2016). In a comparative study, Peter Geschiere analyzed the ambivalent trust among family members who try to protect one another against witchcraft but also fear that one of them might be a witch. For example, the Maka of Cameroon believe that witches live in people's bellies and may change at night into spirits and animals to fly to a gathering of witches. The witches indulge in a cannibalistic feast to which participants contribute a family member. The victim will die the following day, unless a healer identifies the witch and succeeds in forcing him or her to lift the spell. This belief inserts mistrust in households and families. The knowledge that a family member may be devoured by witches is terrifying and all the more so if the witch is suspected to live in the household (Geschiere 1997, pp. 43–49, Geschiere 2013, p. 4).

Mourning a dead or missing person is thus a manifestation of attachment and trust. Attachment and trust have made the Mothers of the Plaza de Mayo do everything humanly possible for their disappeared loved ones, short of revenge. They held street protests during the dictatorship, endured repeated intimidation, and continued to risk falling victim to enforced disappearances, even after some of them were abducted, tortured, and assassinated. They opposed amnesty laws and presidential pardons and demanded truth and justice. The Grandmothers of the Plaza de Mayo tirelessly sought their stolen grandchildren and gave the impetus to DNA testing. These mothers and grandmothers inscribed the history of the disappearances into Argentine history.

People's care for the loved person's human remains is a consequence of the social bond cultivated during their lifetime together, which is often extended to group members and may be generalized to any human being. Carrying out culturally prescribed mortuary rituals and cooperating as a group to find disappeared persons express attachment and trust, which shows that the ways bereaved individuals cope with losses is influenced but not defined by social or national mourning.

8.4 Oscillatory mourning of the dead and the disappeared by the bereaved

Mourning is about coping with primary losses, either death or disappearance, and secondary losses, such as giving new meaning to one's existence and facing life's demands in the absence of the loved person. I draw here on the Dual Process Model of Coping with Bereavement, developed by Stroebe and Schut (1999), which I extend from mourning a death to mourning a disappearance. Mourning is not a linear process, according to these psychologists, but the bereaved's attention oscillates between two dimensions of personal mourning, namely, loss-oriented coping with primary losses and restoration-oriented coping with secondary losses. The term "restoration" doesn't imply that the bereaved's coping is successful, such as finding a new partner, but simply that mourners have to deal with challenges that they may or may not overcome. Even when bereaved persons cannot reconcile themselves with a human loss, they still need to carry on with their lives. People give a different individual weight to loss- and restoration-oriented coping. Some may be immersed in sorrow and only rarely find distraction, while others are busy running a single-parent household and avoid loss-oriented memories about the deceased. People may also suffer from emotional overload when the dual demands of loss and restoration are too great to carry, for instance, in the case of a dramatic drop in income and living standard (Stroebe and Schut 2016). Oscillated personal mourning doesn't necessarily lead to closure because the bereaved may settle into active and emotionally stable bonds with the deceased or disappeared loved ones.

Social and national mourning is also characterized by oscillatory movements between loss orientation and, what I have called, recovery orientation because I reserve the term "restoration orientation" for personal mourning (Robben 2014). Social mourners may find comfort in coping with their losses together and can organize themselves to pursue humanitarian and political goals. Whether searching relatives are personally grieving permanently over the disappearance of their loved one, suffering from impeded mourning, or resigning themselves to disappearances as the inevitable cost of a social revolution – as happened in Argentina – they may still unite their protest voices against the state.

How Argentine family-based and human rights organizations tried to achieve their objectives differed between and within these organizations. Internal disagreements had far-reaching consequences for the members because the loss-oriented and recovery-oriented oscillations of social mourning influenced their personal mourning, as is illustrated by the following conflict.

In March 1985, an Argentine judge ordered the opening of three anonymous graves in the city of Mar del Plata. The graves contained the skeletal remains of three disappeared persons. The relatives of two of them favored the exhumation, but the mother of the third person, who was presumably her daughter, was against. She belonged to a faction of the Mothers of the Plaza de Mayo that rejected forensic exhumations as a government ploy to individualize the mourning of what was regarded as a collective loss that deserved social mourning. Hebe de Bonafini, the family-based organization's president, stated that the Mothers "don't accept either anthropologists or scientists from anywhere else in the world to come and tell us that the packages of bones are our children" (Gorini 2008, p. 308). The Argentine Forensic Anthropology Team entrusted with the exhumations respected the mother's wishes and withdrew from the gravesite (Robben 2018, p. 209).

The disagreement about forensic exhumations ran so high in 1986 that the Mothers of the Plaza de Mayo split into two groups. Both associations continued to demand truth and justice from the Argentine state, but one group collaborated with forensic anthropologists to find their disappeared children and bury the remains, while the other group opposed the exhumations and sought psychological counseling to help them with their individual bereavement and cope with the emotional cost of giving up the search.

Dependent on the government in charge, Argentina's national mourning oscillated between attention to primary losses or loss orientation and secondary losses or recovery orientation. The national loss orientation was directed at the disappeared, the perpetrators, forensic exhumations, and the active remembrance of the dead and disappeared. The national recovery orientation dealt with the tensions in post-authoritarian Argentina, in particular the coexistence of the military and civil society, the memorialization of the violent past, and the reparation of losses suffered by ex-disappeared, bereaved relatives, and political refugees. Some governments focused their policies more on loss orientation than on recovery orientation, and vice versa. Due to these oscillations, the bereaved and their organizations came to mistrust the state, a suspicion that had been set in motion by the military regime.

Before handing over power, the transitional military government called in April 1983 on the Argentine people to forget about the violent past and look toward the future. This was at a time of rising street protests by the human rights movement and the labor unions. The junta admitted that the disappeared were an open wound in Argentine society that could not heal without resolving the fate of the disappeared and decided to pronounce them dead: "it must be absolutely clear that those who appear on the lists of the disappeared and who are not in exile or in hiding, are considered dead in legal and administrative terms, even though the cause and occasion of their unexpected death or the place of their burial cannot yet be determined" (Militar 1983, p. 13). In addition, the transitional military government issued in September 1983 a Law of National Pacification that freed officers and guerrillas from being prosecuted for violent acts committed between 1973 and 1982. With these loss-oriented and recovery-oriented measures, the departing dictatorship hoped that the searching relatives would mourn the death of the disappeared, and the Argentine people would reconcile over a violent past that was dividing society.

The democratically elected government of Raúl Alfonsín was installed in December 1983. The Argentine Congress immediately derogated the junta's amnesty law intended to pacify the country, and the government created a truth commission to examine the fate of the disappeared. These two loss-oriented measures were taken to calm the human rights movement. The government also tried to appease the military with the recovery-oriented proposal to prosecute only commanding officers because the lower ranks had only obeyed orders. This national mourning strategy backfired. The truth commission concluded in September 1984 that there were at least 8960 disappeared persons. They were all dead, as the military had claimed in April 1983, but there were 172 kidnapped babies and infants that were probably living in families of military and police officers (Robben 2005, p. 321).

The human rights and family-based organizations were shocked. They emphasized that there were 30 000 disappeared and that the government should actively search for the stolen children. Furthermore, an opinion poll revealed that a majority of the Argentine people wanted to bring all perpetrators to trial, high- and low-ranking, military and police. In an additional loss orientation, the organizations kept the remembrance of the disappeared alive with street marches and eyewitness accounts of torture and assassination. The Alfonsín government gave in to the public pressure and adjusted its national mourning policies away from its earlier recovery orientation. It focused now principally on documenting the military's crimes against humanity, exhuming anonymous graves, and prosecuting all suspected perpetrators. The recovery orientation was reduced to undoing repressive administrative measures by the military dictatorship, such as the reinstatement of dismissed state officials and employees of banks, hospitals, schools, and universities. The state's national mourning came to resemble the social mourning of the human rights movement that supported loss- over recovery-oriented measures.

The prosecution of the military reached its high point with the conviction of five junta members who had ruled Argentina between 1976 and 1982, including the infamous General Videla and Admiral Massera, who were given life sentences. Encouraged by this trial, hundreds of officers were accused of gross human rights violations. However, the prosecution of officers who had followed orders was unacceptable to the armed forces, while President Alfonsín feared that the prospect of hundreds of lengthy trials and appeals would destabilize the budding democracy. In 1986 and 1987, he succeeded in passing two laws through Congress that gave amnesty to the indicted officers, except if they had been involved in the kidnapping of babies and small children. These amnesty laws were a notable shift from loss orientation to recovery orientation.

President Alfonsín was replaced in July 1989 by President Carlos Saúl Menem, who decisively embraced a recovery-oriented strategy, determined to reduce the attention to loss orientation and finally reconcile Argentina "to heal without much ado the bleeding wound of the Argentine body" (Pisani 1990, p. 7). Vice-President Eduardo Duhalde added: "We have to occupy ourselves with the human rights of the living to be able to bury the past, and dedicate ourselves 24 hours a day to the present and the future" (Granovsky 1989, p. 6). Menem issued a presidential pardon in October 1989 that benefited hundreds of officers and former guerrillas. Moreover, he pardoned the incarcerated junta commanders in December 1990, despite massive street protests and opinion polls that showed little support. Finally, after nearly a decade of resistance by the human rights movement, the Argentine Congress adopted in 1992 and 1994 reparation laws that offered financial compensation to former political prisoners and relatives of the disappeared.

The human rights movement was outraged by the government's reparation policies and the state's impunity of the perpetrators. Yet, it failed to mobilize substantial protest crowds because the Argentine people accepted the official shift from loss-oriented to recovery-oriented national mourning. Memory became now a major focus of the human rights movement's social mourning and no longer the loss-oriented remembrance of the disappeared through street demonstrations and public testimonies. The recovery-oriented memorialization was undertaken to turn Argentina's enforced disappearances and the military's state terrorism into indisputable historical facts that were impressed on the Argentine people with annual commemorations, memorials, and memory sites. Again, the Mothers of the Plaza de Mayo were divided over this oscillatory change to restoration orientation, as they had over the forensic exhumations. The two associations continued with their weekly marches before the presidential palace in Buenos Aires, but the group around Hebe de Bonafini argued that memorialization interred the active remembrance of the disappeared into ritualistic commemorations and petrified sites of memory. The other group and most human rights organizations supported the move from remembrance to memorialization.

Unexpectedly, Argentina's social and national mourning shifted in 1995 from recovery orientation to loss orientation after retired Navy Captain Adolfo Scilingo admitted to having thrown dozens of disappeared Argentines into the Atlantic Ocean. Scilingo's confession resulted in an oscillation from recovery-oriented memorialization to loss-oriented remembrance and retribution. The relatives of the disappeared came to the shocking realization that the remains of their disappeared loved ones would never be found, and the human rights movement renewed its efforts to prosecute perpetrators. President Menem tried to stay the course of social peace by discrediting Captain Scilingo, but he could not stop the public outcry.

The state's national mourning reached its tipping point in 1998 when Argentina's Army Commander, General Balza, declared that babies and infants had been routinely separated from their captured parents and given up for adoption. The military could now be prosecuted on new charges. General Videla, Admiral Massera, and dozens of officers were detained for kidnapping. The human rights movement's opposition to the state's national mourning policies grew through the years. The amnesty laws of 1986 and 1987 were successfully contested in several court cases and finally overturned in 2005 by Argentina's Supreme Court. In 2007, the Supreme Court also declared the presidential pardons of 1989 and 1990 as unconstitutional. The revived criminal trials began in 2006. General Videla was convicted in 2010 once more to a life sentence. A court ruled in 2005 that Admiral Massera was incapable to stand trial due to poor health. He died in 2010. By March 2021, 45 years after the military coup d'état of 1976, 1025 persons were serving their sentences in prison or under house detention, and 618 persons were still under indictment.[3]

Social and national mourning became balanced processes by a continued recovery-oriented memorialization and a resurgent loss-oriented remembrance. The Argentine state approved several memorialization proposals from the human rights movement: a Memory Park (1998) containing a memorial wall with the names of the disappeared; a national Day of Memory (2002); a Memory Institute

(2002); a memorial museum at a former Navy torture center (2004); and around 200 memory sites in the city of Buenos Aires by 2009. Nevertheless, the Mothers of the Plaza de Mayo, presided by Hebe de Bonafini, continued to oppose the memorialization efforts: "The Mothers do not want a monument that becomes a cemetery to bemoan our dead" (Vecchioli 2000, p. 53). This group persisted in the weekly marches at the Plaza de Mayo that kept the remembrance of the disappeared alive. Other manifestations of active remembrance were the street happenings by the children of the disappeared that exposed the domiciles of perpetrators. These happenings aimed at ostracizing them from their neighborhoods and to attract media attention. In the same period, there were crowd protests that demanded the prosecution not only of the military and police but also of companies that had collaborated with the dictatorship.

This summary of the mutual influences of personal, social, and national mourning in Argentina and the oscillations between loss orientation and restoration/recovery orientation in each of them, demonstrates that humanitarian forensic exhumations must not focus purely on the bereaved relatives and their culturally distinct mortuary rituals but require a comprehensive understanding of the oscillating dimensions of mourning. Conflicts within social movements about the desired direction of social mourning and political changes in the state will affect how people cope with their primary and secondary losses and how their personal coping with bereavement will influence their involvement and resistance to the oscillations of social and national mourning.

8.5 Conclusion

Forensic humanitarian work is conducted under the assumption that bereaved people need to conduct grief work to loosen the emotional tie to the dead and achieve closure and that the relatives and friends of missing persons will be unable to mourn as long as they cannot bury their human remains. This chapter has argued instead that people may transform their relationships with the deceased or missing victims of political violence into enduring bonds. The ways in which people relate to the dead and the disappeared is culturally dependent. Ending the relationship is not a universal requirement for the bereaved's mental and physical health but only one of many forms of mourning.

Forensic humanitarian practitioners are sensitive to cultural variations in caring for the dead and the bereaved but should also acquire knowledge about people's notions of trust and attachment to carry out effective humanitarian work. How corpses are exhumed and what will be done with the human remains have different consequences for the bonds of the living and the dead. Although attentive to the conflicting interests of various stakeholders, current forensic humanitarian practices require a better understanding of personal, social, and national mourning as different processes of coping with violent death and disappearance. Mourning by the bereaved should not be conflated with the mourning process of a community or a state. People's personal mourning is defined by their intersubjective relationship with the dead or disappeared and the oscillation between loss-oriented and restoration-oriented coping with bereavement, whereas communities, and especially states, have social and political concerns in mourning the dead and the missing and are characterized by oscillations between loss orientation and recovery orientation.

Mourning the dead and searching for the disappeared are manifestations of social attachment and trust. People trust that their loved ones will not abandon them when they die or are missing because of their deep attachment. The living are expected to be loyal to the dead. They trust that their relatives and friends will mourn them, bury them, attend their funeral, and remember the times spent together, just as disappeared persons trust that people will search for them. To be mourned is a human right because the dead, the disappeared, and the bereaved have the right to continue their relationship after death or disappearance and enact the trust that was nurtured between them during their lives together.

Notes

1. The term "forensic humanitarianism" has been coined by Moon (2014).
2. This statement is accompanied by a graphic representation of the stages of coping with a disappearance, namely, denial, anger, guilt, and grief. It resembles the highly influential but debunked stage model of mourning developed by Elisabeth Kübler-Ross (Stroebe et al. 2017).
3. Procuraduría de Crímenes contra la Humanidad. 2021. A 45 años del golpe de Estado, suman 1025 las personas condenadas por crímenes de lesa humanidad en 254 sentencias. Https://www.fiscales.gob.ar/lesa-humanidad/a-45-anos-del-golpe-de-estado-suman-1025-las-personas-condenadas-por-crimenes-de-lesa-humanidad-en-254-sentencias/; accessed on August 30, 2021.

References

Almirón, F. (1999) *Campo Santo*. Buenos Aires: Editorial 21.

Bowlby, J. (1997 [1969]) *Attachment and Loss*. Vol. 1: Attachment. London: Pimloco.

Broch-Due, V. and Ystanes, M. (eds.) (2016). *Trusting and Tribulations: Interdisciplinary Engagements with Intimacy. Sociality and Trust*. New York: Berghahn.

Cordner, S. and Tidball-Binz, M. (2017). Humanitarian forensic action: its origins and future. *Forensic Science International* **279**: 65–71.

Damousi, J. (1999a). Private loss, public mourning: motherhood, memory and grief in Australia during the inter-war years. *Women's History Review* **8**(2): 365–378.

Damousi, J. (1999b). *The Labour of Loss: Mourning, Memory and Wartime Bereavement in Australia*. Cambridge: Cambridge University Press.

Diago, A. (1988). *Hebe: memoria y esperanza*. Buenos Aires: Ediciones Dialéctica.

Edelman, L.I. and Kordon, D.R. (1995). Trauma y duelo. Conflicto y elaboración. In: *La impunidad: una perspectiva psicosocial y clínica* (eds. D.R. Kordon, L.I. Edelman, D.M. Lagos, and D. Kersner), 101–110. Buenos Aires: Editorial Sudamericana.

Erikson, E.H. (1963). *Childhood and Society*, 2 e. New York: W.W. Norton and Company.

Feitlowitz, M. (1998). *A Lexicon of Terror: Argentina and the Legacies of Torture*. New York: Oxford University Press.

Ferrándiz, F. (2019). Unburials, generals, and phantom militarism: engaging with the Spanish Civil War Legacy. *Current Anthropology* **60**(Supplement 19): S62–S76.

Freud, S. (1917) (1955). Mourning and Melancholia. In: *The Standard Edition of the Complete Psychological Works of Sigmund Freud*, Vol. 14, 243–258. London: Hogarth Press.

Geschiere, P. (1997). *The Modernity of Witchcraft: Politics and the Occult in Postcolonial Africa*. Charlottesville: University Press of Virginia.

Geschiere, P. (2013). *Witchcraft, Intimacy, and Trust*. Chicago: University of Chicago Press.

Giddens, A. (1991). *Modernity and Self-Identity*. Cambridge: Polity Press.

Gorini, U. (2008). *La otra lucha: historia de las Madres de Plaza de Mayo*, Vol. 2 (1983–1986). Buenos Aires: Grupo Editorial Norma.

Granovsky, M. (1989). ¿La Argentina era una fiesta? *Derechos Humanos* **6**(24): 6–7.

Hertz, R. (2018 [1905-1906]). A contribution to the study of the collective representation of death. In: *Death, Mourning, and Burial: A Cross-Cultural Reader* (ed. A.C.G.M. Robben), 2 e, 19–33. Oxford: Wiley Blackwell.

Jalland, P. (2010). *Death in War and Peace: Loss and Grief in England, 1914-1970*. Oxford: Oxford University Press.

Janz, O. (2009). Death and mourning in the Memory of World War I in Italy. In: *Memories and Representations of War: The Case of World War I and World War II* (eds. E. Lamberti and V. Fortunati), 273–286. Amsterdam: Rodopi.

Junta Militar (1983) *Documento Final de la Junta Militar sobre la Guerra contra la Subversión y el Terrorismo*. Http://www.memoriaabierta.org.ar/materiales/documento_final_junta.phpwww.institutomemoria.org.ar. (accessed February 26, 2015).

Kastenbaum, R.J. (1977). *Death, Society, and Human Experience*. St. Louis: The C.V. Mosby Company.

Keller, H. (2014). Introduction: understanding relationships – what we would need to know to conceptualize attachment as the cultural solution of a universal developmental task. Chapter 1. In: *Different faces of attachment: Cultural variations on a universal human need* (eds. H. Otto and H. Keller), 1–24. Cambridge, UK: Cambridge University Press.

Kidron, C.A. (2020). The 'Perfect Failure' of communal genocide commemoration in Cambodia: productive friction or 'Bone Business'? *Current Anthropology* **61**(3): 304–334.

Kordon, D.R., Edelman, L.I., Lagos, D.M., Nicoletti, E., et al. (eds.) (1988). *Psychological Effects of Political Repression*. Buenos Aires: Sudamericana/Planeta.

Kwon, H. (2006). *After the Massacre: Commemoration and Consolation in Ha My and My Lai*. Berkeley: University of California Press.

Laqueur, T.W. (2015). *The Work of the Dead: A Cultural History of Mortal Remains*. Princeton: Princeton University Press.

Larsson, M. (2009). A disenfranchised grief: post-war death and memorialisation in Australia after the First World War. *Australian Historical Studies* **40**(1): 79–95.

Möllering, G. (2006). *Trust: Reason, Routine, Reflexivity*. Oxford: Elsevier.

Moon, C. (2014). Human rights, human remains: forensic humanitarianism and the human rights of the dead. *International Social Science Journal* **65**(215–216): 49–63.

Mosse, G.L. (1990). *Fallen Soldiers: Reshaping the Memory of the World Wars*. Oxford: Oxford University Press.

Nelson, C. (2008). *Dancing with the Dead: Memory, Performance, and Everyday Life in Postwar Okinawa*. Durham: Duke University Press.

Pichel, M. (1985). El testigo de la semana: Iris Etelvina de Avellaneda. *El Diario del Juicio* **2**: 2–3.

Pisani, S. (1990). Instó Menem a una definitiva reconciliación. *La Nacion* **17**, June, 1, 7.

Quinn, N. and Mageo, J.M. (eds.) (2013). *Attachment reconsidered: Cultural perspectives on a Western theory*. New York: Palgrave Macmillan.

Robben, A.C.G.M. (2005). *Political Violence and Trauma in Argentina*. Philadelphia: University of Pennsylvania Press.

Robben, A.C.G.M. (2012). The human right to mourning: social trauma and transitional justice in post-conflict Argentina. In: *Human Rights and Conflict: Essays in Honour of Bas de Gaay Fortman* (eds. I. Boerefijn, L. Henderson, R. Janse, and R. Weaver), 483–497. Cambridge: Intersentia.

Robben, A.C.G.M. (2014). Massive violent death and contested national mourning in post-authoritarian Chile and Argentina: a sociocultural application of the dual process model. *Death Studies* **38**(5): 335–345.

Robben, A.C.G.M. (2015). Exhumations, territoriality, and necropolitics in Chile and Argentina. In: *Necropolitics: Mass Graves and Exhumations in the Age of Human Rights* (eds. F. Ferrándiz and A.C.G.M. Robben), 53–75. Philadelphia: University of Pennsylvania Press.

Robben, A.C.G.M. (2018). *Argentina Betrayed: Memory, Mourning, and Accountability*. Philadelphia: University of Pennsylvania Press.

del Rosario de Cerruti, M. (1984). Reportaje a Hebe Bonafini: 'No vamos a claudicar'. *Madres* **1**(1): 2.

Rosenblatt, A. (2015). *Digging for the Disappeared: Forensic Science after Atrocity*. Stanford: Stanford University Press.

Siebrecht, C. (2014). The female mourner: gender and the moral economy of grief during the First World War. In: *Gender and the First World War* (eds. C. Hämmerle, O. Überegger, and B. Bader-Zaar), 144–162. London: Palgrave Macmillan.

Silverman, P.R. and Klass, D. (1996). Introduction: what's the problem? In: *Continuing Bonds: New Understandings of Grief* (eds. D. Klass, P.R. Silverman, and S.L. Nickman), 3–27. Washington, DC: Taylor and Francis.

Stroebe, M. and Schut, H. (1999). The dual process model of coping with bereavement: rationale and description. *Death Studies* **23**: 197–224.

Stroebe, M. and Schut, H. (2016). Overload: a missing link in the dual process model? *Omega* **74**(1): 96–109.

Stroebe, M., Schut, H., and Boerner, K. (2017). Cautioning health-care professionals: bereaved persons are misguided through stages of grief. *Omega* **74**(4): 455–473.

Tidball-Binz, M. (2013). Global forensic science and the search for the dead and missing from armed conflict: the perspective of the International Committee of the Red Cross. In: *Forensic Science: Current Issues, Future Directions* (ed. D.H. Ubelaker), 337–365. Oxford: Wiley-Blackwell.

Ubelaker, D.H., Shamlou, A., and Kunkle, A.E. (2019). Forensic anthropology in the global investigation of humanitarian and human rights abuse: perspective from the published record. *Science and Justice* **59**(2): 203–209.

Valentine, C. (2006). Academic constructions of bereavement. *Mortality* **11**(1): 57–78.
Vecchioli, V. (2000). "Os trabalhos pela memória". Um esboço de campo dos direitos humanos na Argentina através da construção social da categoria de vítima do terrorismo de estado. Unpublished Master's thesis. Museu Nacional da Universidade Federal do Rio de Janeiro, Rio de Janeiro.
Walter, T. (1996). A new model of grief: bereavement and biography. *Mortality* **1**: 7–25.
Weiss, R.S. (1993). Loss and Recovery. In: *Handbook of Bereavement: Theory, Research, and Intervention* (eds. M.S. Stroebe, W. Stroebe, and R.O. Hansson), 271–284. Cambridge: Cambridge University Press.
Winter, J. (1995). *Sites of Memory, Sites of Mourning: The Great War in European Cultural History*. Cambridge: Cambridge University Press.
Zambernardi, L. (2020). Western attitudes toward soldiers' death: from the early modern period to the present. *Mortality*. Published online: 23 December.

CHAPTER 9

Whose humanitarianism, whose forensic anthropology?

Jaymelee J. Kim[1] and Adam Rosenblatt[2]

[1]*Forensic Sciences Program, Department of Justice Sciences, University of Findlay, Findlay, OH, USA*
[2]*International Comparative Studies, Duke University, Durham, NC, USA*

9.1 Introduction

Anthropologists brought Minik, Qisuk, Atangana, Nuktaq, Aviaq, and Uisaakassak from Greenland to New York in 1897 for study and display at the American Museum of Natural History. Within two months, the Indigenous captives had contracted tuberculosis; the child, Minik, was orphaned upon the death of his father, Qisuk. Through an elaborate charade, anthropologists staged a burial of Qisuk to appease the Inughuit. In reality, scientists dissected, defleshed, and displayed Qisuk's remains after death (Harper 2000; Harper 2002; Weaver 2002). Qisuk's life was shaped by myriad forms of violence – displacement, captivity, disease, colonialism, and scientific racism. In death, he remained deeply situated in what Scheper-Hughes and Bourgois (2004, p. 19) describe as the violence continuum, or "a multitude of 'small wars and invisible genocides' conducted in the normative social spaces of public schools, clinics, emergency rooms, hospital wards, nursing homes, courtrooms, public registry offices, prisons, detention centers, and public morgues". Those responsible for social spaces of museums and living exhibits committed violence *after* Qisuk's death through technologies of dissection and display and promotion of a colonial logic that objectified and dehumanized Qisuk and his family.

The deceased continue to participate in the culture and lives of survivors and descendants. They can experience violence, commit violent acts, or sometimes be wielded as instruments of violence, for example, when perpetrators carry out "necroviolence" – the erasure or destruction of dead bodies – for the pain they know it will cause to the living (De León 2015, p. 69). Much of this continuum

Anthropology of Violent Death: Theoretical Foundations for Forensic Humanitarian Action, First Edition.
Edited by Roberto C. Parra and Douglas H. Ubelaker.

exists in normative spaces overlooked by those positioned to render it visible. For instance, when working in the medical examiner's office, anthropologists can use training and experience to extrapolate part and parcel of someone's behavior, health history, and living conditions – serial healed rib fractures, long-healed amputated limbs, bone porosity from malnutrition, and significant antemortem tooth loss (edentulous does *not* imply old, at least not in some regions, but perhaps does imply something about access to dental care). Myriad antemortem conditions may present, but the medico-legal system and those signing death certificates specifically want to know if anthropologists can extract information particular to the cause and mechanism of death. From Scheper-Hughes and Bourgois's (2004) point of view, in this public space, it has been normalized not to interrogate the violence experienced through systemic and structural barriers to medical care, housing, or food. The deceased, in this sense, continue to encounter erasure and marginalization; they participate unwillingly in silencing narratives of power. Here we ask, what is the role of forensic anthropologists in documenting violence on a continuum? How can a reimagined forensic anthropology – especially one that calls itself *humanitarian* – tell fuller, more transformative stories about the living and the dead?

Reframing forensic anthropology's responsibility to recognize the continuum of violence stands to influence approaches to local and international casework, research, and public outreach. Increasing global expectations of humanitarian forensic intervention, while appearing inclusive in definition, also narrowly rely on mass *physical* violence – when in reality, those in power harness other forms of violence to target, marginalize, and eradicate groups. At the same time, if considering the participation of the dead in the violence continuum, we may find ourselves close to entering humanitarian, *non-forensic* intervention that still draws on the skills typically found among forensic specialists, which surely can make some uncomfortable. This article embraces the evolving expectations of forensic interlocutors and the chance to reexamine the boundaries of "forensic" and "humanitarian." It builds on the two basic premises shared in this introduction: that the dead participate in society in diverse ways *and* that the violence they have experienced exists on a continuum.[1] When we ask whose humanitarianism and whose forensic anthropology, we mean: who do these concepts and fields serve, and to what end? Building on the innovations of the human rights/humanitarian tradition, but pushing further still, we offer a different vision of forensic more-than-humanitarianism for the twenty-first century. Already existing outside medico-legal institutions, forensic anthropology, for us, constitutes a range of possible investigative, scientific, and archival practices that people undertake to clarify histories of violence and repair or revise relationships with the dead.[2]

9.2 Positionality of the authors

In what follows, drawing on our research and experiences around burial sites in Uganda's war in Acholiland, the mass institutionalization and anonymous burials of people labeled mentally ill and disabled in the United States, and Canada's genocide in Indian Country using a system of assimilatory forced displacement in a residential school system, we move beyond dichotomous notions of humanitarian or human rights anthropology and expand the bounds of meaningful and thoughtful forensic practice. In doing so, we acknowledge the transformation that forensic humanitarian action and its many diverse practitioners have brought to forensic anthropology and human rights activism. Along with others inside and outside the field, however, we observe that forensic humanitarianism is still carried out within a frame shaped by colonization and by narrow definitions of violence. This frame contributes to the invisibility of some histories and some forms of "preventable suffering" (Soler and Beatrice 2018). We support a dialogue about forensic humanitarianism that is open at its edges to unseen forms of violence and to the re-centering of the dead.

Our research and experience, while overlapping, is also distinct. Jaymelee Kim is a four-field anthropologist engaged in domestic forensic casework: applied, ethnographic, policy, and law research on interventions afforded to survivors of human rights violations (i.e., residential schools, human trafficking, and warfare) and forensic research and capacity-building in Uganda. Adam Rosenblatt is an interdisciplinary scholar whose work has long focused on the intersection of forensic science, human rights, and the care of the dead. More recently, he has been working alongside activists who seek to reclaim and honor burial grounds of marginalized populations in the United States. These include historic African American cemeteries that have suffered from a lack of funding and other forms of structural neglect, as well as the cemeteries around psychiatric hospitals and other disability institutions, which are often anonymous and inaccessible. Kim's casework and research focus on the dynamics between human remains and the living survivors, processes of violence, alternative forms of justice, and interventions for both bodies of the living and bodies of the dead. Whereas Rosenblatt's work now focuses on marginalized cemeteries that people seek to transform into meaningful public spaces, reshaping broader landscapes of memory in the process.[3] Our distinct research agendas have given us ample time to reflect on the justifications, rationales, motivations, and ethics of work that intervene on and around human remains.

We are aware of the persisting colonial legacies of research and practice in our fields, and this informs our decision to discuss deaths on a continuum of violence and to question forensic (un)engagement. We consider that in some contexts, the dead can still serve as "ghost capital" (Berry 2017) to researchers and humanitarians who benefit from interventions of various kinds—exhumation, investigation, research, and publication. In the US, pressing ethical concerns regarding social understandings of race, gender, and oppression continue to undergo heated debate (Bethard and DiGangi 2020; DiGangi and Bethard 2021; Michael et al. 2021; Ross and Pilloud 2021; Ross and Williams 2021), especially as scientists and anatomists continue to disregard the interconnectedness between the living and the dead in their treatment of human remains. Medical researchers once paid graverobbers to bring them cadavers only to be squelched by anatomy acts that questionably legalized the dissection of criminals' bodies among others. In 2021, the University of Pennsylvania and Harvard University admitted that faculty members had kept and used the remains of children who perished in Philadelphia's MOVE bombing in 1985, causing further pain to a family and community that had already been subjected to direct violence, incarceration, and the city's decades-long failure to undo the damage it wrought (see Osder 2013; Stein 2022).

Together, as we work among practitioners and communities of the living and the dead, we have come to see that the burgeoning field of "humanitarian forensic action" may be too ambitious in some places and, in others, too limited in its imagination. Too ambitious in foregrounding humanitarian identification, prioritization of the right to know, or investment in a specific scientific toolkit (perhaps to the exclusion of qualitative methods or alternative notions of evidence). Too narrow in the boundaries, it still places around the "forensic" and the types of violence that trigger a forensic humanitarian response. Together, we interrogate how reconceptualizing "violent death" could move us away from extractive and colonial practices, away from doing harm, and toward the responsibility of advocacy. We ask the reader to consider what sites of violence, what bodies, and what work to identify and care for bodies after violence do not fall under typical notions of forensic human rights or forensic humanitarianism? Who and what is left out of this transition from politically charged forensic human rights to highly internationalized and institutionalized, survivor-centered forensic humanitarian action (promoted by the world's symbol of humanitarian neutrality, the ICRC) (Smith 2017)?

9.3 Reconceptualizing violent deaths

To reconceptualize "violent death," the key term in this volume's title, we take several steps. We do not frame the dead only for the value of the corpus delicti, offering up physical evidence of crimes, nor do they appear only as sources of relief for survivors once their identities and fates have been clarified. Rather, we see the dead as participants situated on a continuum of violence that impacts them and their communities in life *and* death. Our arguments are based on our interactions with people and groups working to render visible the erased and marginalized dead.

There are numerous ways in which the dead can participate in culture and politics posthumously (see, e.g., Verdery 1999). Here we focus on the idea that violence against the remains impacts the living, the dead, and the scenarios in which the tangible remains necessitate action among the living. One key slogan of the disability rights and neurodiversity movements is "nothing about us without us" (Autistic Self Advocacy Network; see Charlton 1998). What if anthropologists were to take that mantra seriously in framing our work, including work with the dead? The slogan speaks to a long history in disability policy and research being shaped without the voices of disabled people, especially when they are living in poverty and/or with additional marginalized identities. "Nothing about us without us" is a demand not just for a seat at the table but also for empowering disabled people to shape the policy and research agendas that affect them most (See Milton 2019). How then do those who have died, often through combined acts of physical, slow, and structural violence, gain a seat at the table? How do they participate? How do forensic anthropologists deny, ignore, or shape and reshape that participation? And what are the repercussions?

Recently, humanitarian forensic anthropologists have begun to discuss intersections of violence. For example, the suffering experienced by the thousands of immigrants who die crossing the "violent borders" (Jones 2017) every year has been documented in forensic work along the US–Mexico borderlands (Anderson and Spradley 2016; Martinez et al. 2018; Spradley and Gocha 2020). In this way, the violence in life that culminated in a desperate attempt to cross clandestinely into the United States led to a violent death – be it from *coyotes* leading individuals into the borderlands or the unforgiving climate of the desert itself.

In a similar vein, forensic anthropologists have been discussing structural violence manifest in skeletal remains. Structural violence, often considered an invisible violence that does harm through denial of resources, such as healthcare, is often written on the bodies of people from marginalized groups (Scheper-Hughes and Bourgois 2004; Farmer 2004). In cases of human rights violations or disaster, often these more subtle but life-threatening forms of violence continue for extended periods of time. Living in a marginalized state can present in the skeleton through stress markers and pathological conditions – which have been interrogated in remains from central and South America, from the United States (Goad 2020; Beatrice and Soler 2016; Soler and Beatrice 2018; Beatrice et al. 2021), and in diverse archaeological contexts (Tremblay and Reedy 2020). Contextual information in casework in Detroit suggests slow deaths from exposure and lives impacted by painful health conditions until death in extreme poverty (Moore and Kim 2022). Indirectly, this scholarship suggests that "violent" deaths may not fall under traditional assumptions of overt brutality from one person enacted upon another or mass physical violence. Doretti and Burrell (2007, p. 46) describe the gray spaces of human rights forensic anthropology and the need to find "a middle ground on which to carry out investigations, a search that includes negotiations of roles, positions, politics, and funding requirements." In attempts to find this middle ground, we suspend a priori assumptions about investigative and identification needs through considering the dead as participants to be listened to, as their lives, death, and afterlife shape communities.

9.4 The dead as articipants[4] in forensic anthropology

Here, to consider whose humanitarianism and whose forensic anthropology, we draw on our fieldwork to present three brief scenarios at the nexus of complex forms of violence, interactions of the living with the dead, and potential humanitarian forensic action. Violence continues as spirits of the improperly buried dead call for justice; descendants react to continued physical violence against Indigenous remains; and the historical erasure of the disabled dead continues at MetFern Cemetery and other places like it.

9.4.1 The case of Acholiland, Uganda: Violent deaths and disturbing pirits

The situation in Uganda has all the traditional components of violent death with human remains leveraged in diverse ways for political gain. Uganda has a long history of war, and as such, unmarked, mass, and otherwise problematic graves have been populated over decades. The most recent conflict, a war between the rebel group the Lord's Resistance Army (LRA) and the government of Uganda, ended in 2006. For over 20 years, the LRA swept through northern Uganda, kidnapping boys to indoctrinate as child soldiers and girls into sexual slavery as soldiers' "brides." The LRA attacked government forces and civilians alike; military forces on both sides allegedly tortured and killed countless individuals. In response, the government seized private land, converting parcels into overcrowded and undersecured internally displaced persons (IDP) camps, which became targets of violence – via direct attacks, disease, and malnutrition. Total war led to the collapse of infrastructure, extreme loss of life at the hands of both forces, and decimation of resources such as cattle and crops and destruction of educational or medical facilities.

The conflict predominantly took place in northern regions of the country occupied by the Acholi people; the Acholi are one of more than 50 ethnic groups in the country with distinctive beliefs, language, and practices. The colonial spread of Christianity, advances in technology, and globalization also shape behaviors and beliefs. Cosmological perspectives frequently offer a syncretistic mixture of "traditional" beliefs, Christian frameworks, and scientific understanding. These are important factors when considering the multitude of factors that influence whether or not the dead are considered to be properly or improperly buried (Elgerud and Kim 2020).

Kampala, the capital city of Uganda, is situated in traditional Bagandan (not Acholi) territory. Being the capital city, many of the scientists, medical officers, and government officials who would otherwise be interested in forensic intervention are *not* Acholi. They do not share Acholi beliefs about the social lives of the dead and are frequently completely unaware of them. Acholi survivors describe the deceased as though they continue to act in the world that seems preposterous to some of their Ugandan counterparts of other ethnic origins. Consistently, survivors state that the spirits of the dead participate in social experiences through possession, visions, crop failure, and illness. As one Catholic elder at Bucoro explains, "at times the school children also get possessed by the spirits. That manifests as being strangled by what you don't see" (Interview, July 2017).

Restless spirits frequently contribute to ongoing violence. A protestant man who lived in what was once an internally displaced persons camp states that "these spirits, when angered, can cause unexpected illness that could lead to death" (Interview, July 2017). One *rwot*, or clan chief, also describes how spirits, angered by improper burial rites, could impact a whole community; he says, "you will see a community that is not healthy . . . because they are being disturbed by spirits of their relatives who were killed during the war" (Interview, June 2016).

Because the etiology of illness and death may be attributed to spirits who die violent deaths *or* without proper interment, the spirits of the dead can also be manipulated by intentional improper deposition of the remains. For example, a woman from Pella Wicere shares an experience in which "clan members wanted the woman to go away from that family. They decided that since she is disrespectful they will bury her child like that [in a specific way] so that the woman will never be able to conceive again" (Interview, July 2017). Many of the "improper burials" shown to us by survivors of the conflict are those of individuals who died of disease and lack of access to healthcare. Analysis of the remains may show evidence of long-healed torture or malnutrition or any other number of pathological conditions, but would not show the evidence of massacre frequently sought by judicial investigations. A noticeable number of problematic remains are of those with known identities, but having a known identity does not prevent the spirits from participating in the lives of survivors. Do these deaths from the indirect violence of displacement, disease, and malnutrition merit the recognition of a violent death and intervention using the skills of forensic anthropology? Do the circumstances of death call for documentation to reinforce the Acholi narrative of suffering in the historical record? So often, overt violence such as torture and murder dominate them yet is accompanied by protracted forms of violence that go unnoted. Forensic anthropologists are beginning to address structural violence as a key area for further research and intervention (see Byrnes and Sandoval-Cervantes, 2022). But sometimes the distinction between these phenomena and direct, physical harm – the traditional concern of forensic anthropology – seems overdrawn. The voices and experiences of Acholi survivors in Uganda remind us that a continuum connects all of this suffering and impacts how the dead participate in the lives of the living.

9.4.2 The case of c̓əsnaʔəm, British Columbia, Canada: Violence against the dead

"We're allowed to burn here?" I looked at the barrel fire thinking that I had grown used to the sound of chopping wood without ever really questioning where the wood came from. It seemed like the city police might have an issue with a fire. "No one said anything about it?"

"We told them it was a sacred fire."

"I see." I gave a knowing look and appreciated the fire that kept us warm. Likely, the need to stay warm in the chill night would not be enough of a reason to allow the protestors to keep the fire going. Acceptance of the fire as sacred by law enforcement was telling, highlighting the vast lack of understanding that remained on the part of authorities and underscoring the notion of "the other." To be fair, in a much more metaphorical way, the fire was sacred, as it kept warm those who stood vigilant over the violated dead.

As I heated my hands, my gaze drifted to the chain link fence that was once intended to protect the construction site from trespassers, but now delineated the physical space occupied by the living from that which was occupied by the dead. Flags adorned the fence from Indigenous nations who had made the pilgrimage to the site in solidarity with those affected by the grave desecration, reminiscent of a memorial. Let me be clear, the dead were not worshipped. That anthropological term of ancestor worship, as many scholars over the years have pointed out, is problematic at best despite its persistence in the lexicon. Instead, Ingold (2000, p. 112) explains the relationship between the living and the dead as "deeply embedded in everyday practice". The deceased may communicate information, observe behaviors of the living, provide guidance, or take action – all of which have the power to shape the perceptions, mental health, physical health, and actions of the living. In such cultures, the spirits of the dead do not act as passive guardians, but as participants. These dead participants are perceived very differently – and take different actions – than the restless dead in

Acholiland. Their cause of death and manner of burial were not a factor in their restlessness. Yet the continued fascination outside researchers have with Indigenous bodies adds another dimension to the violence experienced by the living and the dead (as was the case with the savagery experienced by Minik Qisuk at the hands of anthropologists).

I had arrived in British Columbia asking about human rights violations and the bodies of thousands of First Nations children buried at their schools. Like the people buried at MetFern Cemetery, Indigenous children were confined to institutions in both the United States and Canada in the nineteenth and twentieth centuries. Canada employed compulsory residential schools for the explicit assimilation of Indigenous children. Lifeways, language, cultural norms, and facets of identity that deviated from Euro-American and Euro-Canadian norms were strictly prohibited. While the start of the residential schools predates the 1948 Convention on the Prevention and Punishment of the Crime of Genocide in the eyes of the law, the design of the schools is well understood to be an act of genocide under Article 2.E., "Forcibly transferring children of the group to another group." Reports and evidence of widespread physical and sexual assault permeate the narratives of the United States and Canadian schools, with evidence of medical experimentation at some (Mosby 2013; MacDonald et al. 2014).

Institutionalized for their Indigeneity, cemeteries across Canada, overgrown and forgotten by the government, hold the remains of those who lived and died at the school. However, my informants pointed me in the direction of c̓əsnaʔəm, which despite its 5000-year time depth and its 1933 recognition as a historic site, was being excavated for construction. At first glance, this was not related to the residential schools, but, like that of the residential schools, it was a scenario in which the dead participate in life. The conflict rooted in the future of the urban graves in many ways clarified the entanglement of the living and the dead in the continuum of violence.

The firelight flickered, casting shadows into the dark void of the moonlit land. From this vantage point, the open graves could not be seen. The fact that graves resided in a historically recognized Indigenous burial site had not prevented investors from unearthing and scattering bones, creating a political deadlock between First Nations, who sought to halt the attacks on the dead, and the provincial government.

The interactions between the living and the dead were complicated. Some of those engaged with more "traditional" spiritual practices could see them – the spirits – suffering because their remains were being violated in death as they so often were in life. Several sang as they drummed, walking the perimeter and cleansing the area. Some fell ill from the spiritual disturbance. Cedar branches, with what Euro-Americans likely would call prayer, could be used to cleanse the soul of the living. As one who grew up among the Woodland Indians, this particular practice, common among many peoples of the Pacific Northwest, was unfamiliar to me. But as ethnic groups came and went, the ceremonial events changed, and diverse practices could be seen. Like the "sacred fire," they were, well, mostly welcome, serving a purpose. Others retained cosmological views in which the dead ceased to exist. Rather, the concerns for the remains were rooted in a sense of responsibility to ensure that authorities observed the legal protections while also painfully aware of desecration and "transitional justice" occurring in tandem.

At the same time, Indigenous peoples grapple with the long-term impacts of ongoing colonialism and the erasure of Indigenous experiences of malnutrition, disease, and mental anguish in the residential schools. For many, but certainly not all, of the Indigenous whose family members were laid to rest in that cemetery, this moment was a confluence of the past, the present, and the future. The dead, the living, and the future generations inhabit a single universe. There is no doubt that the perceived actions of the dead and the actions taken against them have real and meaningful impacts on the survivors.

9.4.3 The case of MetFern Cemetery, Massachusetts, USA: the violence of erasure and the forensics of disability

The small stone grave markers at MetFern Cemetery sit in a small clearing in the woods, with a large red oak standing in its midst. A hiking and mountain biking trail winds its way past, down the hill from condominiums that stand on the grounds of a former psychiatric hospital. Nearly 300 people were interred between the years of 1947 through 1979 at this burial ground in Waltham, Massachusetts, a large suburb of Boston. Before death, these children and adults lived as inmates within a complex of disability institutions, including the Metropolitan State Hospital, a psychiatric asylum, and the Walter E. Fernald School, the United States' first institution for youth with social and intellectual disabilities.[5] MetFern is one of the hundreds of institutional cemeteries of its kind where the graves are either unmarked or otherwise made anonymous.

MetFern cemetery is a landmark of a dark and overlooked chapter of violent American history. The Fernald School was founded by the anti-slavery abolitionist and physician Samuel Gridley Howe. Like other reformers of the time, such as Dorothea Dix, he was seeking a more humane model for the care and education of intellectually disabled people than the confinement in homes and jails that was the norm. The Massachusetts School for Idiotic and Feeble-Minded Youth opened in Boston in 1948, the first publicly funded school of its time. In the late 1880s, it moved to Waltham and was renamed after its superintendent, Walter E. Fernald, in 1925 after his sudden death the year before. Metropolitan State, which opened in 1930 to treat people with mental and physical illnesses, "was considered the most modern mental health facility in the country" (Town of Lexington Historical Commission, n.d.).

The rise of American eugenics in the 1920s both dramatically increased the population of these institutions and transformed their logic. Eugenics reshaped science, policy, and public opinion around the belief that the disabled and mentally ill were fundamentally defective, their abilities – intelligence especially – fixed for life. Institutions filled with disproportionate numbers of immigrants and especially their children (Green 2021), "promiscuous" women and others who "embarrassed" their families (Appleman 2018, pp. 439–440; see Palomba n.d.), and poor children – many of them born to immigrant families – who were seen as potential burdens at a regular school (Penney and Stastny 2010). The solution was "a combination of institutionalization, incarceration in penal institutions, and surgical sterilization" (Appleman 2018, p. 438).

Disability, "disabled persons," impairment, and mental illness are already contested terms and concepts that vary significantly based on context and discursive power. Because school administrators, medical doctors, and others could exert such wide discretion over who belonged in an institution, the terms "disability institutions" and "disabled dead," used in this chapter, become yet more fraught, since speaking a foreign language, poverty, or resisting authority at school could results in a wide range of diagnoses that sent people to institutions. Here we use all of these terms, and the lumping together of diagnoses and conditions traditionally associated with disability and mental illness, via a central tenet of critical disability studies – that disability labels and spaces meant to separate those who are labeled disabled from the rest of society function to construct a norm of able-bodied, functioning, ideal lives, and bodies on the other side (see Davis 2017). In other words, while their experiences may have differed greatly, everyone we refer to as the "disabled dead" in this chapter did, in some way, experience the disabling power of their society – in death, in their anonymous graves, as in life.

Eugenics changed the institutions into places for the permanent removal of those who were labeled disabled and mentally ill from society; the goals of learning and independence were more or less abandoned. These institutions also offered perfect conditions of hierarchy, surveillance, and impunity to predators of various kinds. Many children at the Fernald School were physically and sexually abused (D'Antonio 2004). The school's most publicized episode of abuse was the experiments conducted on at least 70 boys from Fernald, who were told they were in a "Science Club." The studies, a partnership between Quaker Oats and the Massachusetts Institute of Technology, were described to the children's families as merely an effort to improve nutrition, with no mention of the radioactive elements scientists were putting into the students' oatmeal and delivering via injection to later test their absorption of iron (D'Antonio 2004, pp. 55–58). In later decades, through activism by families and disability organizations as well as prominent exposés of the Quaker Oats experiment and other abuses, the Fernald

School transitioned to focus on care for intellectually disabled adults in on-site group residences.

The realities at Metropolitan State Hospital also quickly diverged from its founding ideals "to provide humane care and treatment for the mentally ill and to be a center for service to the community," as Massachusetts Governor Frank G. Allen put it at the facility's grand opening in 1930 (Gray 2018–2021). As psychiatrist Allen Frances writes, "The mental hospitals established by the states in the 19th century had the best of intentions and the worst of consequences. . . The 20th century witnessed a rapid and thorough degradation of the system, with cattle-car overcrowding and system-wide patient neglect" (Frances 2019). Many factors fueled this unraveling, including the Great Depression and decades of lack of funds that, among other things, kept staff members overwhelmed, resentful, and with high rates of turnover. Overcrowding quickly became the norm, with solitary confinement and sedation becoming standard ways of managing an untenable situation.

As for the people buried in MetFern Cemetery, either they had no one to claim their bodies or their families were too poor to pay for burial elsewhere. Most of these people's bodies now rest under simple stone blocks bearing no name but rather a number and "C" for Catholic or "P" for Protestant – with the two populations buried on separate sides of the small cemetery. Gann Academy High School students and their teachers who have been researching the lives of these individuals have found that even these small indicators of their humanity can be inaccurate, erasing the identities of at least two Jewish individuals and one who is identified as "Mohammedan" in the archives, though his Armenian roots suggest he may be a misidentified Armenian Orthodox Christian (Green et al. n.d.). The little stone markers, marked with numbers instead of names, are agents of anonymity, but this does not mean they are all alike. Rosenblatt's field notes record signs of individuation via both human and non-human presences: "C-43 is surrounded by anthills"; "P-8 fell over at one point, but has been set back up straight. The outline from where it lay previously is still visible in the grass."

Often, MetFern is a quiet place. Metropolitan State Hospital closed in 1992, as part of the broader movement toward deinstitutionalization that started in the 1960s (Appleman 2018, pp. 452–458). Some of its residential buildings were converted into condominiums. Local activists fought for a large portion of the grounds to remain open space, where there is now a network of trails and a dog park. The Fernald School is a ruin, with its former stately buildings and overgrown lots whose future is hotly debated (Fisher 2020).

People walking past the cemetery on the trail occasionally notice the sign marking it as a cemetery and stop to look around. They may even leave some coins or a stone on a small pedestal at the center of the cemetery, where candles, small statues (Jesus, the Buddha, and an angel), and origami cranes form a makeshift altar. Before the COVID-19 pandemic, the disability organization the Arc of Massachusetts held annual memorial ceremonies at MetFern. Organizers read the names of every person buried in the cemetery and handed out flowers for attendees to place on the grave markers.

Since 2017, disability historian Alex Green has researched the lives of people buried at MetFern as well as the history of the cemetery and of the institutions connected to it. He has worked both independently and with former colleagues and students at Gann Academy, a private Jewish high school that sits on the grounds of the Metropolitan State Hospital complex. Thanks to this collective work, families who did not know where their kin were buried have been able to locate the graves and hold small memorial services there, reconnecting with their loved ones. In May 2021, Rosenblatt attended a service for John Scott, buried under marker C-154. His three siblings and former teacher at the Fernald School gathered while Adam Walden, an autistic musician studying at Boston's Berklee School of Music, played the cello.

While a site like MetFern is clearly significant for survivors and their families, preservationists, public historians, and disability activists to memorialize and interpret, these projects may seem outside of the realm of forensic humanitarianism or human rights.[6] Nothing found at these cemeteries will be used in court proceedings focused on the abuse and neglect institutionalized people have experienced. On the grounds of Central State Hospital in Milledgeville, Georgia, home to what Mab Segrest calls "the largest graveyard of disabled people in the world" (its six cemeteries hold the remains of around 25 000 people), incarcerated laborers were forced to toss 2000 numbered markers for patients into the woods to make mowing easier (Segrest 2020, p. 6; Monroe 2015). Whether they look like open fields or more recognizable cemeteries, these places are still far from being widely visited and commemorated as "sites of conscience" or places to remember historical atrocities (though see Steele et al. 2020).

Yet the questions we raise about the boundaries of forensic humanitarianism and "violent death" point toward a different possibility: a practice at the transformative edges of the forensic. The forensics of disability at MetFern and places like it is a recovery effort aimed at histories and people whose lives have been sidelined by both human rights culture and forensic anthropology, as we discuss below. Without formal intervention, this "citizen forensics" (See Cruz-Santiago 2020) has been undertaken by ordinary people without claims of technical expertise in archaeology or forensic science. They seek to "make the bones speak" – or let the dead participate – in ways that do not involve digging up bodies but do seek to expose hidden and disregarded evidence of violence. In an e-mail he shared with Rosenblatt, Alex Green writes:

> There is a kind of archaeological memorialization that can occur if we go into these spaces and turn these burials back on themselves by finding names, telling stories, and reconnecting the relatives of survivors with their loved ones and their ancestors. Each step of this work reverses the core tenets of disregard that led these people to be treated in life and buried in death in such a fashion, and while we cannot undo those indignities, we can engage in a kind of retributive act in which we deny the people in power the very things they thought they controlled into finality. They believed these burials were an end because their thinking was eugenically linear ... but we can bend that history into a loop and refuse the finality of what they did (Green, personal communication).

"Cemetery citizens" such as Green recognize the dead as participants in history and in the lives of the living – even, sometimes, as their kin (Rosenblatt, forthcoming). To the extent that the dead participate, it is different from what Kim observed in Acholiland. Rosenblatt has not spoken to anyone who sees the dead causing injuries, infertility, or possessing people. Instead, the grassroots efforts reinsert the dead into the social fabric and into history through acts of care and through "reuniting" the dead with living family members who may not know the final resting place of their kin. What Rosenblatt has witnessed among the quiet graves at MetFern, then, is both a challenge to the kinds of expertise that is usually associated with forensic humanitarianism and an equally important correction as to whose histories of violence and whose graves are considered worthy of a human rights investigation.

9.5 What's missing from human rights

The rise of forensic humanitarianism has expanded the terrain of forensic intervention and the methods associated with the response to mass violence in key ways, moving beyond a narrow focus on evidence for criminal trials. However, it has also retained and even reinforced boundaries around what kinds of violence "count" for a humanitarian response, reinforced assumptions about death and relationships, and declared whose missing persons – whose bodies – require urgent attention. Forensic humanitarianism did not emerge sui generis. It carries with it the histories of humanitarian and human rights practices that came before and the troubled legacies of their uneven, flawed imaginings.

Forensic anthropologists have begun to interrogate the structural violence of those denied access to healthcare, exposed to the elements, or migrating to escape malnutrition and poverty (see Byrnes and Sandoval-Cervantes, 2022). The US–Mexico border crisis is a particularly salient example of the dead participating in the social, political, and personal tensions associated with immigration in the United States. In Uganda, angered spirits may torment the living if their remains are not properly interred. Among the Musqueam, destruction of physical remains – yet another form of erasure that stirs the spirits who compel the living to advocate – is but one piece of colonial mechanization. The erasure of the disabled dead persists, and those dead become the stimulus for community mobilization as well as a form of placemaking – taking burial grounds that were designed to be hidden and anonymous, places of shame and erasure, and reconfiguring them as public spaces, spaces where a lineage connects the dead confined in institutions to living disability advocates (see Rosenblatt, forthcoming).

Using the law as a starting point, we also have relied on specific notions of *who* is marginalized in the eyes of the law and *which* types of violence to prioritize. The violence continuum necessitates examining policies and laws that often accompany and outlast overt violence. Not all of these interventions need to be "forensic" in the traditional sense, though they may be undertakings forensic anthropologists are well trained to pursue. This presents an opportunity to open pathways for the participation of the dead in the social world, the construction of history, and practices of care. The 1948 Universal Declaration of Human Rights was a direct response to World War II and the Nazi Holocaust; as contributor to this volume, Claire Moon posits, "the UDHR might be seen as an expression of what we owe the dead, or as a promise made by the living to the dead" (Moon 2018). But to which of the dead were these promises made?

The first group of people the Nazis began murdering – and thus, perhaps, the first group of the dead to whom we might owe something – was disabled people, starting with children. The so-called "Children's Campaign" was carried out in secret from 1939 to 1941, but the murders continued after its official end. They also quickly expanded to include adult disabled people, many of whom had already been forcibly sterilized but were nevertheless put to death as the Nazis sought to "cleanse the present and erase the past" by eliminating "life unworthy of life" (Friedlander 2000, p. 62). In Germany alone, according to Hugh Gregory Gallagher, over 200 000 people were murdered by physicians under Nazi euthanasia programs. In Poland, the murder of psychiatric hospital patients was part of a "hidden genocide" that left an estimated 20 000 dead.[7] The murders of these people, most of them taken from asylums and other disability institutions in Poland, served as "an experimental ground for researching and testing the most effective methods to kill people on an industrial scale" – including the first use of mobile gas vans that preceded the gas chambers at concentration camps (Nasierowski 2006, p. 52, 59).

In the United States, long before the rise of the Third Reich in Germany, practices of institutionalization and forced sterilization of the Indigenous and impoverished people permeated social practices – and eventually influenced Nazi ideology. For instance, in the 1930s, the removal of over 500 families from what is now Shenandoah National Park was "considered by some to be a humanitarian act" (Horning 2015), despite firsthand accounts of forced sterilization, institutionalization in mental health facilities, and deliberate removal of children of the Appalachian poor. Diverse socially acceptable, yet anathemic policies, practices, and beliefs throughout human history foreground the eventual development of international human rights law.

On December 8, 1948, the United Nations adopted a broad, utopian vision for a global order based on the inherent dignity of the individual person under a Universal Declaration of Human Rights. The day after, on December 9, the same body adopted the Convention on the Prevention and Punishment of the Crime of Genocide. The latter is a more direct response to Nazi atrocities and the promise of "never again"; in a broken world, it focuses on the prevention and punishment of the most terrible of crimes. The convention defines specific acts of violence that legally constitute genocide, and it specifies four identity categories that can be victims of genocide: national, ethnic, racial, and religious. Disability, which served as testing ground for the Nazis – showing them the willingness of civilians to embrace genocidal logics and honing their methods of industrialized killing – was never really considered.[8] For all that the new human rights declarations and treaties were a response to the Holocaust, then, they also helped institutionalize the forgetting of the origins and scope of eugenics and bureaucratized mass murder, of power over disabled lives and deaths.

The foundations of human rights law in many ways created a narrow scope through omission. This legacy lives on in human rights institutions today. The United Nations Convention on the Rights of Persons with Disabilities was adopted in 2006, a late entry into the human rights canon for a group of people estimated to represent fifteen percent of the world's population (a number that is increasing due to aging and other factors, and which also jumps upward dramatically when one considers that nearly all of us will experience at least some form of temporary disability over the course of our lives; see World Health Organization 2021). A year later, in 2007, The UN adopted the Declaration on the Rights of Indigenous People, a late recognition – that is not legally binding – for deep histories of persisting colonial violence across the globe.

Beyond the declarations and conventions that make up the legal framework of human rights, a "human rights culture" (Friedman 2011), in which forensic human rights and humanitarian anthropology is rooted, offers its own dynamics of inclusion and exclusion. The overlapping fields discussed in this article – transitional justice, human rights, science and technology studies, forensic humanitarianism, and the published research that accompanies them – constitute not only "technologies of repair" (Wagner 2008, p. 256) but also ways of designating some histories, some places, some violences, and some graves as part of human rights history.

Studying absence is complex, and the exclusion of forms of violence or omission of specific marginalized groups is worthy of more sustained investigation than we offer here. But we know of no transitional justice process that has focused on the disabling effects of mass violence or reparations for disabled people. Byrnes and Muller (2017), describing an emergent "bioarchaeology of impairment and disability," cite "an ethical imperative to investigate the lived experience of disabled people in the past, but this perspective has not yet permeated the world of humanitarian and human rights forensic anthropology. We see no forensic humanitarian investigation that highlights findings related to disability (though some forensic anthropologists have been trained using the remains of people who died at carceral institutions with large populations of disabled people). To date, none of the books or journals about forensic humanitarian action have considered disability; even a special journal issue about transitional justice "from the margins" has no disability-related content.[9] Forensic anthropologists are late to engage in an interrogation of "violence" and these complex relationships humans maintain in life and in death. This is in part due to the forensic community often rejecting these questions as factors outside the scope of positivist science or irrelevant to the legal infractions anthropologists are asked to scrutinize (see, e.g., Soler and Beatrice 2017; Winburn and Clemmons 2021).

9.6 The continued expansion of forensic anthropology

Forty years ago, anthropology and archaeology forayed into the work of witnessing on behalf of national and international human rights investigations, plunging anthropological methods into novel contexts and diverse communities. The field application brought anthropologists out of the laboratory, pushing them to engage with archival research and interaction with survivors – both of which are not typically found in traditional U.S. domestic casework. Human rights investigations in Argentina from 1984 onward transformed notions about how forensic science could be applied in the world stage; Clyde Snow and the scientists who formed the Equipo Argentino de Antropología Forense (EAAF, known in English as the Argentine Forensic Anthropology Team), conducted historical and document research, interviewed witnesses, and pursued excavation, identification, and repatriation of the disappeared. This approach quickly became known as forensic human rights anthropology and has spread via EAAFs continued work in over 40 countries. The terminology of "human rights anthropology" reflected its association with the violence that galvanized new human rights networks in the late twentieth century (See Keck and Sikkink 1998; Moyn 2012). Organizations such as Physicians for Human Rights (PHR) used the human rights framework as the main vocabulary for explaining and publicizing forensic investigations (in PHR's case, in the former Yugoslavia, Rwanda, Iraq, and elsewhere) and other activities around the globe. Deaths via gross human rights violations – mass violence, genocide, ethnocide, and extrajudicial killings – grounded this form of applied anthropological investigation.

Over time, the human rights/humanitarian model of forensic investigation has expanded to include not only deaths due to armed conflict but also disaster and displacement. While forensic anthropologists and archaeologists had previously engaged in disaster and violence recovery work, 9/11 pushed forward anthropological involvement beyond establishment of biological profile (Mundorff 2012). Similar to how the EAAF broadened the scope of forensic anthropology, so too has disaster victim identification as more anthropologists engage with other responders in on-scene recovery, triage, scene management, and quality control (Mundorff 2014). In the United States, post-9/11, medical examiner consultation with anthropologists increased, generating interest across disciplines in the contributions of anthropology to the investigation of violent deaths.

The increased involvement in violent death investigation has urged anthropologists to confront ethical and psychosocial concerns for survivors going through the protracted identification process or the politicalization of human remains. For each new setting in which forensic anthropologists can make real contributions to documenting violence (in its many forms) and responding to suffering, the ethical questions – "gray spaces and endless negotiations," in Doretti and Burrell's (2007) words – multiply. For this reason, some practitioners have always resisted the expanding scope of forensic anthropology – and might still argue, for example, to relegate the work we have described in cemeteries at residential schools and disability institutions as solely archaeological, too ethnographic, or better suited to historic preservation – not forensic anthropology. As a field, however, forensic anthropologists have unique influence over what forms of violence are understood as wrongful, preventable, and worthy of the "public forum" that the word forensic demands. Looking back at the transformations in forensic anthropology over the past 40 years, then, we ask – as a political and ethical question, not one based in disciplinary boundaries or resource scarcity – what can or should the field be 40 years from now? Whose forensic anthropology should it be, employing what notions of violence? Whose humanitarianism will shape its priorities? Since forensic humanitarianism does not stand somewhere outside of science's long entanglement with marginalizing some dead bodies and enacting further violence against others – from Minik, Qisuk, Atangana, Nuktaq, and Uisaakassak to the numbered graves at MetFern to the contemporary treatment of victims and survivors of the MOVE bombing – can we now open the field to the many ways in which the dead may still act in the world as victims and agents of violence, and everything in between?

Notes

1. For examples of interaction of the dead and living, see Verdery (1999), Baines (2010), Kim (2014), Kim and Hepner (2019), and Crocker et al. (2021).
2. For a wide and fascinating range of methods designated as forensic, see Forensic Architecture (n.d.).
3. Lisa Y. Henderson, who has spearheaded the reclamation of three African American cemeteries in Wilson, North Carolina, used this term in an interview. Rosenblatt prefers it to the more common terms "abandoned" or "neglected," which too often lead people to believe that it is descendants and mourners – rather than systemic racism and inequality – that is to blame for the state of burial grounds of the marginalized dead. "Degraded" seems to ask more pointedly *who* degraded these spaces.
4. Scholars have long debated the "agency" of human remains and how mortuary practices and the treatment of dead bodies confer personhood upon them (Hallam et al. 1999; Hallam and Hockey 2001; Prior 1989; Rosenblatt 2010). Some studies emphasize how human remains may be endowed or ascribed with "will" by surviving community members (Gell 1998; Harper 2010). Anthropologists, geographers, and thanatological scholars have also contributed to discussion studies of postmortem agency, or the role and significance imposed upon bodies and body parts by the living also have merited debate among Tung (2014), Young and Light (2013), and Heng (2020).
5. We use the term "inmates" here following disability historian Alex Green and his research team, who note, "our conversations with former inmates make it clear that they view their time at the institutions as carceral, and they see themselves as having been inmates" (Green n.d., "Editor's Note").
6. We recognize that in this piece we are not doing justice to the distinction between the humanitarian and human rights traditions or the distinct organizations and legal frameworks that shape them. This is in part because the distinction between human rights and humanitarian priorities in forensic investigations after mass violence – if, in fact, they are possible to distinguish – remains contested in the field. Despite attempts (especially by the ICRC) to place a long and complex history under the banner of "forensic humanitarian action," the field has always included organizations whose missions and rhetorics invoked both humanitarianism and human rights and whose activities fell under the domain of those two areas of international law (see Rosenblatt 2019).
7. The term "hidden genocide" appears early in the Institute of National Remembrance (IPN) report on the killing of psychiatric patients in the Warta and Pomerania regions of Poland (Gut n.d.). Nasierowski provides the estimate of 20 000 murders of psychiatric patients (2006, pp. 50–61).
8. See Ford (2014); Philippe Sands writes of Rafael Lemkin making a "passing mention" of disabled people in his *Axis Rule in Occupied Europe*, though even this requires significant digging (Sands 2016, p. 182).
9. See Rooney and Ní Aoláin, 2018. For some emergent discussions, see Disability Rights International (2021) and Rosenblatt (2018).

References

Anderson, B.E. and Spradley, M.K. (2016). The role of the anthropologist in the identification of migrant remains in the American Southwest. *Academic Forensic Pathology* **6**(3): 432–438.

Appleman, L.I. (2018). Deviancy, dependency, and disability: the forgotten history of eugenics and mass incarceration. *Duke Law Journal* **68**(3): 417–478.

Baines, E. (2010). Spirits and social reconstruction after mass violence: rethinking transitional justice. *African affairs* **109**(436): 409–430.

Beatrice, J.S. and Soler, A. (2016). Skeletal indicators of stress: a component of the biocultural profile of undocumented migrants in southern Arizona. *Journal of Forensic Sciences* **61**(5): 1164–1172. doi: 10.1111/1556-4029.13131.

Beatrice, J.S., Soler, A., Reineke, R.C., and Martínez, D.E. (2021). Skeletal evidence of structural violence among undocumented migrants from Mexico and Central America. *American Journal of Physical Anthropology* **176**(4): 584–605. doi: 10.1002/ajpa.24391.

Berry, D.R. (2017). *The Price for Their Pound of Flesh: The Value of the Enslaved, from Womb to Grave, in the Building of a Nation*. Boston: Beacon Press.

Bethard, J.D. and DiGangi, E. (2020). Letter to the editor—moving beyond a lost cause: forensic anthropology and ancestry estimates in the United States. *Journal of Forensic Sciences* **65**(5): 1791–1792. doi: 10.1111/1556-4029.14513.

Brown, S. (2021) Mass. locked up people with mental illness for decades. Now advocates want their stories told. WBUR (September 27). https://www.wbur.org/news/2021/09/27/bill-commission-state-hospital-mental-illness

Byrnes, J. and Muller, J. (2017). *The Bioarchaeology of Impairment and Disability: Theoretical, Ethnohistorical, and Methodological Perspectives*. Switzerland: Springer.

Byrnes, J. and Sandoval-Cervantes, I. (eds.) (2022). Marginalized in Death: A Forensic Anthropology of Intersectional Identity in the Modern Era. Lanham, MD: Lexington Books.

Charlton, J.L. (2000). Nothing About Us Without Us Disability Oppression and Empowerment, 213: University of California Press.

Crocker, R.M., Reineke, R.C., and Ramos Tovar, M.E. (2021). Ambiguous loss and embodied grief related to mexican migrant disappearances. *Medical Anthropology* **40**(7): 598–611.

Cruz-Santiago, A. (2020). Lists, maps, and bones: the untold journeys of citizen-led forensics in Mexico. *Victims and Offenders* **15**(3): 350–369. doi: 10.1080/15564886.2020.1718046.

D'Antonio, M. (2004). *The State Boys Rebellion*. New York: Simon and Schuster.

Davis, L. (2017). Introduction: disability, normality, and power. In: *The Disability Studies Reader* (ed. L. Davis), 1–14. New York: Routledge.

De León, J. (2015). Land of Open Graves: Living and Dying on the Migrant Trail. Berkeley: University of California.

DiGangi, E.A. and Bethard, J.D. (2021). Uncloaking a lost cause: decolonizing ancestry estimation in the United States. *American Journal of Physical Anthropology* **175**(2): 422–436.

Disability Rights International (2021) Transitional justice and disability in the Americas: accountability for serious and pervasive human rights violations (webinar). https://www.facebook.com/watch/live/?ref=watch_permalink&v=1655360851316517

Doretti, M.D. and Burrell, J. (2007). Gray spaces and endless negotiations. In: *Anthropology Put to Work* (eds. R.G. Fox and L. Field), 45–64. Oxfordshire: Routledge.

Downs, J. (2012). *Sick from Freedom: African-American Illness and Suffering During the Civil War and Reconstruction*. Oxford: Oxford University Press.

Elgerud, L.M.M.K. and Jaymelee, J.K. (2020). Mapping the intangible: forensic human rights documentation in post-conflict Uganda. *The International Journal of Human Rights* **25**(4): 1–22.

Elgerud, L. and Kim, J.J. (2020). Mapping the intangible: forensic human rights documentation in post-conflict Uganda. *The International Journal of Human Rights* **24**(4): 594–615.

Farmer, P. (2004). An anthropology of structural violence. *Current Anthropology* **45**(3): 305–325.

Fisher, J. (2020) Waltham eyes moving public works to fernald property. Patch https://patch.com/massachusetts/waltham/waltham-eyes-moving-public-works-fernald-property (accessed November 23, 2021).

Ford, A.R. (2014). A race apart: genocide and the protection of disabled persons under international law. *Review of Disability Studies* **5**(2).

Forensic Architecture (n.d.) Investigations, Forensic Architecture. https://forensic-architecture.org/ (accessed December 15, 2021).

Frances, A. (2019). *Dungeons and back alleys: the fate of the Mentally Ill in America. Psychiatric Times* https://www.psychiatrictimes.com/article/dungeons-and-back-alleys-fate-mentally-ill-america.

Friedlander, H. (2000). *The Origins of Nazi Genocide: From Euthanasia to the Final Solution.* Chapel Hill: University of North Carolina Press.

Friedman, L.M. (2011). *The Human Rights Culture: A Study in History and Context.* Chicago: Quid Pro Books.

Gallagher, H.G. (2009). Holocaust: the genocide of disabled peoples. In: *Century of Genocide: Critical Essays and Eyewitness Accounts* (eds. S. Totten and W.S. Parsons), 3 e, 207–232. New York and London: Routledge.

Gell, A. (1998). *Art and Agency.* Oxford: Clarendon Press.

Goad, G. (2020). Expanding humanitarian forensic action: an approach to US cold cases. *Forensic Anthropology* **3**(1): 50–59.

Gray, J. (2018–2021) History. Metropolitan State Hospital. https://www.metstate.com/history (accessed December 14, 2021).

Green, A. (2021) The purple folder: preliminary findings on the disabled dead at MetFern cemetery. Unpublished manuscript.

Green, A. (2022). Truth, reconciliation and disability institutionalisation in Massachusetts: an interview with Alex Green. In: *Sites of Conscience and the Unfinished Project of Deinstitutionalization: Place, Memory and Social Justice* (eds. E. Punzi and L. Steele): UBC Press.

Green, A. (n.d.) Editor's Note. MetFern Cemetery website. http://www.metferncemetery.org/process.

Green A. *et al.* (n.d.) About the MetFern Cemetery. metfern.org

Gut, A. (n.d.) Eutanazja – ukryte ludobójstwo pacjentów szpitali psychiatrycznych w Kraju Warty i na Pomorzu w latach 1939-1945. [Euthanasia - the Hidden Genocide of Patients of Psychiatric Hospitals in the Warta Region and Pomerania, 1939-1945.] Instytut Pamięci Narodowej [Institute of National Remembrance]. https://ipn.gov.pl/pl/aktualnosci/585, Eutanazja-ukryte-ludobojstwo-pacjentow-szpitali-psychiatrycznych-w-Kraju-Warty-i.html (accessed October 28, 2020).

Hallam, E. and Hockey, J. (2001). *Death, Memory and Material Culture.* Oxford: Berg.

Hallam, E., Hockey, J., and Howarth, G. (1999). *Beyond the Body: Death and Social Identity.* London: Routledge.

Harper, K. (2000). Give Me My Father's Body: The Life of Minik, the New York Eskimo. New York: Simon and Schuster.

Harper, K. (2002). The Minik affair: the role of the american Museum of natural history. *Polar Geography* **26**(1): 39–52.
Harper, S. (2010). The social agency of dead bodies. *Mortality* **15**(4): 308–322.
Henderson, L. (2021) Interview with Adam Rosenblatt, February 9.
Heng, T. (2020). Interacting with the dead: understanding the role and agency of spirits in assembling deathscapes. *Social and Cultural Geography* **27**: 1–24.
Horning, Audrey J. (2015) The displaced. National Parks Service. https://www.nps.gov/shen/learn/historyculture/displaced.htm (accessed June 10, 2022).
Ingold, T. (2000). The Perception of the Environment: Essays on Livelihood, Dwelling and Skill. New York: Routledge.
Jones, R. (2017). *Violent Borders: Refugees and the Right to Move.* London and Brooklyn: Verso Books.
Keck, M.E. and Sikkink, K. (1998). *Activists Beyond Borders: Advocacy Networks in International Politics.* Ithaca: Cornell University Press.
Kim, J.J. (2014) They made us unrecognizable to each other: human rights, truth, and reconciliation in Canada. Doctoral dissertation for the University of Tennessee-Knoxville.
Kim, J.J. and Redeker Hepner, T. (2019). Of justice and the grave: the role of the dead in post-conflict uganda. *International Criminal Law Review* **19**(5): 1–26.
Kim, J.J., Elgerud, L., and Tuller, H. (2020). Forensic archaeology and anthropology sensitization in post-conflict Uganda. *Forensic Science International* **306**: 110–062.
MacDonald, N.E., Stanwick, R., and Lynk, A. (2014). Canada's shameful history of nutrition research on residential school children: the need for strong medical ethics in Aboriginal health research. *Paediatrics & Child Health* **19**(2): 64–64.
Martínez, D.E., Reineke, R.C., Rubio-Goldsmith, R., and Parks, B.O. (2014). Structural violence and migrant deaths in Southern Arizona: data from the Pima County Office of the Medical Examiner, 1990–2013. *Journal on Migration and Human Security* **2**(4): 257–286.
Michael, A., Bengtson, J., Blatt, S., and Genes, R. (2021). Ancestry, and identity in forensic anthropology: historical perspectives and contemporary concerns. *Forensic Genomics* **1**(2): 41–46.
Milton, D. (2019). Beyond tokenism: Autistic people in autism research. *The Psychologist* **32**: 2–3.
Monroe, D. (2015). Asylum: inside Central State Hospital, once the World's Largest Mental Institution. *Atlanta Magazine* https://www.atlantamagazine.com/great-reads/asylum-inside-central-state-hospital-worlds-largest-mental-institution.
Moon, C. (2018). Politics, deathwork, and the rights of the dead. Humanity (blog). http://humanityjournal.org/blog/claire-moon/ (accessed March 27, 2021).
Moore, M.K. and Kim, J. (2022). Marginalization, death, and decline: the role of forensic anthropology to document the osteology of poverty in Detroit, Michigan in the 21st Century. In: Marginalized in Death: A Forensic Anthropology of Intersectional Identity in the Modern Era (eds. J. Byrnes and I. Sandoval-Cervantes): Lexington Book.
Mosby, I. (2013). Administering colonial science: nutrition research and human biomedical experimentation in Aboriginal communities and residential schools, 1942–1952. *Histoire sociale/Social history* **46**(1): 145–172.
Moyn, S. (2012). *The Last Utopia: Human Rights in History,* Reprint e. Cambridge: Harvard University Press.
Mundorff, A.Z. (2012). Integrating forensic anthropology into disaster victim identification. *Forensic Science, Medicine, and Pathology* **8**(2): 131–139.

Mundorff, A.Z. (2014). Anthropologist-directed triage: three distinct mass fatality events involving fragmentation and commingling of human remains. In: *Commingled Human Remains: Methods in Analysis, Recovery and Identification* (eds. B. Adams and J. Byrd), 365–388. San Diego: Academic Press.

Nasierowski, T. (2006). In the abyss of death: the extermination of the mentally Ill in Poland during World War II. *International Journal of Mental Health* **35**(3): 50–61.

Osder, J. (2013). Director, Let the Fire Burn.

Palomba, A. L. (n.d.). Below the surface: a special report. https://below-the-surface.github.io/main.html (retrieved November 19, 2021).

Penney, D. and Stastny, P. (2010). *The Lives They Left Behind: Suitcases from a State Hospital Attic*: Bellevue Literary Press.

Prior, L. (1989). The disposal of dead persons. In: *The Social Organisation of Death*, 153–174. London: Palgrave Macmillan.

Rooney, E. and Ní Aoláin, F. (eds.) (2018) Special issue: transitional Justice from the margins: intersections of identities, power and human rights. *International Journal of Transitional Justice*, **12**(1).

Rosenblatt, A. (2010). International forensic investigations and the human rights of the dead. *Human Rights Quarterly* **32**: 921.

Rosenblatt, A. (2015). *Digging for the Disappeared*. Stanford: Stanford University Press.

Rosenblatt, A. (2018). Autism, advocacy organizations, and past injustice. *Disability Studies Quarterly* **38**(4), Article 4. doi: 10.18061/dsq.v38i4.6222.

Rosenblatt, A. (2019). The danger of a single story about forensic humanitarianism. *Journal of Forensic and Legal Medicine* **61**: 75–77.

Rosenblatt, A. (forthcoming) (2023).). Cemetery Citizens: Reclaiming Buried Pasts to Remake the Present: Stanford University Press.

Ross, A.H. and Pilloud, M. (2021). The need to incorporate human variation and evolutionary theory in forensic anthropology: a call for reform. *American Journal of Physical Anthropology* **176**(4): 672–683.

Ross, A.H. and Williams, S.E. (2021). Ancestry studies in forensic anthropology: back on the frontier of racism. *Biology* **10**(7): 602.

Sands, P. (2016). East West Street: On the Origins of Genocide and Crimes Against Humanity. New York: Alfred A. Knopf.

Scheper-Hughes, N. and Bourgois, P. (eds.) (2004). Violence in War and Peace: An anthology. Mountaineers Books. Oxford: Blackwell.

Segrest, M. (2020). *Administrations of Lunacy: Racism and the Haunting of American Psychiatry at the Milledgeville Asylum*. New York: The New Press.

Smith, L.A. (2017). The missing, the martyred and the disappeared: global networks, technical intensification and the end of human rights genetics. *Social Studies of Science* **47**(3): 398–416.

Soler, A. and Beatrice, J.S. (2017). Expanding the role of forensic anthropology: migrant death investigation in Southern Arizona. In: Sociopolitics of Migrant Death and Repatriation: Perspectives from Forensic Science (eds. K.E. Latham and A.J. O'Daniel), 120–128. Switzerland: Springer.

Soler, A. and Beatrice, J.S. (2018). Expanding the role of forensic anthropology in a humanitarian crisis: an example from the USA-Mexico border. In: *Sociopolitics of Migrant Death and Repatriation* (eds. K.E. Latham and A.J. O'Daniel), 115–128. Cham: Springer.

Spradley, K. and Gocha, T.P. (2020). Migrant deaths along the Texas/Mexico border: a collaborative approach to forensic identification of human remains. In: Forensic Science

and Humanitarian Action: Interacting with the Dead and the Living (eds. R.C. Parra, S.C. Zapico, and D.H. Ubelaker), 535–548.
Steele, L., Hibberd, L., Yeh, F., and Djuric, B. (2020). Parramatta female factory precinct as a site of conscience: using institutional pasts to shape just legal futures. *University of New South Wales Law Journal* **43**(2): 521–551.
Stein, M.N. (2022). "The blood of innocent children": race, respectability, and "true" victimhood in the 1985 MOVE Police Bombing. *Souls* **22**(2-4): 160–184.
Town of Lexington Historical Commission (n.d.). Area AA/AE - Metropolitan State Hospital. Area Surveys. https://www.lexingtonma.gov/historical-commission/comprehensive-cultural-resources-survey/pages/area-surveys (retrieved November 19, 2021)
Tremblay, L.A. and Reedy, S. (eds.) (2020). *The Bioarchaeology of Structural Violence: A Theoretical Framework for Industrial Era Inequality*. Cham: Springer Nature.
Tung, T.A. (2014). Agency,'Til death do us part? Inquiring about the agency of dead bodies from the ancient Andes. *Cambridge Archaeological Journal* **24**(3): 437–452.
Ubelaker, D.H. (2008). Issues in the global applications of methodology in forensic anthropology. *Journal of Forensic Sciences* **53**(3): 606–607.
Ubelaker, D.H. (2018). A history of forensic anthropology. *Journal of Physical Anthropology* **165**: 915–923.
Verdery, K. (1999). The Political Lives of Dead Bodies: Reburial and Postsocialist Change: Columbia University Press.
Wagner, S.E. (2008). *To Know Where He Lies: DNA Technology and the Search for Srebrenica's Missing*. California: University of California Press.
Willis, G.D. (2021). Mundane disappearance: the politics of letting disappear in Brazil. *Economy and Society* **50**(2): 297–321.
Winburn, A.P. and Clemmons, C.M. (2021). Objectivity is a myth that harms the practice and diversity of forensic science. *Forensic Science International Synergy* **3**: 100196.
Winburn, A.P., Marten, M.G., Walkup, T., Plasencia, E., et al. (2022). Theorizing social marginization for forensic anthropology: insights from medical anthropology and social epidemiology. In: Marginalized in Death: A Forensic Anthropology of Intersectional Identity in the Modern Era (eds. J. Byrnes and I. Sandoval-Cervantes): Lexington Book.
World Health Organization (2021) Disability and health. https://www.who.int/news-room/fact-sheets/detail/disability-and-health (accessed December 9, 2021).
Young, C. and Light, D. (2013). Corpses, dead body politics and agency in human geography: Following the corpse of Dr Petru Groza. *Transactions of the Institute of British Geographers* **38**(1): 135–148.

CHAPTER 10

Battlefields and killed in action: tombs of the unknown soldier and commemoration

Laura Wittman

Department of French and Italian, Stanford University, Stanford, CA, USA

10.1 Introduction

Among war memorials, the Tomb of the Unknown Soldier stands out for its commemoration of an anonymous soldier and, even more, for its choice to represent this anonymity via a single, concrete body, whose parts were retrieved from the battlefield, recomposed, and reburied. Invented in the wake of World War One, it bears an uncanny, reverse resemblance to contemporary but more traditional forms of commemoration. These include local plaques or steles with lists of names but no buried bodies, vast military cemeteries with seemingly countless identical grave markers, as well as ossuaries where the bones of the many nameless lost are gathered together in one tomb. In these latter instances, names and bodies are kept separate (or identical abstract markers with names make specific bodies disappear), such that the timelessness of the former makes up for the decay of the latter.[1] These commemorations respond to the unprecedented obliteration of combatants' bodies in modern warfare via a compensation that depends on forgetting the living link between social and emotional identity, on the one hand, and embodiment or concrete lived life, on the other. The Tomb of the Unknown Soldier rejects such compensation by foregrounding an indissoluble link between physical suffering and anonymity: the body in this Tomb, and its suffering, are unique and irreplaceable, and no naming, no number of markers and plaques, can make up for the loss of existential embodied identity that war forces upon so many, reducing them – in the words of many World War One writers – to "animals" or "cannon fodder."[2]

Anthropology of Violent Death: Theoretical Foundations for Forensic Humanitarian Action, First Edition.
Edited by Roberto C. Parra and Douglas H. Ubelaker.

The Tomb of the Unknown Soldier is therefore uniquely ambivalent with respect to the sort of heroism nations usually seek to ascribe to the killed in action. The Tomb wants them to be heroes, to be sure, but without abdicating their individuality and especially their expression in the body: through its joys, its sufferings, its situatedness – through that feeling of being *in* the world that is unique to each individual.[3] It continues to speak to us for the past 100 years, I contend, for this very reason, in particular since its invention during the last "Great War" has given way to wars that are increasingly morally fraught and politically contested, that is, wars in which personal heroism might differ significantly from heroism mandated by the state.[4] This is the twentieth- and twenty-first-century Western context of what Giorgio Agamben, drawing on Michel Foucault's notion of biopolitics, calls "bare life," which is essentially the declaration by political powers that they, and only they, determine the meaning of embodied life, which is, on its own, mute, meaningless, and mere matter. But bare life, as Foucault famously shows in the case of sexuality and mental illness, and Agamben in the case of sacrifice, retains a transgressive power that must constantly be held at bay. It seeks to declare and explore its own internal, self-generated meanings; through it, the individual may explore some of his or her most intimate and unique ways of being. As such, bare life bears a special relationship to trauma and PTSD, which, amidst many debates about their nature, undeniably involve a disjunction, a blockage, even a rift, between the concrete, embodied experience of suffering, and its recollection, verbalization, and social meanings. Bare life is powerful then, but disruptive, and often suppressed by society (Foucault 1965; Agamben 1998). Unsurprisingly, the trauma of combatants became a major focus in psychoanalysis during World War One, even as governments sought to minimize it; as we will see shortly, the Unknown Soldier seeks to heal trauma and thereby offers some insights into its nature that are still relevant today.[5] In the rest of this chapter, I will explain how the Tomb of the Unknown Soldier in some of its earliest instances at once foregrounds and contains bare life, in particular through its emphasis on the soldier's mutilation. Here, embodied identity and the reality of trauma emerge provocatively at times and at others are appropriated by external authorities. I will conclude with some remarks on what makes the difference between more healing and more alienating uses of this type of memorial.

10.2 Tomb of the unknown soldier

Though the British, the French, and the Italian governments each claimed precedence in inventing the Tomb of the Unknown soldier, archival investigation shows that the idea was floated by soldiers themselves in all three nations well before the war ended and likely without mutual influence. Numerous historians evoke the practice of improvised burials on the battlefield itself, often for bodies of comrades whose identity could be verified.[6] Makeshift crosses or sticks and sometimes rifles with helmets on top were often all that was left to mark the presence of a body, and it is haunting to read how much effort was spent, in dire circumstances, to ensure the separate burial of each body, and a certain respect of its integrity, which the mass grave would have betrayed. If we consider the radical minimalism of early Tombs of the Unknown soldier – a slab in the ground at Westminster in England and at the Arc de Triomphe in France, a coffin embedded into the much larger Vittoriano complex in Italy – we can see how "the" Unknown echoes the many unknowns, and their tombs, which had been left in no man's land. Yet at the same time, such minimalism is surrounded in all cases by much louder national and political claims. I will focus more on the Italian case in what follows, because in it we see a starker contrast between the soldier's embodied suffering and meanings superimposed upon it, linked to Italy's situation, postwar, as a particularly precarious and recent nation.

The Italian Unknown Soldier was inaugurated on November 4, 1921 (a year after the British and the French ones, due to logistical delays), with a ceremony that was hailed then and continues to be described in recent newspaper accounts, as the last time all Italians genuinely came together with real consensus. The Vittoriano, which surrounds it, was designed in 1895 to celebrate Italian unification but was not completed until 1935 under Fascism, and it was and still is a controversial representation of the Italian state. Beneath the ornate depiction of the goddess Roma and the equestrian statue of King Victor Emmanuel II, the Tomb of the Unknown is a simple slab with the curt inscription "Ignoto Militi." The link between the political cohesion above and the shared suffering below is clear but never articulated explicitly, allowing different types of consensus to coexist without conflict becoming too apparent. The Unknown Soldier was extraordinarily popular, and in many ways, the government felt forced to create a tomb for him and to respond to a widespread desire for memorials to turn their back on past commemorations, which celebrated the nobility, generals, heroes, and other exceptional people. But this subversive quality could here be contained by a more traditional frame.

The crowds at the 1921 inauguration in Rome were immense (and required complex crowd control maps and personnel), but they should not make us think everyone present agreed on what they were commemorating. For the government, the Unknown Soldier's anonymity indicated his absolute obedience and his willingness to sacrifice even his identity to Italy. Consensus came from the identicalness of all of Italy's sons in their common sacrifice to the Patria. Instead, for veterans and their families, in popular culture and in literature, the Unknown Soldier's anonymity was not an accident of war but an existential condition: it reflected an inherent truth not only of modern warfare on a mass scale but also of modern life in large, alienating cities, dependent on working conditions divorced from the land and community. Consensus came from the common experience of the tragic reduction of humans to cogs in the machine of Western war and progress. In other words, the authorities cast the Tomb of the Unknown Soldier as bellicist. In contrast, much of the population and many intellectuals insisted that the Unknown Soldier was anti-bellicist, exposing the cost of war as well as its economic underpinnings and calling for an end to all wars. In the words of Henri Barbusse:

> "A father [read: A politician] has no moral right to use the heroic death of his son to add bluster to his personal prestige [. . .] or to support a politico-commercial doctrine which, consciously or not, would provoke new massacres."[7]

This contrast is nowhere more clear than in governments' complete refusal to acknowledge that the Unknown Soldier, for all that each nation had its own, also showed far more drastically than any previous memorial that sacrifice at war looks the same no matter which nation you die for. To paraphrase the satirical words of Blaise Cendrars, in his *La vie et la mort du soldat inconnu,* how do we know the Unknown Soldier under the Arc de Triomphe (or for that matter in the Vittoriano) is not a German, a Jew, a 'Nègre,' or even a woman? In a literal sense, Cendrars is exaggerating, because in each nation a great deal of care was taken to find one body with enough of a uniform left to indicate Frenchness or Italianness, but with very little otherwise to determine identity. From an ideological and philosophical perspective, however, Cendrars is asking a pertinent and provocative question: Is the anonymity and the consensus celebrated by different nations the same? If so, how can it still be nationalistic, especially in a bellicist sense? What differentiates one nation's Unknown Soldier from another nation's (Cendrars 1995, pp. 29–33)?

These questions become even more pertinent if we consider that between 1921 and the present, the popularity of the Unknown Soldier has been extraordinarily consistent, but his anonymous body has received radically divergent interpretations. In the late 1930s, Mussolini could celebrate through the Unknown Soldier Italy's dead in its colonial war in Ethiopia, whereas in 1945, the same Unknown Soldier came to represent the partisans' "non-military" sacrifice to free Italy from Fascist oppression. Never mind the fact that Germans also had an Unknown Soldier Memorial, inaugurated in 1931. Damaged in World War Two, it was restored in 1993 as an overtly pacifist memorial. There are Unknown Soldier Memorials in almost every nation of the world, no matter what its ideology. Hence, for example, Saddam Hussein erected a massive monument to the Unknown Iraqi Soldier in 1982 in the context of the war against Iran, but Canada inaugurated its Unknown Soldier in 2000, and New Zealand repatriated an Unknown Soldier from France as recently as 2004. There is even a Memorial to the Unknown Deserter, inaugurated in Potsdam in 1990. Very provocatively, in 1998, Michael Verhoeven chose to entitle *The Unknown Soldier* his documentary about the controversial late 1990s "Wehrmacht Exhibition," which explored both the participation and the dissent of "common soldiers" in the "final solution." In the United States, the Unknown Soldier Memorial at Arlington Cemetery, inaugurated in 1921, did not become controversial until after the Vietnam War, when it sparked debate about who – families or the government – owned the dead bodies of soldiers; still, it remains a core element of presidential inaugurations and was used most recently by Joe Biden to pay homage to the military as well as to show public grief that echoed the people's need for mourning in response to the COVID-19 pandemic.[8]

10.2.1 We cannot then but ask

How can the same memorial receive such opposite political interpretations? How can it appear, in turn, bellicist and pacifist? And why insist on recycling this particular type of memorial, with its disturbing emphasis on the corpse, instead of inventing a new one for each new cause? The flexibility and endurance of the Unknown Soldier suggest that its core is a quintessentially modern confrontation with death that is still with us and cannot be subsumed to any specific political or religious agenda. A different kind of mourning is at work here, which is not eliminated by nationalism but remains implicit within it. This becomes most apparent, first, when we put the Unknown Soldier into a much longer history, not limited to 1918–1921, allowing us to compare its multiple reinterpretations of his body and its bare life across time and into our present. Second, and more important, the monuments themselves are only a small part of how the character of the Unknown Soldier, and the quality of his embodied life, were imagined. To explore the psychological and spiritual power of this anonymous corpse, we have to consider how, from the beginning, in Europe and America, the Unknown Soldier was also the protagonist of imagined biographies, satirical cartoons, popular fiction, avant garde poems, philosophical plays, and sociological studies, which would continue to be published throughout the twentieth century. These materials, which include works by major authors such as d'Annunzio, Ungaretti, Giono, and Cendrars, but also involve war diaries and correspondence, and photographical testimonies, show that the experience of existential anonymity, far more than that of obedience or nationalist pride, is fundamental to the memorial's appeal across time and national boundaries. Journalists, writers, and filmmakers transform anonymity from a passive condition to an active questioning of the supremacy of civic, cultural, and linguistic identity. They fundamentally claim that an Unknown Soldier's anonymity transcends nations, just as his sacrifice transcends religious dogma and its military appropriations. For them, the memorial allows the soldier to be a hero without demonizing the enemy, and it allows mourners to claim that his sacrifice was not in vain without reducing its purpose to a political agenda (see Cendrars 1918; d'Annunzio 1918, 1942 [hereafter *Prose*]; d'Annunzio 1947, pp. 564–571; Comento meditato a un discorso improvviso, in: d'Annunzio 1947, pp. 495–563; d'Annunzio 1921, d'Annunzio 1995; Giono 1971; Ungaretti 1969).

10.3 Mutilated victory

I have discussed these materials at length elsewhere. Here, I will concentrate on the most radical aspect of the memorial – its anchoring of anonymity in a single body – and its symbolic genesis, which is tied to the work of the veteran, nationalist, and poet Gabriele d'Annunzio. The term "mutilated victory" was coined by d'Annunzio to decry Italy's loss of territories in Dalmatia after World War One; the phrase also denounced the thing Massimo d'Azeglio is famously credited with complaining about, "Italy has been made, but we have not yet made Italians."[9] It was an extremely popular phrase that echoed throughout the Fascist era, visually associated with the mutilated statue, the Nike of Samorthrace – and with the Unknown Soldier, whose broken body signified a precarious, perhaps irremediably broken, unity of Italians. From this perspective, it is very interesting to compare the language used in official documents to discuss this body, with both popular press accounts, and more literary evocations.

At this point, you may have asked yourself: how did they find the anonymous body of a soldier to bury in the memorial, in 1921, three years after the war had ended? The answer is one that the government wanted people to both know and not to know. What they wanted people to know was that a military commission worked for months, gathering bones from the 11 great Italian battlefields, so that 11 whole bodies could then be put in 11 identical coffins; then, in a grand and very public ceremony at Aquileia on October 27, 1921, one coffin was chosen at random from the 11 to become *the* Unknown Soldier. What the government definitely did not want people to know was what was really inside the coffins and how difficult it had been to reconstruct anything like a whole body from the shattered remains that could be disinterred. There exist some extremely rare images of this process, published by Augusto Tognasso, who was part of the military commission in charge of finding a body. His book, created for a group of veterans who funded its limited publication, consists mostly of photographs, with only six or so pages of text, that document all the bones that were found; it is presented as an homage to all those who were *not chosen* to be the Unknown Soldier (Tognasso 1922).[10] Here we see the horror of the battlefield come alive again, because the remains are mutilated and often one body cannot even be separated from another.

The Italian State actually forbade citizens from attending the exhumations and fairly successfully prevented newspapers from photographing or describing them. The only exceptions were the local newspapers near the battlefields, *La voce dell'Isonzo, Il Giornale di Udine,* and *La Patria del Friuli,* which published maps and informed citizens of when the commission was digging in their area. An interesting detail is that d'Annunzio was invited by the authorities to attend exhumations, but the archives of the Ministry of the Interior reveal that they did so because they were afraid he would show up anyway, unannounced, perhaps with angry veterans in tow – they were afraid he would create more publicity if they did not invite him. He did not show up, but as we will see, he was busy writing texts that emphasized the suffering body of soldiers.[11]

The language used in official documents tries to make us forget the concreteness of exhumations. For example, in its official approval of the Unknown Soldier, the Italian Senate established his role as "the symbol of the collective virtue of our people," while the Chamber of Deputies insisted on how "the absolute suppression of individuality, [. . .] demonstrates, in the end, that to have been Italian and to have fallen for Italy is a great enough title for supreme honors and eternal veneration, above and beyond any other sign of identification." The documents say that a commission will find the anonymous body of a soldier, but it does not even use the word *exhumation*. The newspapers generally echoed the abstract vocabulary of humble sacrifice used by the government, in particular when they described the Unknown Soldier's bones magically rising up from the battlefield to find themselves in the glory of Rome or when they talked about his "transfiguration" or his "apotheosis" – theological terms that refer to the redemption of the body in Catholicism and thus imply that the Unknown Soldier's broken body is now whole again, intact, and eternal.[12] This idea of transfiguration is visually present in the memorial because the intact body of Roma seems to rise up from the Unknown Soldier's tomb.

Nonetheless, sometimes the newspapers resisted such abstraction. The Socialists in particular emphasized in *Avanti!* that "shredded bones" do not make a hero but reveal only "a human body, shredded by other humans, like him in shreds." Major dailies like *La Tribuna* and *Il Corriere della sera* did not go quite that far, but they did repeat a quote from one of the witnesses to the exhumations, which became famous:

> The last [body], gathered from near the Timavo, was truly the expression of martyrdom; with its broken legs and its head punctured by projectiles, it inspired so much pity to the Research Commission that its members fell to their knees.

Similarly, the poet Ada Negri published a poem in *Il secolo illustrato* entitled "The Unknown Hero Returns," which emphasized "at the center of his forehead the great and bloody stigmata" and the "shrapnel holes and burns" in his uniform.[13] But more than anyone, it was d'Annunzio who insisted that the corporeality and mutilation of soldiers not be forgotten. In his *Notturno,* he wrote, for example:

> "I lie all night against the barbed wire that blocks off the hill. I count the corpses. They are all caught up in the iron thorns, compressed by the twisting and broken metal wires, they hang between posts like thieves poorly nailed to their crosses, they twist like animals caught in snares."
> "They have no eyelids, they have no lips. I see frozen naked eyes. I see frozen naked teeth."
> "I see the blood dripping down the wood and the iron, thickening, blackening, viscous like bird-trapping glue."
> "There is no more dew, there is no more dawn for the world (D'Annunzio, 1921, pp. 66–67, 98–99)."

Much of the *Notturno* was written by d'Annunzio in 1916, after he had a plane accident – he was famous for his flying feats of dropping anti-German leaflets on German camps. In that accident, he lost one eye, and in order not to lose sight from his other eye as well, he was immobilized in the dark, eyes bandaged, for many months. He thus had to write on strips of thin paper that accommodated only a few lines at a time. But his blindness became the foundation for highly tangible memories of the war. Structured as a litany for his deceased comrades, the *Notturno* evokes them via the modulations of a few stark images: the moment of death, witnessed or imagined not only as heroic but also as a complete breakdown of paradigms; the dissolution of each comrade's body as it is mirrored in d'Annunzio's own physical sensations of metamorphosis; the attempt to halt this decay by associating the purity of bones with the "sibylline" words written on white strips of paper in the dark; and finally the traumatic confusion of living and dead bodies that no amount of writing can erase.[14]

Going directly against the abstract rhetoric of the Italian government, d'Annunzio imagines that broken bones grow new flesh and are given over to suffering again and again:

> "As I write in the darkness, my thoughts break and my hand stops. [. . .]
> I shiver in fear. And I stop moving, my whole body rigid, and I dare not trace a single sign in the darkness.
> [. . .] Then only my bones exist, only my skeleton bandaged with flesh. And in my skeleton there is a sudden coagulation of life.
> Life precipitates, thickens like blood which is no longer fluid. It is a horrible weight. [. . .]
> My suffering is vile and powerless" (D'Annunzio 1921, 66–67, 98–99).

In the "Annotazione," a postface to the *Notturno* published only in 1921, d'Annunzio made his critique of the official Unknown Soldier Memorial explicit while at the same time indirectly claiming he was one of the original sources for the idea.

> "While in sadness I transcribed the example of the nameless peasant who entered the ford dropping to his knees in the midst of the current, and, sacrificing himself, sculpted his sacrifice into the water, inside the basilica of Aquileia, a mourning mother was choosing between the eleven nameless coffins the one to be buried in the monument.
> [. . .]
> And why wasn't the Great Sufferer's coffin enveloped by the flag of the Timavo, the flag I keep, the one once named "the shroud of sacrifice," "the foot soldier's banner," the one draped across the coffins of my dead of Fiume, lined up against the earth?
> At first, the image of only one dead hero was incised upon it; now it bears the image of all the dead, as all those who died for the *Patria* and in the *Patria* resemble each other just as Giovanni Randaccio in his stone ark resembles the unknown soldier gathered inside four boards (D'Annunzio, 1921, pp. 333–334)."

Let me unpack this a little. At the outset, it is important to know d'Annunzio planned to publish the final version of the *Notturno* on the very day of the Italian Unknown Soldier Memorial's inauguration, November 4, 1921. He did not succeed in finishing it on time, but major extracts were published on that day in the *Illustrazione italiana,* right next to the magazine's photo spread of the memorial's inauguration. In the passage from the *Notturno*'s postface that I just quoted, d'Annunzio connects the Unknown Soldier to his own writings and rituals of remembrance via three key references. The image of the peasant soldier comes from the earlier, 1916, portions of the *Notturno,* which, in 1921, he transcribed just as the Unknown Soldier was chosen from among the 11 candidates; this peasant could be among them, he implies. The "dead of Fiume" refers to d'Annunzio's paramilitary takeover of that city in 1919–1920, which was meant to highlight Italy's mutilated state and to call for its redemption; this redemption, he insists, has still not taken place. Finally, Randaccio was a war hero and friend of d'Annunzio's, whose death in 1917 was the occasion for the invention of new forms of commemoration; these, d'Annunzio demands, should be the model for the Tomb of the Unknown Soldier. I will explain these three references in turn, focusing mostly on the last one, in which mutilation becomes central.

As regards the first, d'Annunzio invented in the *Notturno* an image that would become recurrent in Italian culture, that of the "miles patiens," as Paolo Valesio has termed him, that is, the "peasant soldier" in his uniquely humble suffering. This Italian peasant who accepts death by drowning in order not to reveal to the enemy that the river can be forded is close to the Unknown Soldier not only because his sacrifice is anonymous but also because of his social class, which separates him from officers or career military men and connects him to the earth.

This image of the "peasant-soldier" was also all over the Italian press at the time (Valesio 1978, 1990).

As regards the dead of Fiume, second, d'Annunzio is describing here his use of a tattered Italian flag in mourning them; it was known as the "Banner of Randaccio" or also "the foot soldier's banner," and I will tell you about its origins in a minute. At Fiume, it was used regularly not only to mourn and to commemorate but also as a relic upon which loyalty was sworn and as an incitation to anarchy and subversive symbolic action. Its most significant use was right after the Italian government finally shelled Fiume during the so-called "Bloody Christmas." The banner was draped first over the caskets of d'Annunzio's troops, but then, a few days later after d'Annunzio surrendered, it was used to mourn both his troops and their Italian opponents.[15] This flag and d'Annunzio's use of it were very famous, as seen, for instance, in a two-page photo of it in *L'illustrazione italiana*. What is really remarkable about connecting this flag to the Unknown Soldier is that in this photo, the flag commemorates paramilitary fighters, who took over Fiume against the government's will – most of them were veterans, to be sure, but the official take on them was that they were "deserters." Moreover, the aviation officer who officially proposed the Unknown Soldier Memorial in Italy, Giulio Douhet (an admirer of d'Annunzio's feats of aviation), was himself court martialed and suspended for a year for opposing General Cadorna's disastrous strategy at Caporetto. In his veterans' newspaper, *Il Dovere*, where he proposed the Tomb, Douhet also defended those unjustly accused of being deserters – a huge problem for Italians in the wake of the horrible defeat at Caporetto. So, the point is, for the State, the Unknown Soldier had to be absolutely obedient in his anonymity, but for Douhet and d'Annunzio, there was an even greater courage that consisted of disobeying unjust leaders.

The most important thing about this flag takes me to the third reference in d'Annunzio's text: the death and commemorations of his comrade Randaccio. The origins of this flag are mythical almost as much as those of the Shroud of Turin, which is one of its models. D'Annunzio first fought with Randaccio and his company in the ninth battle of the Isonzo, in November 1916. D'Annunzio and Randaccio were almost killed, but ultimately their success was celebrated in the newspapers with images of Randaccio, a tattered Italian flag wound around his chest, about to reach the summit, followed by d'Annunzio. Less than a month later, Olga Levi, d'Annunzio's Triestine lover, gave him an oversized Italian flag so that he might plant it somewhere on the summits of the battlefield, whence it might be seen from Trieste. In May 1917, d'Annunzio joined Randaccio's company again in the tenth battle of the Isonzo. On May 28, Randaccio was wounded as he desperately tried to capture the summit of the mountain once again. D'Annunzio laid him upon the flag, and he was taken to the Monfalcone hospital, where he died. The bloodied flag covered his coffin at his funeral in Monfalcone on May 30, as celebrated both in the *L'illustrazione italiana* and in the *Domenica del Corriere*. Images also showed the monument erected to Randaccio's heroism on the mountain where he was mortally wounded: the location is important because it is near the mysterious sources of the Timavo river. As this river runs underground for over 40 kilometers, in this highly contested border zone, its sources, eventually known to be three, were as alluring as those of the Nile. Their defense made Randaccio a mythological hero. The association between Randaccio and the Unknown Soldier that d'Annunzio insists upon is comforted by the Unknown Soldier's connection to the Timavo: water from the Timavo river was used to bless his coffin at the inauguration.

A month after his death, Randaccio was reburied at Aquileia – the same place where the Unknown Soldier was chosen among the 11 possible candidates four years later. D'Annunzio gave his funeral oration, "La corona del fante," and the bloody tattered flag was unfurled over the coffin again. This reburial, complete with close-ups that show the flag, was also extensively covered in *L'illustrazione italiana*. The repetition itself, and the obsessive media focus on it, suggest the presence of trauma: Randaccio's body, made more present and concrete by the suffering visible in the bloody flag, does not seem to want to stay buried. But to return to d'Annunzio's commemoration of Randaccio, as important as his gestures was the text that accompanied them. The oration was included in a booklet entitled *La riscossa*. Published in May 1918 by the Print Secretary's Office, that is, by the military, it was widely distributed among Italian soldiers; it was also simultaneously published in English translation as *The Rally* and distributed to British soldiers as well.

In a key passage, d'Annunzio claims that Randaccio represented "the foot soldier" and that to honor him in death was to honor all dead foot soldiers:

> "But this day cannot be mine, comrades. This can only be the votive day of the martyr of Aquileia, the day sacred to the hero of the Timavo. [. . .]
> Giovanni Randaccio [. . .] was a son of the earth, a creature of the soil and of the rock, of the mud and of the dust. [. . .] he was the true maker of victory. In sum, he was the foot soldier.
> He was like you [. . .] [His] heroism was a flash of lightening. [. . .] Yours is like your bones, it is the internal core, it is always there; [. . .]
> "you are all heroes," Giovanni Randaccio cried out to you [. . .]
> You, people of the fields, people of different trades, people of the workshop and of the office, peasants, workers, bourgeois from every walk of life and in every profession, grown wild like those who wait in caves, [. . .] stooping in the filthy burrows that smell of sewer and grave, [. . .] you, people foul and heavy beneath the earth, you in that moment were but a swift flame, a splendid soul, as on Resurrection Day."[16]

We find here three elements central to the Unknown Soldier. First, the naming of "il fante" or "the foot soldier" as representative of all true heroes, in which "operaio della vittoria" ("maker of victory") is a prelude to Douhet's assertion that the Unknown Soldier was "il vero vincitore" ("the true winner"). And we know Douhet was an admirer of d'Annunzio and in particular of his rebelliousness. Second, the soldier is associated not just with the peasant ("gente dei campi," or "farmers," noticeably the first category mentioned) but also with a list of vocations (more than professions) that tries to be encyclopedic while excluding precisely those who would normally be heroes, the nobility. And this list is absolutely a key trace of how important d'Annunzio and his commemorations were in Italy at the time. When the Minister of War Rodinò presented the Unknown Soldier proposal to the Italian Parliament on July 28, 1921, he echoed word for word d'Annunzio's 1917 oration for Randaccio, giving the same unusual (and a little archaicizing) list of vocations.[17]

Third, to return to the oration, the soldier's humility and courage are represented by his bones and by a reading of them that eschews transcendence and purity in order to emphasize a kind of resurrection that is inseparable from the earth, the mud, the mass grave, and even the sewer. The importance of this humble and primal chorality is attested to by the fact that d'Annunzio had already, in a rather new show of humility brought on by the war, evoked it in an entry from his war diaries dated 1915 and published in 1916. Here he identified with a soldier sitting next to him in the trenches.

> "We are both here on the bench, one next to the other. It seems our destinies are about to be linked, intertwined. He is young, and I am no longer young. Both of us could be dead before noon on Tuesday: a fistful of scorched flesh, a few blackened bones, some shriveled cartilage, a crushed skull with a few gold teeth sparkling in the sludge."
> "We return here to the mud of the trenches, in which the bones of comrades become indistinguishable from each other. Most important, this chorality is once again not "from above," tied to abstraction and purity, but "from below", a descent into the chthonic and into common mutilation."[18]

For d'Annunzio, then, a common embodied suffering, felt viscerally as "scorched flesh," is what the Unknown Soldier Memorial should commemorate. This is made even more clear in one of d'Annunzio's most famous political speeches, delivered from the balcony of the Campidoglio on May 4, 1919 – a few months before he marched on Fiume. On this occasion, he again unfurled the oversized flag, which bore the "blood and lymph" ("sangue e sanie") of Randaccio, over the balcony, announcing:

> "This, Romans, this, Italians, this, comrades, is the flag of this hour.
> The sublime image of the soldier who leaned his head upon it has remained impressed in it.
> And it is the image of all the dead; for all who have died for the *Patria* resemble each other."

"It is the shroud of sacrifice.
[. . .] I will lower this flag, until Fiume is ours, until Dalmatia is ours.
Every good citizen should lower his flag, until Fiume is ours, until Dalmatia is ours."[19]

Among many other newspapers, Douhet's *Il Dovere* celebrated d'Annunzio's gesture at the Campidoglio. This was well before any official proposals for any Tomb of the Unknown Soldier, in Italy or elsewhere. It is thus particularly significant that d'Annunzio not only sees the flag as an image of "the soldier" and thus of "all the dead" but also insists on how this image was produced, calling it "the shroud of sacrifice." This refers to Shroud of Turin – the cloth in which Christ was purportedly wrapped at the deposition, on which a sort of living painting of his body can be seen. It was also thought that the image of his face had remained imprinted on the veil used by a woman to wipe it when he was on his way to Calvary: this object – of which many versions have existed throughout history – is known as the veil of the Veronica. As we will see shortly, d'Annunzio refers to this image also.

The crucial thing here is the impression of one body, and even more one face, that leaves its trace on the fabric. With the Banner of Randaccio as with the Shroud of Turin, the point of such an image is not visual correctness but physical continuity: we do not see suffering here, but rather we touch it, and the traces of one dead body ultimately allow us to touch all the dead. It is clear that such tactile continuity between the living and the dead is a rejection of the separation between bodies and names or between existential anonymity and its political and social meanings; as such, it is also a prelude to healing from a trauma that is similarly embodied. One last example shows how key, for d'Annunzio and many of his readers, was the insistence on tactile, visceral identification, on the part of the living, with the embodied, mutilated dead of World War One. In his "La Chiesa di Doberdò," published in *L'ardente* of July 1, 1921, d'Annunzio described a bombed church that served as a hospital; to show how it was filled not only with the wounded but also with the dead, whose bodies were too torn apart to be identifiable visually as bodies, he evoked "the battered peeling pierced helmets, one on top of the other, grey like ashes, the leather inside macerated in sweat, infused with blood." In his diary entry of September 24, 1916, when he visited Doberdò, which is clearly the inspiration for his later published text, d'Annunzio noted: "The christ – The shoes the helmets remains of the dead – The Christ carrying the cross – the VIth station over the main altar Leaning on the wall the stretchers spotted with blood."[20]

This entry contracts and anticipates remarkably the power of the Banner of Randaccio a year before Randaccio's death. Helmets and shoes emphasize the pathos of bodies reduced to objects as well as insist on the importance of physical traces of suffering for they are blood-soaked "remains." These are associated with the sixth station of the Cross, when Christ is vilified on the way to his crucifixion – the very opposite of transfiguration. Most telling, however, this sixth station is associated with the blood-stained stretchers leaning on the wall, which reminds us that this station is also that of the "veil of the Veronica." In all of these images, what is once again central is the fleshiness of suffering and the need for a remembrance of it that bears its direct physical traces. To sum up, then, what d'Annunzio shows us is that the Unknown Soldier's enduring appeal – across time and nations and across political divides – is a lot less about ideology than it is about what the philosopher Edith Wyschogrod calls "carnal generality." This is not abstract knowledge of a shared human condition, but the direct embodied experience of the continuity of my flesh and that of the other. When such continuity is with the flesh of an other who has been mutilated, often beyond human recognition, the experience of carnal generality is bound to be horrific, perhaps even traumatic Wyschogrod (1973, 1985, 1998).

10.4 As an Epilogue

Recent works on the cultural history of how trauma has been constructed and reconstructed in the past 100 years address the thorny question of whether repeating trauma can be a way to heal it, or whether, on the contrary, repetition condemns us to endless mourning. Ruth Leys, in particular, argues that this is not an either/or question, but rather that each era of crisis reinvents the complex link between trauma and its representations, which is also to say the link between the suffering body and its social, institutional, and political meanings.[21] Based on her investigation, but also on recent work with veterans with PTSD, and in light of what is revealed by the creation of the Unknown Soldier (as a monument as well as a character, even an archetype), I propose that as long as the repetition is *embodied*, it can heal. That is, we can heal if we can re-experience trauma with our whole person, without mind–body dissociation, and with the help of another person with whom we can also feel carnal generality. The uniqueness of suffering as situated in one individual and one body must not be abstracted into universals, but rather made present. The Unknown Soldier offers many insights into how such bringing of suffering into presence can take place. We have focused one striking example, which includes both the use of memorial objects that retain a physical connection to the traumatized body and their embeddedness into a story and a ceremony. The story and the ceremony, which call for actual readers and embodied attendance, respectively, confirm the symbolic power of such objects for the community. In Italy and elsewhere, after the initial inaugurations, ceremonies for the Unknown Soldiers gradually removed such objects from view (d'Annunzio's flag disappeared, for instance), but periodically popular sentiment, expressed by veterans in particular, seeks to bring it back: in England, a flag whose purpose was very similar to the the Banner of Randaccio, the flag of Father David Railton, who used it to wrap soldiers' bodies, was returned to the British Unknown Soldier's Tomb in 2006 (it had been removed as obsolete in 1953). Notably, the context at the time was the coalition invasion of Iraq, which had started in 2003.[22] The Tombs of the Unknown Soldier bring suffering into presence in a number of other ways as well, which make the existential experience of being incarnate more real: they include the use of photographs, such as Tognasso's, which I alluded to above, as well as of reenactments in fiction, theater, and film, which I document in my book, *The Tomb of the Unknown Soldier.* In the end, however, the uniqueness of carnal generality – the complex expression of a commonness that cannot be made abstract or even completely verbalized – demands new and creative forms of expression in response to new traumas. The Tomb of the Unknown Soldier can inspire us, but its specific symbolic objects are not necessarily to be copied directly. As we seek ways to express grief and to heal in the wake of COVID-19 then, the Unknown Soldier invites us to consider what can be added to memorials where countless white flags symbolize the dead, to reduce abstraction and give place to a more embodied suffering. From this perspective, it is striking how ubiquitous the masks that cover the individual faces of patients and caregivers have become in recent commemorative art[23]: though masks might seem initially to be a strange suppression of the individual identity that is being remembered, the Unknown Soldier shows us that they are also an enactment of carnal generality; they are symbolic objects, like the tattered flag that wrapped bodies of soldiers, that bear the physical traces of suffering and create an embodied link between the dead and us, the mourners.

Notes

1. On the abstraction of names, see Sherman (1998). He cites a French senator who spoke of having known personally many of "the names" (not the persons) whose memorial he was inaugurating. For bodies and names, see: Ingersoll and Nickell (1987, pp. 199–225) and Laqueur (1996, pp. 123–141).
2. On embodiment and the Unknown Soldier, see Wittman (2011). More recently, on the French Unknown Soldier, see Gauthier (2014). On Unknown Soldiers all over the world, see Cochet and Grandhomme (2012). For an exploration of animality, see Bonadeo (1989).
3. On the feeling of being in the world and its existential component, from a psychiatric and philosophical perspective, see Ratcliffe (2008). On the importance of the body in soldiers' testimonies, in correspondence and via other materials, see: Leed (1979) and Winter (1995). The French war memorial at Péronne, France, for which Winter was a key advisor, incorporates corporeality into its architecture itself, but putting the museum objects in trenches and graves dug into the floor rather than in raised display cases.

4. Most recently, on this theme, see Samet (2021).
5. See Leed (1979, pp. 3–4) for general remarks on trauma during World War One; for a history of the term, with a chapter on the World War One era, see Leys (2000).
6. For images of improvised battlefield burials in France, see Fonck (2004); for Italian versions, Dogliani (1996, pp. 377–389). For the complex story of how the British, French, and Italians all claimed to have invented the memorial first, even as it existed on the battlefield before any official memorial was proposed, see Wittman (2011, Ch. 1, "A Unanimous Idea"). The same chapter gives archival and newspaper sources for the details of the Italian creation and inauguration that follow.
7. Barbusse is cited in Winter (1995, p. 182).
8. On post-1921 uses of the Unknown Soldier memorial in Italy, see Ridolfi (2003). On students in 1940 France, see Tandonnet (2009). On 1935 rallies by the Croix-de-Feu, see Le Naour (2018, p. 64). A reminder of the peace rallies held in Rome earlier in 2003 is in "Italy Holds State Funeral for 19 Troops," *New York Times*, November 18, 2003. On the British Memorial to Innocent Victims of Oppression, Violence, and War, see Ezard (1996), "A Tribute to Civil Victims of War and Tyranny," *Guardian*, October 11, 1996. On its use to mourn after the events of September 11, 2001 in New York and Washington, see Boggan and Hughers (2001), "Like a River of Grief, Widows and Children Flowed Past a Memorial to Mass Murder," *Independent*, November 30, 2001. On the Potsdam Memorial to the Unknown Deserter, see the following: City of Potsdam (n.d.), "Greens Win Permission to Display Monument to Unknown Deserter," *International News*, September 21, 1989; Kinzer (1993). On the "Wehrmacht Exhibition" and the related film, see Fawcett (2002); Brenner (2007). The United States is the only country to have added more bodies to its Unknown Soldier Memorial, adding three more to the one buried in 1921: one each after World War Two, the Korean War, and the Vietnam War. It was only in 1988 that controversy erupted over the suggestion that the authorities had a good idea of who the Vietnam Unknown Soldier might be and that DNA testing should be done; it was, amid much controversy, and he was identified as Lieutenant Michael Blassie. For the basic story, see "From Tomb of Unknown to Grave of Lieut. Blassie," *New York Times*, July 12, 1998. For a discussion of the philosophical implications of this identification of the Unknown Soldier, see Naas (2003). For the Unknown Soldier Memorial in Iraq, see Al-Khalil (1991) and Rosie DiManno, "Hunt for the Disappeared Leads to Hellish Tunnels," *Toronto Star*, April 21, 2003. On Canada, see Delisle (2005). On New Zealand, see Helen Tunnah, "Soldier's Name Secret Forever," *New Zealand Herald*, November 6, 2004.
9. On the "new Italian," the canonical phrase is attributed to Massimo D'Azeglio, as he is most often cited: "having made Italy, it remains to make the Italians." In reality, D'Azeglio (1966), vol. I, at 17: "The Italians have wanted to make a new Italy, but themselves remain the old Italians." This, along with D'Azeglio in relation to Italians' creation of their own national past, is discussed in Adrian Lyttelton, "Creating a National Past: History, Myth, and Image in the Risorgimento," in Russell Ascoli and von Henneberg (2001), pp. 27–74.
10. Tognasso was a mutilated veteran himself and was part of the commission of soldiers who performed exhumations and chose one appropriate body from each battlefield. The book does not indicate the name of the photographer, but we gather it was Tognasso himself, perhaps in collaboration with other soldiers, during the work of the commission. This book is rare enough that only four libraries in Italy have a copy. It was reprinted in 1962 in Milan by the Tipografia Zanoli, in an "edizione fuori

commercio," this time "A favore della Casa militare veterani guerre naz. Umberto 1. e della erigenda Casa del combattente in Bovisa."

11. On d'Annunzio being invited to Rome, see Bernardi (1962). On his invitation to participate in exhumations at the Timavo; this is also mentioned in Miniero (2008), p. 187. D'Annunzio was also invited to participate in the choosing ceremony at Aquileia (Bernardi 1962, 1137). "Lo spirito di d'Annunzio si aggirava intorno ai convenuti, ma il vate [...] non comparve" (Miniero 2008, *Da Versailles*, p. 188).

12. "Per la tomba del soldato al Pantheon," initially published in Il Dovere, August 24, 1920, reproduced in Douhet (1931, pp. 424–433). Quotes are, respectively, from pp. 424, 426, 427, 431. Semeria's critique of "apotheosis" as a fair term is in Corriere d'Italia of November 2, 1921.

13. Timavo: *Corriere della Sera*, Oct 28, 1921, and *La Tribuna*, October 27 and 30, 1921. Negri's poem, in *Il secolo illustrato*, November 1, 1921, imagines the soldier telling his young sister to stop wearing the clothes of mourning.

14. For the reference to the Sybil, see d'Annunzio (1921, p. 5).

15. Thus, on September 12, 1919, it was used to consecrate the taking of Fiume and then on October 7, 1919, to bury the two aviators who were the first to die for the cause of the city. Later it was unfurled during a trip by d'Annunzio to Zara, asserting the spread of Fiume's "fires." He also brought it out during a referendum regarding Fiume's National Council, to indicate his refusal to abide by their rules. At the end of the Fiuman enterprise, it was used to commemorate those who died when the city was finally shelled by Italians during the "Bloody Christmas": first on December 27, 1920, when they mourned d'Annunzio's troops and then, more significantly, after d'Annunzio surrendered, on January 2, 1921, and on January 3, 1921, when they mourned both d'Annunzio's troops and their Italian opponents.

16. The publication of *La riscossa* was done at the behest of the Duke of Aosta, who wished to have it distributed to all the soldiers of the Third Army; see Martinelli, *La guerra di d'Annunzio*, 166. For the date of the volume, see Andreoli, *Il vivere inimitabile*, 545. The actual book has no date printed in it, while the only publication data are as follows: "Edizione fuori commercio a cura del Sottosegretariato per la Stampa," "Casa Editrice d'Arte Bestetti & Tuminelli Milano"; the English volume, *The Rally*, with the translation by Magda Sindici, is physically identical to the Italian one and bears the same publication data. For the quote, see d'Annunzio (1918), pp. 160–162. I use a modified version of Sindici's translation. For a list of documents about Randaccio and d'Annunzio, see Wittman, Ch. 1, "The Origins of the Unknown Soldier."

17. Rodinò also says his proposal follows "il sogno del Poeta" or "the Poet's dream" but does not mention d'Annunzio by name; arguably this was not necessary in 1921.

18. The diary entry is from d'Annunzio (1942), pp. 64–66.

19. "Dalla ringhiera del Campidoglio," on "terre irredente," is in d'Annunzio (1947), pp. 883–884. It was also published in 1919 in his d'Annunzio (1919). See d'Annunzio (1995, p. 37).

20. The diary entry for d'Annunzio's visit to Doberdò is in d'Annunzio (1976, pp. 870–871).

21. See Leys (2000) and Young (1995). For more recent mourning and trauma, Tick (2005).

22. Neil Hanson, "Flying the Flag for the Padre Once More: The flag that covered the Unknown Warrior – a potent symbol literally steeped in blood – must be restored to its rightful place, says Neil Hanson," *Daily Telegraph*, November 10, 2006; Cassandra Jardine and Richard Savill, "Wootton Bassett: A Very British Way of Mourning," *Telegraph*, July 7, 2009.

23. For flags on the Washington, DC. Mall, see *National Geographic*'s recent coverage: https://www.nationalgeographic.com/culture/article/epic-covid-19-memorial-national-mall-one-stunning-photo; for examples of art with masks: https://www.lamag.com/culturefiles/coronavirus-murals/; https://www.cbsnews.com/news/massive-mural-of-doctor-who-died-of-covid-19-honors-frontline-workers-in-new-york-city/; https://www.nationalgeographic.com/magazine/article/danny-wilcox-frazier-on-photographing-covid-19-in-detroit.

References

Agamben, G. (1998). *Homo Sacer: Sovereign Power and Bare Life (translated by Daniel Heller-Roazen).* Stanford: Stanford University Press.

Al-Khalil, S. (1991). *The Monument: Art, Vulgarity, and Responsibility in Iraq.* Berkeley: University of California Press.

Bernardi, M. (1962). Gabriele d'Annunzio e il Milite Ignoto. Quaderni dannunziani (Gardone, Fondazione 'Il Vittoriale degli Italiani') **22–23**: 1127–1132.

Boggan, S. and Hughers, J. (2001) Like a river of grief, widows and children flowed past a memorial to mass murder. Independent, November 30.

Bonadeo, A. (1989). *Mark of the Beast: Death and Degradation in the Literature of the Great War.* Lexington, KY: University Press of Kentucky.

Brenner, P. (2007) *The Unknown Soldier* (review of film by Michael Verhoeven). http://www.filmcritic.com/misc/emporium.nsf/reviews/The–Unknown–Solider.

Cendrars, B. (1918). *La vie et la mort du soldat inconnu. Cahiers Blaise Cendrars. H. Champion, Paris.* Translated by Magda Sindici (1918) as *The Rally Casa.* Milan: Editrice d'Arte Bestetti & Tuminelli.

Cendrars, B. (1995). La vie et la mort du soldat inconnu. *Honore champion.*: 175.

City of Potsdam (n.d.) *Platz der Einheit, Bassinplatz Squares and the Dutch Quarter.* http://www.potsdam.de/cms/beitrag/10032561/287369/1.

Cochet, F. and Grandhomme, J.-N. (2012). *Les Soldats Inconnus de la Grande Guerre: la mort, le deuil, la mémoire.* Saint-Cloud: Soteca.

D'Annunzio, G. (1918). *La riscossa.* Milan: Casa Editrice d'Arte Bestetti and Tuminelli.

D'Annunzio, G. (1921). *Notturno.* Milan: Garzanti.

D'Annunzio, G. (1942). Le tre redazioni di un taccuino di guerra di Gabriele d'Annunzio (A. Bruers). Milan: Mondadori.

D'Annunzio, G. (1947). 'Il sudore di sangue' Prose'. La penultima ventura. Milan: A. Mondadori.

D'Annunzio, G. (1947). 1922. Il libro ascetico della giovane Italia. Milan: Mondadori.

D'Annunzio, G. (1976). *Taccuini.* Milan: Mondadori.

D'Azeglio, M. (1966). *Things I Remember (I miei ricordi).* London/New York: Oxford University Press.

D'Azeglio, M. (1995). *Siamo spiriti azzurri e stelle: Diario inedito (17–27 agosto 1922).* Florence: Giunti.

D'Annunzio, G. (1919). *Contro uno e contro tutti.* Rome: Presso La Fionda.

D'Annunzio, G. (1942). Agli uomini milanesi per l'Italia degli italiani.' Prose di ricerca, di lotta, di comando, di conquista, di tormento, d'indovinamento, di rinnovamento, di celebrazione, di rivendicazione, di liberazione, di favole, di giochi, di baleni. Milan: Mondadori.

D'Annuzio, G. (1995). *Siamo spiriti azzurri e stelle: Diario inedito (17–27 agosto 1922).*

Delisle, J. (2005). For king and country: nostalgia, war, and Canada's "Tomb of the Unknown Soldier". *Dalhousie Review* **85**(1): 15–32.
Dogliani, P. (1996). Redipuglia. In: *I luoghi della memoria; Simboli e miti dell'Italia unità* (eds. M. Isnenghi and E.A. Perona). Rome: Laterza.
Douhet, G. (1931). *Le Profezie di Cassandra: raccolta di scritti*. Genova: Lang e Padano.
Ezard, J. (1996). A tribute to civil victims of war and tyranny. *Guardian*, October 11.
Fawcett, G. (2002). The Wehrmacht Exhibition. *History Today* **52**(4): 2–3.
Fonck, G. (2004) Le soldat inconnu. Vol. 1. Les démarches. Autoédition, Reims.
Foucault, M. (1965). *Madness and Civilization: A History of Insanity in the Age of Reason*, (translated by Richard Howard). New York: Pantheon Books.
Gauthier, A. (2014) 1914–1918: La prise en charge des morts pour la France et l'invention du Soldat Inconnu. Collection L'éveil De La Mémoire. Un Autre reg'art, Albi.
Giono, J. (1971). *Le grand troupeau*. In: *To the Slaughterhouse* (ed. R. Ricatte). Paris: Gallimard. Translated by Norman Glass, as (2004). Peter Owen and Dufour Editions, London and Chester Springs.
Ingersoll, D.W. and Nickell, J.N. (1987). The most important monument: the tomb of the unknown soldier. In: *Mirror and Metaphor: The Material and Social Constructions of Reality* (ed. G. Bronitsky). Lanham: University Presses of America.
Kinzer, S. (1993). Berlin Journal; The War Memorial: To Embrace the Guilty, Too? The New York Times.
Laqueur, T.W. (1996). Names, bodies, and the anxiety of erasure. In: *The Social and Political Body* (eds. T.R. Schatzki and W. Natter). New York: Guilford Press.
Le Naour, J.-Y. (2018). *Le Soldat Inconnu*. Paris: Fayard.
Leed, E.J. (1979). *No Man's Land: Combat and Identity in World War I*. Cambridge: Cambridge University Press.
Leys, R. (2000). *Trauma: A Genealogy*. Chicago: University of Chicago Press.
Miniero, A. (2008). *Da Versailles al Milite ignoto: Rituali e retoriche della vittoria in Europa (1919–1921)*. Roma: Gangemi.
Naas, M. (2003). History's remains: of memory, mourning, and the event. *Research in Phenomenology* **33**: 75–96.
Ratcliffe, M. (2008). *Feelings of Being: Phenomenology, Psychiatry and the Sense of Reality*. Oxford: Oxford University Press.
Ridolfi, M. (2003). *Le feste nazionali*. Bologna: Il Molino.
Russell Ascoli, A. and Von Henneberg, K. (eds.) (2001). *Making and Remaking Italy: The Cultivation of National Identity around the Risorgimento*. Oxford and New York: Berg.
Samet, E. (2021). *Looking for the Good War: American Amnesia and the Violent Pursuit of Happiness*. New York: Farrar, Straus, and Giroux.
Sherman, D. (1998). Bodies and names: the emergence of commemoration in interwar France. *American Historical Review* **102**(2), 443–446, 455.
Tandonnet, M. (2009). *1940, un autre 11 novembre: Étudiant de France, malgré l'ordre des autorités opprimantes, tu iras honorer le soldat inconnu*. Paris: Tallandier.
Tick, E. (2005). *War and the Soul: Healing Our Nation's Veterans from Post-Taumatic Stress Disorder*. Wheaton, Ill: Quest Books.
Tognasso, A. (1922). *Ignoto Militi*. Milan: Tipografia Magnani.
Ungaretti, G. (1969). *Vita d'un uomo: Tutte le poesie*. Milan: Mondadori.
Valesio, P. (1978). Pax Italiae and the literature of politics. *Yale Italian Studies* **2**: 143–167.
Valesio, P. (1990). Ungaretti and the Miles Patiens: Dannunzian Genealogies. *Stanford Italian Review* **8**(1–2): 103–137.

Winter, J.M. (1995). *Sites of Memory, Sites of Mourning: The Great War in European Cultural History*. Cambridge/New York: Cambridge University Press.

Wittman, L. (2011). *The Tomb of the Unknown Soldier, Modern Mourning, and the Reinvention of the Mystical Body*. Toronto Italian Studies: University of Toronto Press, Toronto.

Wyschogrod, E. (1973). The Phenomenon of Death: Faces of Mortality. Harper Colophon Books. New York: Harper and Row.

Wyschogrod, E. (1985). *Spirit in Ashes: Hegel, Heidegger, and Man-Made Mass Death*. New Haven: Yale University Press.

Wyschogrod, E. (1998). *An Ethics of Remembering: History, Heterology, and the Nameless Others*. Chicago: University of Chicago Press.

Young, A. (1995). *The Harmony of Illusions: Inventing Post-Traumatic Stress Disorder*. Princeton: Princeton University Press.

CHAPTER 11

Mass grave protection and missing persons

Melanie Klinkner

Department of Humanities and Law, Bournemouth University, Bournemouth, UK

11.1 Introduction

Missing persons cases are a global phenomenon that exists on a shocking scale. People go missing during armed conflict, migration, as a result of systematic human rights abuses, disasters, or organized crime. The 2021 Global Report compiled by the International Commission on Missing Persons (ICMP) paints stark and often harrowing pictures: the many missing persons cases arising from migration hotspots and routes in the Middle East and North Africa (MENA) region (Hamadeh 2021); missing persons as a result of trafficking, particularly in relation to women and children from African states (Decker 2021); hundreds of unresolved missing persons cases as a legacy of armed conflict in the Balkans (McDonald-Gibson 2021); the remarkable activism of mothers and relatives in spurring on the development of frameworks for investigation, legislative developments, and redress in Latin America (Cruz-Santiago 2021); and the impact of natural disasters, such as the 2004 tsunami, amidst a plethora of causes for people going missing in Asia (Tae-Ung 2021).

Places, circumstances, and reasons may all differ. But in all cases, there is likely to be a family or community suffering from anguish and grief as a result of their loved ones going missing. They need answers and have the right to know what happened to those that went missing. This requires first and foremost clear actions on behalf of the State who has obligations primarily to protect individuals and resolve the fate of missing and disappeared persons.

Anthropology of Violent Death: Theoretical Foundations for Forensic Humanitarian Action, First Edition.
Edited by Roberto C. Parra and Douglas H. Ubelaker.

The same can be said about mass graves: they too exist on a shocking scale. And habitually they are identified with conflict and gross human rights violations, typically in countries and communities already ravaged by poverty and inequality. Yet, the discovery of suspected mass graves in Kamloops, British Columbia, and elsewhere in Canada – unrelated to COVID-19 mass burials – has made global headlines (Honderich 2021). They are the shocking legacy of government-run residential schools that operated for more than a century and were designed to systematically assimilate Indigenous children and destroy Indigenous cultures and languages. Importantly, mass graves can be found across the globe and throughout various human histories. This recent discovery in Canada triggered a variety of emotions, reactions, and questions, including a call by the United Nations Special Rapporteurs for a full and prompt investigation (UN Human Rights Office of the High Commissioner 2021).

This chapter charts the importance of mass grave protection in the quest to address and, where possible, solve missing persons cases. With reference to a collaborative, legally led project resulting in *The Bournemouth Protocol on Mass Grave Protection and Investigation* (Klinkner and Smith 2020), this chapter firstly outlines who the missing in mass graves are likely to be. In other words, what is the intersection between missing persons more broadly and mass graves more specifically?

Secondly, the chapter clarifies the legal framework in relation to who suffered harm and, therefore, has legitimate interests, before examining how those interests are protected by international law.

Thirdly, the chapter then examines practical elements for protection to ensure an effective investigation can safely follow. Further, it sets an agenda for strengthening mass grave protection through considering the potential of mapping efforts and for "closing" existing blind spots in law and practice.

The chapter concludes with an emphatic endorsement for protection, though arguably the answers to the question "what form of protection?" requires continuous collaborative efforts involving all stakeholders and experts to ensure culturally appropriate and victim-sensitive and acceptable protection.

11.2 Missing persons in mass graves: a worldwide phenomenon

People of all ages go missing for a variety of reasons. They include poor mental health, loss of documentation, miscommunication, lost contact with relatives, new relationships, removed by, or traveled with a parent, runaway and absconding, but they also result from domestic abuse or seeking asylum, refugee status, or migration generally (Shalev Greene and Collie 2021).

Of concern to this chapter are those missing for reasons more akin to the following three broad categories:

1. Natural or manmade disasters.
2. War, conflict, systematic human rights abuses, and enforced disappearance specifically (ICMP 2021; Dulitzky 2019).
3. Migration and trafficking (Laczko et al. 2019; Grant 2016).

Each of these three categories may result in mass graves. But what do we understand to be a mass grave? Mass graves may arise for differing reasons and may exist as a result of body disposal where the reason for the death was suspicious or the burial improper or both (Klinkner and Smith 2021; UNSC 1994). Over the years many definitions have been proffered, but during a recent collaborative study for the purpose of creating unifying guidelines for the protection and investigation of mass graves, the following definition was adopted, whereby a mass grave denotes a site or defined area containing a multitude (more than one) of buried, submerged, or surface scattered human remains (including skeletonized, commingled, and fragmented remains), where the circumstances surrounding the death and/or the body disposal method warrant an investigation as to their lawfulness (Klinkner and Smith 2020, p. 4).

This definition has since been adopted by the former UN Special Rapporteur on extrajudicial, summary, or arbitrary executions in her report (UNGA 2020). Importantly, from a legal perspective, there is this potential dual unlawfulness in relation to mass grave; not only is it the way those buried died that might be breaching law, but it is also the method of disposal that could be unlawful.

Returning to the three categories of reasons for persons going missing – how might they relate to mass graves?

As demonstrated by the pandemic, the first category can result in the creation of mass burials. And the practice of mass burial in those contexts may be appropriate, so long as it is conducted as a "methodical, multistage, and multidisciplinary procedure, which should be performed cautiously by skilled and pre-trained personnel" (Perera and Briggs 2008, p. 8). In times of a pandemic, therefore, mass burials may be a suitable method of "body disposal." Mass burials in this context mean that the dead are buried together, but importantly with the proviso that these burials adhere to standards and allow for future exhumation and, with it, future return of human remains. Crucially, in situations where a State adopts mass burials as a method of body disposal, identification of those buried as well as their dignified burial should be safeguarded. There may be circumstances in which identification might not be ascertained. Where such identification is not possible, all records to facilitate future identifications must be kept.

This is important: because if a mass burial is not appropriately conducted by respecting the rights of those buried and the rights of the family members, then it might constitute a mass grave. Furthermore, two further concerns may arise:

firstly, that states might use the pandemic as a pretext for hiding other human rights violations where individuals are unlawfully killed and then disposed of in a mass grave. The second charge is that states may have insufficiently protected individuals from the impact of the pandemic, which could result in the breach of their human rights. In both cases, a mass burial might in fact be a mass grave for those buried may have died a suspicious death.

The second category identified above for causing people to go missing (that is, through war, armed conflict, and systematic human rights abuses) is most typically linked to mass graves. Such mass graves are truly sites of tremendous human suffering and the phenomenon is ubiquitous. Described by Rosenblatt as "an underground map of atrocity that stretches across the planet's surface" (2015, p. 32), the numbers involved are staggering and testify to suffering across all continents: in Cambodia 309 mass grave sites with an estimated total of 19000 grave pits have been recorded (Yale University 2021). These linked to the events of the 1970s and Pol Pot's attempt at creating an agrarian utopia, decimating Cambodia's population by a third in the process.

In Iraq, over 200 mass graves have been found in the territory formerly controlled by Islamic State of Iraq and the Levant (ISIL), containing up to 12 000 victims (UNAMI/ OHCHR 2018). This, on top of the crimes and sites linked the Saddam Hussein era of human rights abuse and violence.

In the Balkans, and Srebrenica in Bosnia specifically, 17 000 sets of human remains from 94 graves and 337 surface areas have been recovered, with 6982 individuals identified (ICMP 2021). The events surrounding the Srebrenica massacres have since been recognized under international law as genocide.

Guatemala is still grappling with the 36-year civil war in which 200 000 people, mainly indigenous civilians, were killed, many confined to secret cemeteries and graves (Guatemala Commission for Historical Clarification 2013).

Rwanda's landscape is littered with mass graves, with the 2021 commemorations seeing 64 bodies buried at the Mugina genocide memorial (National Commission for the Fight Against Genocide 2021). Of course, many more examples can be cited. The point here is to point to the scale of the challenge. According to the UN Special Rapporteur on extrajudicial, summary, or arbitrary executions in her 2020 report, "the number of sites from the 20th century alone exceeds tens of thousands" (UNGA 2020, para. 6).

As far as mass graves arising out of migration are concerned, their governance is often complicated by the sea as a migratory route or the crossing of borders and deserts, resulting in protracted state responsibility. Migration is one of the core international societal challenges, with many migrants going missing en route to safety and a better life (IOM 2021). The IOM's Missing Migrant Project tracks the number of missing migrants and fatalities across the world. Their figures, however, do not include the many missing persons who have not been recovered, recorded, or reported, some of which may have fallen victim to trafficking.

Akin to the issues reported by De Léon in his examination *The Land of Open Graves. Living and Dying on the Migrant Trail* (2015), stretches of sea are turning into seas of hidden graves. And arguably some of those deaths, burials, surface scattered, or submerged bodies may qualify as mass graves. Insufficient investigations, if there are any, result in fewer identifications and the repatriation of remains, while increasing the number of hidden graves at sea or "official clandestine graves" on land where authorities have not sought to identify human remains, and instead have simply buried them.

In addition, there is increased recognition of an overlap, though empirically perhaps still unsubstantiated, between migration and enforced disappearance (Council of Europe 2016). The UN Human Rights Council Working Group (2017) observes that migration may be triggered by a person's fear of forced disappearance in his or her home country; migrants may disappear during the journey or in the destination country, or after being unlawfully returned. Relatives may migrate in order to search for disappeared members of their families and may themselves be abducted. Migrants may face abduction for political reasons, disappear in the context of smuggling or trafficking, or through disorganized or clandestine detention and deportation. From enforced disappearance, the link to extrajudicial killings resulting in the disposal of bodies in mass graves is alarmingly close.

The consequences for the families (whether in the originating country, destination country, or still on the move) are dire: the ambiguity of their loss may amount to immense suffering.

And the common denominator for the phenomenon of missing persons and mass graves is the harm suffered – by the dead prior to their death and the families. Those buried in the graves can be men, women, or children; they can be civilians, migrants, or armed combatants. But for each body, there is a family in anguish. From their notion of harm suffered, many further needs arise: the return of loved ones for dignified commemoration, the realization of justice for victims, their families, and affected communities, not only in terms of perpetrator accountability but also for commemoration purposes. Protecting mass graves from this point alone, therefore, appears morally compelling. The next section of the chapter will examine the legal protection of mass graves and the missing persons contained therein.

11.3 The legal framework for mass grave protection

11.3.1 Missing persons and international norms

The preceding section pointed to the notion of harm suffered by missing persons and their families and this harm, in turn, is likely to result from breaches of (at time concurrent) rights. Fundamentally, they include the right to life, the right not to be subjected to torture or degrading treatment as well as the right to a family life. These find codification in international legal instruments, such as the Universal Declaration of Human Rights (Articles 3 and 12) and the International Covenant on Civil and Political Rights (Articles 6, 7, and 17). Other international codifications in the Convention Against Torture and Other Cruel, Inhuman, or Degrading Treatment or Punishment or the Convention on the Rights of the Child with its provision on the right to receive essential information concerning the whereabouts of an absent member of the family (Article 9(4)) can be cited in support. Of particular note due to their specific relevance and alignment with missing persons are the International Convention for the Protection of all Persons from Enforced Disappearance, which defines enforced disappearance, as well as the Rome Statute for it criminalizes enforced disappearance as a form of crime against humanity.

The issue of missing person also finds resonance in regional human rights mechanisms, such as the European Convention on Human Rights (notably Article 5 on the right to liberty and security of the person), the Kampala Convention (the Convention for the Protection and Assistance of Internally Displaced Persons in Africa with its provision for placing, inter alia, tracing obligations on the state, as contained in Article 9), and the Inter-American Convention on Forced Disappearance of Persons. Furthermore, during armed conflict, international humanitarian law (the Geneva Conventions I–IV and their additional Protocols) seeks to ensure that people do not go missing (No author 2017; see also ICRC 2009, 2020). Of particular note in the context of armed conflict is Rule 117 of the ICRC's customary international humanitarian law study, which safeguards accounting efforts for missing persons: "Each party to the conflict must take all feasible measures to account for persons reported missing as a result of armed conflict and must provide their family members with any information it has on their fate" (Henckaerts and Doswald-Beck 2005, rule 117).

The point to note here is that while States and relevant state authorities cannot guarantee that a missing person will be found or indeed be reunited with their family, they are obliged to put measures and efforts in place to do so. This equates to the duty to conduct an effective investigation. Therefore, in addition to seeking to prevent persons from disappearing, UN Human Rights Committee General Comment 6 stipulates that "States should establish effective facilities and procedures to investigate thoroughly cases of missing and disappeared persons in circumstances, which may involve a violation of the right to life" (UNHRC 1982, p. 4).

Moreover, as clarified by the UN Human Rights Committee in its General Comment 31, the general duties arising for states are far-reaching:

> States Parties are required [. . .] to respect and to ensure the Covenant rights to all persons who may be within their territory and to all persons subject to their jurisdiction. This means that a State party must respect and ensure the rights laid

> down in the Covenant to anyone within the power or effective control of that State Party, even if not situated within the territory of the State Party. [. . .] [T]he enjoyment of Covenant rights is not limited to citizens of States Parties but must also be available to all individuals, regardless of nationality or statelessness, such as asylum seekers, refugees, migrant workers and other persons, who may find themselves in the territory or subject to the jurisdiction of the State Party. This principle also applies to those within the power or effective control of the forces of a State Party acting outside its territory, regardless of the circumstances in which such power or effective control was obtained, such as forces constituting a national contingent of a State Party assigned to an international peace-keeping or peace-enforcement operation (UNHRC 2014, para. 10).

This long quotation neatly connects the discussion of law with the rationales for persons going missing in the previous section: for state duties as part of international human rights law clearly extend to situations of disaster, conflict-related peace-keeping operations, migration, and refugees.

11.3.2 Mass graves and international norms

For mass graves, as for missing persons, an equally compelling case can be made for comprehensive protection. While the context, significance, and impact of any given mass grave may differ from place to place, individual to individual, and community to community, the need to know the fate and whereabouts of loved ones and to have mortal remains returned for dignified commemoration is seemingly universal.

Mass graves contain evidence that is essential to the realization of justice and accountability goals at multiple levels: for victims, affected communities, states in transition, and the international community. In addition to the compelling needs to protect missing persons and their human remains, the evidential content makes mass graves vulnerable to disturbance, destruction, or relocation, where abusive States and/or perpetrator groups seek to evade legal responsibility and scrutiny for their actions. According to Van Schaack, "[m]ass graves are particularly vulnerable to destruction as they provide strong evidence of crimes against humanity and other international crimes" (2019, p. 2). Such disturbance and destruction can present problems for investigators, including significant contamination of evidence and commingling of body parts.

The practice of mass grave disturbance or destruction, including the relocation of bodies to secondary and tertiary sites as a means of avoiding detection, is evidenced in Srebrenica, amply documented in the judgment of, for example, the case *Prosecutor v Karadžić* (2016) before the International Criminal Tribunal for the Former Yugoslavia. Such attempts by perpetrators to conceal their crimes seem worryingly prevalent, with forensic experts noting that "[i]n our experience working on mass graves in the Balkans, Guatemala, and Iraq disturbance is a common occurrence as perpetrators hide and destroy evidence" (Wright and Hanson 2016, p. 608).

For families of the missing – who need to know the fate and whereabouts of loved ones and to receive mortal remains for burial and dignified commemoration – the effects of this can be devastating: many are confronted with the prospect that a body will never be found, or they receive incomplete remains for reburial. The protection of mass grave sites is therefore essential to the achievement of State responsibility, perpetrator accountability, and the return of human remains, and it is guaranteed by international law.

The Bournemouth Protocol on Mass Grave Protection and Investigation brings international legal norms together in a unifying way from which then guidelines for practice are deduced. Fundamentally, the Protocol reflects human rights standards in an inclusive way to ensure the families' needs (of those that might be in mass graves) are met. The Protocol, derived from a collaborative research project with the participation of experts from across the globe (Klinkner and Smith 2021a), is anchored in international law to help meet those needs because it proffers a unifying legal approach to mass grave protection and investigation by bringing together the branches of international human rights law, international humanitarian law as well as international criminal law. Reference is also made to disaster victim identification efforts and disaster management efforts.

The rights of individuals and corresponding duties of a State may be numerous in relation to mass graves. They are mostly congruent with those discussed above in relation to missing persons (the right to life; the right to be free from torture and inhumane treatment). The guarantor or duty bearer is the State with its obligation to protect, and in case of breaches, investigate, search, and identify.

Reflecting the complex nature of mass graves and the careful coordination of multiple needs and stakeholders, the Protocol follows seven chronological stages of the mass grave investigation: first discovery of the site and the availability of safe reporting procedures; the challenges of site access (including where land is privately owned); issues that relate to the protection of the site – both physically and digitally; the investigation of the site, including overall and operational responsibility, potential team composition and communication channels for both victims' families and the media; the forensic identification of human remains; the collection and use of evidence from the mass grave at trial; the return of remains and artifacts to family members; additional avenues of justice for families; to aspects of commemoration and memorialization. Through this approach, each aspect of mass graves, from their discovery to their commemoration as final resting places, is situated not only in the law but also in the bigger picture of multiple, potentially divergent, victims' needs, legal considerations, and practical challenges.

11.3.2.1 The investigative duty

As outlined in relation to missing persons, central to protection measures and investigation is the duty of the state, for investigations are contingent on the preservation of the various lines of inquiries. With reference to the case of Da Silva (before the European Court of Human Rights, regarding an investigation into a police shooting) what does an effective investigation entail?

As a precondition, those in charge of and carrying out the investigation have to be independent, since independence is critical for the public's confidence in the investigation as such (Da Silva 2016, para. 232). Further, an investigation must be "capable of leading to the establishment of the fact" (ibid., para 233); this includes the circumstance that led to the violation and the identification of those responsible as well as, where appropriate, punitive action. To achieve this, the gathering and securing of evidence (involving eyewitness testimony and forensic examinations) is necessary. This is particularly relevant in relation to establishing the cause of death. In fact: "any deficiency in the investigation which undermines its ability to establish the cause of death or the person responsible will risk falling foul of this standard" (ibid., para. 233). That said, the effective investigation is an obligation of means and best effort given the contextual parameters; it is not an obligation of result (ibid., para. 233). Any conclusion from the investigation must be "based on thorough, objective and impartial analysis of all relevant elements" (ibid., para. 234). This is significant because it means that multiple lines of inquiry may need to be pursued. In addition, to ensure the legitimate interest of relatives is safeguarded, there is a requirement to make the investigation accessible to the victim's family (ibid., para. 235). That said, the public disclosure of results and access may however be limited if sensitive or security concerns are attached to their release (ibid., para. 236; for more discussion see Klinkner and Smith 2021a).

But international norms also express requirements in response to the needs arising in relation to the human remains. Some form part of an investigation, others extend beyond but are natural extensions to an effective investigation, as explained in the following.

11.3.2.2 Identification

Once a mass grave is found and an investigation commences, the expectations within the survivor community that human remains are identified and returned are heightened. This is not without controversy, for individuation may not always be possible. However, the International Convention on the Protection of all Persons from Enforced Disappearance stipulates that,

> State Parties shall co-operate with one another and shall afford one another the greatest measure of mutual assistance with a view to assisting victims of enforced

> disappearance, and in searching for, locating and releasing disappeared persons and, in the event of death, in exhuming and identifying them and returning their remains (Article 15).

The requirement to return, wherever possible, human remains to family members is reiterated in Article 24(3) of the Convention and this, of course, then necessitates the relevant storage and identification infrastructure is put in place. The value of DNA analysis as a primary means of identification is recognized in the Minnesota Protocol (Office of the United Nations High Commissioner for Human Rights 2017) or Interpol's Disaster Victim Identification (2018), and Interpol's I-Familia (2021) global database of family DNA held or received by law enforcement agencies and expressed in the UNSC Resolution 2474 (2019) on missing persons, the ICMP Paris Principles (2019, Principle 6) and also domestically, a recent example is Ukraine's Law on the Missing (2019, Articles 21 and 22). Clear provisions for identification and corresponding practice therefore exist.

11.3.2.3 Return of human remains

Efforts to ascertain the identity of the deceased then lead onto the return of human remains. As already mentioned, Article 24(3) of the International Convention on the Protection of all Persons from Enforced Disappearance specifies the return of human remains to the surviving family members. The 2019 Guiding Principles that have been issued in relation to the search for the disappeared expand on this provision by stating that the "return [of human remains] should also involve the means and procedures needed to ensure a dignified burial consistent with the wishes and cultural customs of the families and their communities" (Principle 2(4)). This signifies the connection between the return of remains with the rights of the family to commemoration. In the *Pueblo Bello Massacre v Colombia* case (a case concerning the abduction, killing, and forced disappearance of 37 farmers) the Inter-American Court of Human Rights expressed this by placing further obligations on the state. "When the mortal remains are found and identified, the State must return them to their next of kin as soon as possible, after having proved the relationship genetically, so that they can be honored according to their respective creeds. The State must also cover the burial expenses, in agreement with the next of kin" (2006, para. 273). Here the Inter-American Court points to family relations as genetically proven to safeguard the right to family and private life, for non-return of human remains and burial in an unspecified location would constitute a breach. What exactly constitutes a family for the purposes of missing persons and more broadly in international law remains undefined; family is a concept that relates to societal practice in a specific context. But as espoused by the Inter-American Court, family membership is significant for determining the next of kin as appropriate recipient of mortal remains and issuance of legal status documentation in respect of a missing person (Klinkner and Smith 2020, 2021a; La Vaccara 2019).

11.3.2.4 Pursuit of justice

The purpose of an investigation is not only to reveal the facts; it also forms part of the pursuit of justice. And justice here can mean a number of (overlapping) things: the provision and receipt of information is written large into what is known as "the right to the truth," which encompasses the need of families and societies to know what happened not only to the individual missing persons, but also the broader events that facilitated this. For many, understanding what happens is therefore also an achievement of justice. Moreover, it is seen as a measure to enhance respect for the rule and precondition for a just society when the results of any investigation are authoritatively reported.

Ascertaining the facts through an authoritative investigation can also facilitate access to remedies which can take the form of compensation; restitution; rehabilitation; satisfaction (including the verification of facts and/ or search, recovery, identification, and burial), and lastly guarantees of non-repetition. These remedies have found expression in the Basic Principles and Guidelines on the Right to a Remedy and Reparation for Victims of Gross Violations of International Human Rights Law and Serious Violations of International Humanitarian Law, Principles 19–23 (UNGA 2006) and are pertinent to the subject of mass graves.

Of course, justice is often understood as retributive justice and investigations may reveal not only the commission of violations but also the perpetrators, which can lead to criminal proceedings or, where relevant, extraditions. Many international crimes, such as genocide (Article 5 of the Genocide Convention), torture (United Nations Convention against Torture Articles 2), and enforced disappearances (International Convention for the Protection of All Persons from Disappearance Article 6), but also grave breaches of the Geneva Conventions (Geneva Convention I Article 49; Geneva Convention II Article 50; Geneva Convention III Article 129; Geneva Convention IV Article 146), are prohibited by treaty which means that State Parties are required to enact domestic legislation to provide effective penalties where abuses occur.

What is really important to note here is the recent stipulation in the 2019 Guiding Principles for the search for disappeared persons (UNCED 2019) specifying that "the search for the disappeared person and the criminal investigation of the persons responsible for the disappearance should be mutually reinforcing" (UNCED 2019, Principle 13(1). In other words, what is commonly known as the "humanitarian approach" to identifying and returning missing persons and investigations for criminal purposes should work together and in tandem. The standard of investigation should be able to serve evidential standards required for authoritative identification and the pursuit of further justice avenues.

11.3.2.5 Commemoration

Finally, following investigations, both the original mass grave and any potential new burial and commemoration site may be deserving of protection, as this would be covered through the right to private and family life. The right to freedom of thought, conscience, and religion is also relevant, since the manner of burying the dead can form an essential aspect of religious practice as protected under freedom of thought, conscience, and religion.

Therefore, an excavated mass grave may become a memorial site in its own right, deserving that recognition and potentially long-term legal protection. Conversely, a newly created burial site or place for commemoration will hold great significance for individual and/ or collective commemoration (UNCHR 2005, "Orentlicher Principles," Principle 3) and may also constitute a form of reparation or perhaps symbolize a commitment to non-repetition. Mass graves are a stark reminder of recent history and memory; they may form part of educational materials and national discourse on the past; they may also become a site for community support.

11.4 Practicalities of protection

It is important to stress that the consequences of not protecting and investigating mass graves are significant. Relatives continue to suffer because they do not know what happened to their loved ones, and evidence essential to identification, documentation, and where relevant, prosecution efforts may be contaminated, disturbed, or lost. The careful, considerate, culturally appropriate yet legally compliant, and scientifically robust protection and investigation of mass graves are therefore paramount. How might it be achieved in practice?

As acknowledged in the UN Security Council Resolution 2747, through scientific and technological progress, the investigative processes and successful identification of missing persons have been increased, particularly highlighting "forensic sciences, DNA analysis, satellite maps and imagery, and ground penetrating radar" (UNSC 2019, p. 2). The process of mass grave protection may start with the reporting and recording of sites through geomatics to assist with the collection, storage, analysis, processing, and presentation of geographic data leading to investigations that are multifaceted, lengthy, and expensive processes, requiring significant planning, coordination, resources, official authorization, and political will.

What appears to be absolutely crucial in mass grave protection and investigation efforts is the multidisciplinary approach required, involving much forensic, medico-legal, investigative, and liaison expertise. This in turn highlights the importance of a coordinating role to facilitate this coherent, considered, culturally appropriate, legally compliant, and scientifically robust process. In the *Bournemouth Protocol*, this has found expression through the role of the mass fatality manager who "assumes overall responsibility for the operational management of mass graves including, but not limited to, adherence to jurisdictional agreements and Standard Operating Procedures; maintenance of community liaison, health, safety and well-being on-site; implementation of reporting structures and communication strategy; and co-ordination of the identification and return of human remains process" (Klinkner and Smith 2020, p. 18).

Mass grave protection and investigation will hold inevitable pressures of a highly charged emotional context and expectations have to be carefully managed with the overall investigation process well planned: in fact, meticulous planning, particularly in relation to the actual excavation, is critical for all subsequent phases of the process, including identification efforts, return of human remains, and continued community liaison.

What's more, and immediately discernible though by no means trivial, are overarching considerations that should be afforded to mass grave protection and investigation process and the context in which they are situated, because these overarching principles will impact the practice of all actors and experts alike.

Adopting a *do no harm approach* will actively seek to avoid undermining existing structures and relationships that are essential for community cohesion. It is important to avoid creating inequalities or perceptions of bias or to entrench existing inequalities. It will include clear respect for and, where possible, adherence to cultural sensitivities, beliefs, and norms of victims, and their families to the extent they do not adversely affect the achievement of an effective investigation.

The *physical and emotional safety* of all involved, the relatives and the investigation team alike, are paramount. In the context of mass graves, the safety, dignity, privacy, and well-being of victims and their families should be a key concern for all actors without distinction. This, of course, is also codified in law as rights attached to the families as secondary victims.

That an investigation should be *independent and impartial* is a rather obvious point to make. And yet, since the investigation may relate to an era of (armed) conflict, systematic state-instigated discrimination, or state-sanctioned human rights abuse, it is poignant and relevant: without a non-discriminatory and impartial approach to the mass grave protection and investigation process, the legitimacy of the work may be questioned by the affected community. To enhance public trust, investigations must be independent and impartial and must be seen to be so.

For mass grave investigations to result in identification, it will be critical to acquire personal details and other identifying data, and *confidentiality*, consistent with national legislation, has to be assured. Investigative processes often entail the need for data sharing, but any data sharing should be limited only to those individuals and bodies necessary to ensure the achievement of the objectives of the exhumation process and to the extent agreed by the individual(s) concerned.

Similarly, at all stages of the process (the preliminary investigation, the actual excavation, identification, and return of human remains), *transparency* of processes is key. Clear and ongoing communication will help provide the platform for transparency.

Communication strategies should ideally envisage and accommodate a two-way flow of information between the investigative team and the families, and incorporate regular updates. Finally, all parties involved in the protection and investigation of the mass grave should avoid making commitments to families that they may be unable to keep. This last point links back to the need for an overall coordinating role of the mass fatality manager to ensure that expectations are clearly understood and managed by all involved.

11.5 Protection on a global scale

All of the above may lead to two core deductions: firstly, that there is a substantial body of international norms governing missing persons broadly and mass graves specifically and secondly, that a good deal of legally informed and, with it, victim-aware practice can be gleaned. That assessment is certainly not unreasonable, but the question posed here is: is it comprehensive enough? And it has to be acknowledged that more can be done.

For one, the various spheres of international law and which applies when, can be highly confusing for relatives whose urgent need is to find their loved ones. With the concretization of disaster relief law and a transition of the global compact on migration from soft law toward hard law, more branches of international are likely to be integrated into the existing fabric of rights and obligations. Further, and discussed in the literature, is that a dual approach "humanitarian" *versus* "criminal" is unhelpful, hence the need for universal standards and processes that stand-up to authoritative scrutiny (Tuller and Salado Puerto 2017; Klinkner Smith 2022:forthcoming). Those rather broad-brush concerns aside, there are some more concrete mass grave-specific areas deserving of further attention, presenting an important program of future work and an agenda the Bournemouth mass grave research team is pursuing.

11.5.1 Mapping as a form of protection?

The practicalities surrounding protection and investigation as highlighted are predicated on locating, subsequently protecting, and wherever possible, investigating graves. This is also true of missing persons cases; reporting them is often the first step in solving missing persons cases. But reliable data on missing persons can be difficult to ascertain. The same can be said of mass graves. While we know that mass graves are a global phenomenon, the exact extent of the problem somewhat remains unclear, spurring the then UN Special Rapporteur to urge for mass graves to be "subject to a regularized process of international mapping and recognition" (UNGA 2020, para. 72).

At present, there is no such system of global record keeping of the number of mass graves, nor of the victims in them. Where mapping exists, it has arisen on an *ad hoc* basis to respond to specific contexts and/ or investigations. Moreover, there is presently no guidance available to those engaged in the mapping process to indicate whether and under what circumstances mass grave sites should be recorded and whether this would lend itself to open-source mapping. This gap is leading to a new agenda for research currently underway with the authors of the Bournemouth Protocol exploring the benefits and risks of regularized mapping.

The mapping of mass grave sites may have potential as a form of protection (in and of itself, as well as comprising a precondition for the application of additional forms of protection, such as physical measures). Mapping can also provide educational resources and victim-centered avenues of remembrance and commemoration. Open-source mapping is employed in a number of human rights contexts as a protection and justice-monitoring measure: mapping tools, such as the Environmental Justice Atlas (2021), Airwars (2021), Armed Conflict Location and Event Data Project (2021), and the already mentioned Missing Migrants Project (IOM 2021) have been developed to serve a number of purposes, including to support State accountability efforts, as a form of deterrence, and to provide foundational evidence for legal investigation at a later stage (Martinez-Alier 2021). The various mapping projects seek to address pressing societal challenges, and increasingly, Principles and Guidelines for the good provenance and governance of digital documentation efforts in other human rights contexts are starting to emerge (AAAS 2019).

But, critically and worryingly, the question of the probity of open-source mapping is far from clear and has not been considered. There may be good reasons to keep the location of graves secret in order to protect not only the grave sites themselves but also any informants, witnesses, and investigators, and when formal acknowledgment of a site might prove beneficial for the investigative process.

11.5.2 Understanding the ramifications of existing rights

Inequalities persist (sometimes intergenerationally) in death and have (though not in the context of mass graves, but rather in relation to African America burial grounds) been eloquently labeled "apartheid of the departed" (Lepore 2021, online). When working on the *Bournemouth Protocol* three, arguably interlinked, human rights blind spots in the existing international human rights framework emerged.

The cultural and Indigenous rights surrounding mass graves, while acknowledged, are not necessarily fully understood and warrant attention, particularly where, like in the Canadian example, a policy persisted that sought to systematically assimilate Indigenous children thereby destroying cultures, languages, and possible ties with the land. An Indigenous approach to mass graves may also need to offer legal protection extending to the material artifacts in these graves as they may be important, like human bodily remains, in relation to ancestors as well as may be ancestors themselves; equally the way information is stored or displayed may need consideration. In addition, First Nation, Indigenous, or Aboriginal community borders will not always align with country borders therefore potentially attracting differing protection levels domestically. Similarly, investigations and their outcome are affected by their context of social and religious norms (A. Alberda, personal communication).[1] When investigating in Afghanistan to establish the number of civilians killed in an attack, "[i]t was not possible to clarify this matter further as the social and religious mores of the Afghan population prevented use of the modern forensic investigation techniques, including the exhumation of bodies or DNA analyses, that would be required" (Hanan v Germany 2021, para. 4).

Concerns surrounding the protection of information and individuals' data, particularly as new technologies for identification emerge, are also likely to persist. Emerging technologies require explication in terms of the type of information, for example, new DNA technology reveals, including how that might render itself to exploitation beyond the main identification purpose. The cross-border transfer of this information, its vulnerabilities, third-party involvement, data sharing, and disposition are all areas for continued review, and while this may generally be subject to discussion (Interpol 2021 [I-familia]; Barnert et al. 2021) clearer links to mass grave investigations would be beneficial.

Participatory rights of families are the final point to highlight. While participatory rights are featuring more prominently in international law, their explicit link to mass graves, investigations, and commemoration efforts is ripe for further research and coloratura. The safety of family members participating in the investigation may place some confidentiality requirements and limiting of reporting and data. Conversely, participation during investigations can reveal relevant lines of inquiry. At the same time, participatory rights of the next of kin may not be available to all, leading families of missing persons to proactively engage in search efforts on their own accord and by joining non-governmental organizations (NGOs) that assist with scientific, investigative work, such as forensic groups (Schwartz-Martin and Cruz-Santiago 2016). A growing body of literature on digital evidence and documentation technology for human rights fact-finding efforts has emerged to safeguard the probative value of such efforts before a court of law (UN Human Rights Office of the High Commissioner/ Human Rights Center Berkeley 2020). But the question here is how can the structural divide between a rule of law based, authoritative, independent investigative approach with participatory rights, and the "citizen-forensics" approach be effectively closed.

These are research questions that will help tighten the human rights' framework for better protection and investigation efforts.

11.6 Conclusion: the need to do better

Without doubt, the families of the missing in mass graves, regardless of the reasons for their relative's missingness, are often left in a precarious legal situation. This chapter has sought to lay out the legal framework for the protection of missing persons and corresponding graves. By drawing on the various branches of international law (international human rights law, international humanitarian law, and international criminal law) a tapestry of rights and obligations exist for the protection of missing persons. Central to the quest to solve missing persons cases is the duty to conduct an effective investigation; a duty placed on states. This legal framework can and has been translated into practical guidance for the physical protection of mass graves from their discovery through to commemorative efforts.

Crucial to the successful protection and investigation are multidisciplinary teams that are clearly and consciously directed to facilitate the much-needed victim and community awareness, legal framework, and scientific standard-compliant processes.

Beyond this existing "state of the art" in law and practice, the chapter has probed further to sketch the author's vision of research findings to come. It is important to continually review our handling of mass graves with the aim to ease the struggle of survivors. It is therefore apt to end with an account of Hasan Nuhanović, as someone who has experienced family members going missing and for them to be found and identified many years later: "I've had to fight so long and so hard just to find out what happened, who was responsible, even to establish the Memorial Centre where they are buried. Even after 23 years, our story is still not finished" (Remembering Srebrenica 2021, online).

Note

1. I am immensely grateful for the input of my colleague Dr Alexandra Alberda on this subject (personal communication with Dr Alexandra Alberda, Curator of Indigenous Perspectives, Manchester Museum, March 29, 2021).

References

Additional Protocol I to the Geneva Conventions of August 12, 1949 (adopted June 8, 1977, entered into force December 7, 1979).

African Union (2009). *African Union Convention for the Protection and Assistance of Internally Displaced Persons in Africa ('Kampala Convention')*: the Kampala Convention.

Airwars (2021) https://airwars.org/ (accessed 11 October 2021).

Armed Conflict Location and Event Data Project (2021) https://acleddata.com (accessed 11 October 2021).

Barnert, E., et al. (2021). Using DNA to reunify separated migrant families. *Science* **372**(6547): 1154–1156. doi: 10.1126/science.abh3979.

Convention on the Prevention and Punishment of the Crime of Genocide (adopted December 9, 1948, entered into force January 12, 1951) 78 UNTS 277.

Convention on the Rights of the Child (adopted November 20, 1989, entered into force September 2, 1990) 1577 UNTS 3.

Council of Europe (1950) European Convention for the Protection of Human Rights and Fundamental Freedoms, as amended by Protocols Nos. 11 and 14 (adopted November 4, 1950, entered into force September 3, 1953) ETS 5.

Council of Europe (2016) Missing persons and victims of enforced disappearance in Europe-issue paper. https://rm.coe.int/missing-persons-and-victims-of-enforced-disappearance-in-europe-issue-/16806daa1c (accessed 11 October 2021).

Cruz-Santiago, A. (2021). America. In: *Global Report on Missing Persons 2021* (ed. A. Kleiser), 66–83. The Hague: ICMP.

Da Silva v. United Kingdom (2016) Grand Chamber Judgment, ECtHR Application No. 5878/08 (March 30, 2016).

De Léon, J. (2015). *The Land of Open Graves. Living and Dying on the Migrant Trail*. Oakland, CA: University of California Press.

Decker, A. (2021). Africa. In: *Global Report on Missing Persons 2021* (ed. A. Kleiser), 33–48. The Hague: ICMP.

Dulitzky, A. (2019). The Latin-American flavour of enforced disappearances. *Chicago Journal of International Law* **19**(2): 423–486.

EJAtlas (2021) EJAtlas – Global Atlas of Environmental Justice. https://ejatlas.org/ (accessed 11 October 2021).

Geneva Convention (I) for the Amelioration of the Condition of the Wounded and Sick in Armed Forces in the Field (adopted August 12, 1949) 75 UNTS 31.

Geneva Convention (II) for the Amelioration of the Condition of Wounded, Sick and Shipwrecked Members of Armed Forces at Sea (adopted August 12, 1949) 75 UNTS 85.

Geneva Convention (III) relative to the Treatment of Prisoners of War (August 12, 1949) 75 UNTS 135.

Geneva Convention (IV) relative to the Protection of Civilian Persons in Time of War (adopted August 12, 1949) 75 UNTS 288.

Grant, S. (2016) Dead and missing migrants: the obligations of European States under International Human Rights Law. Report. http://iosifkovras.com/wp-content/uploads/2015/08/Legal-Memo-on-Missing-Migrants.pdf (accessed 11 October 2021).

Guatemala Commission of Historical Clarification (2013) Memory of Silence, Report – Conclusion and Recommendations. https://hrdag.org/wp-content/uploads/2013/01/CEHreport-english.pdf (accessed 11 October 2021).

Hamadeh, N. (2021). Middle East and North Africa. In: *Global Report on Missing Persons 2021* (ed. A. Kleiser), 16–32. The Hague: ICMP.
Hanan v. Germany (2021) Grand Chamber Judgment, ECtHR Application No. 4871/16 (February 16, 2021).
Henckaerts, J.-M. and Doswald-Beck, L. (2005). *Customary International Humanitarian Law, Vol. 1: Rules*. Cambridge/Geneva: Cambridge University Press.
Honderich, H. (2021) Why Canada is mourning the deaths of hundreds of children. BBC News (15 July) online. https://www.bbc.co.uk/news/world-us-canada-57325653 (accessed 11 October 2021).
International Commission on Missing (ICMP) (2019) The ICMP Paris Principles, Annotated Version. https://www.icmp.int/wp-content/uploads/2019/04/icmp-dg-1468-1-W-doc-paris-principles-annotated.pdf (accessed 11 October 2021).
International Commission on Missing Persons (ICMP) (2021) Srebrenica figures as of 1 July 2021. https://www.icmp.int/news/facts-and-figures-on-srebrenica/ (accessed 11 October 2021).
International Committee of the Red Cross (ICRC) (2009) Guiding principles/model law on the missing. https://www.icrc.org/en/document/guiding-principles-model-law-missing-model-law (accessed 11 October 2021).
International Committee of the Red Cross (ICRC) (2020) Accompanying the Families of Missing Persons-A Practical Handbook. https://www.icrc.org/en/publication/4110-accompanying-families-missing-persons-practical-handbook (accessed 11 October 2021).
International Convention for the Protection of All Persons from Enforced Disappearance (adopted January 12, 2007, entered into force December 23, 2010) UN Doc A/RES/61/177.
International Covenant on Civil and Political Rights (adopted December 19, 1966, entered into force March 23, 1976) 999 UNTS 171.
International Organisation for Migration (2021) Missing migrants project. https://missingmigrants.iom.int/ (accessed 11 October 2021).
Interpol (2018) Disaster victim identification guide. https://www.interpol.int/en/How-we-work/Forensics/Disaster-Victim-Identification-DVI (accessed 11 October 2021).
Interpol (2021) I-Familia. https://www.interpol.int/en/How-we-work/Forensics/I-Familia (accessed 11 October 2021).
Klinkner, M. and Smith, E. (2020) The Bournemouth protocol on mass grave protection and investigation. https://issuu.com/bournemouthuniversity/docs/the_bournemouth_protocol_on_mass_grave_protection_ (accessed 11 October 2021).
Klinkner, M. and Smith, E. (2021). From law to policy and practice – collaborative research amidst a pandemic: the creation of the Bournemouth Protocol on Mass Grave Protection and Investigation. *Journal of Legal Research Methodology* **1**(1): 26–49.
Klinkner, M. and Smith, E. (2021a) Academic commentary to the Bournemouth protocol on mass grave protection and investigation. https://issuu.com/bournemouthuniversity/docs/11070_fmc_mass_graves_protocol_academic_commentary (accessed 11 October 2021).
Klinkner, M. and Smith, E. (2022, forthcoming). *Mass Graves, Truth and Justice: Interdisciplinary Perspectives on the Investigation of Mass Graves*. Cheltenham: Edward Elgar.
La Vaccara, A. (2019). *When the Conflict Ends, While Uncertainty Continues: Accounting for Missing Persons between War and Peace in International Law*. Oxford: Pedone/Hart.
Laczko, F., et al. (eds.) (2019). *Missing Migrant Children*, Fatal Journeys, Vol. **4**. Geneva: IOM.

Lepore, J. (2021) When black history is unearthed who gets to speak for the dead? New Yorker (September 27, 2021, online) https://www.newyorker.com/magazine/2021/10/04/when-black-history-is-unearthed-who-gets-to-speak-for-the-dead (accessed 11 October 2021).

Martinez-Alier, J. (2021). Mapping ecological distribution conflicts: the EJAtlas. *The Extractive Industries and Society* **8**: 100883. doi: 10.1016/j.exis.2021.02.003.

McDonald-Gibson, C. (2021). Europe. In: *Global Report on Missing Persons 2021* (ed. A. Kleiser), 50–64. The Hague: ICMP.

No author (2017). Q&A: the ICRC's engagement on the missing and their families. *International Review of the Red Cross* **99**(2): 535–545.

Office of the United Nations High Commissioner for Human Rights (2017) The Minnesota Protocol on the Investigation of Potentially Unlawful Death. https://www.ohchr.org/Documents/Publications/MinnesotaProtocol.pdf (accessed 11 October 2021).

Office of the United Nations High Commissioner for Human Rights (2021) UN experts call on Canada, Holy See to investigate mass grave at indigenous school. Press release (June 4).

Office of the United Nations High Commissioner for Human Rights/Human Rights Center Berkely (2020) Berkeley protocol on digital open source investigations: a practical guide on the effective use of digital open source information in investigating violations of international criminal, human rights and humanitarian law. https://www.ohchr.org/Documents/Publications/OHCHR_BerkeleyProtocol.pdf (accessed 11 October 2021).

Perera, C. and Briggs, C. (2008). Guidelines for the effective conduct of mass burials following mass disasters: post-Asian Tsunami disaster experience in retrospect. *Forensic Science Medicine and Pathology* **4**(1): 1–8.

Prosecutor v Karadžić (2016) Public redacted version of Judgment issued on March 25, 2016, IT-95-5/18-T (March 25, 2016).

Pueblo Bello Massacre v Colombia (2006). Judgment on Merits, Reparations and Costs, Inter-American Court of Human Rights Series C No 140 (January 31, 2006).

Remembering Srebrenica (2021) The Courage to Speak Out: Hasan Nuhanović (June 8, 2018). https://srebrenica.org.uk/survivor-stories/the-courage-to-speak-out-hasan-nuhanovic (accessed 11 October 2021).

Republic of Rwanda-National Commission for the Fight against Genocide (2021) https://cnlg.gov.rw/index.php?id=12 (accessed 11 October 2021).

Rome Statute of the International Criminal Court (adopted July 17, 1998, entered into force on July 1, 2002) 2187 UNTS 3.

Rosenblatt, A. (2015). *Digging for the Disappeared*. Stanford, CA: Stanford University Press.

Schwartz-Marin, E. and Cruz-Santiago, A. (2016). Forensic civism: articulating science, DNA and kinship in contemporary Mexico and Colombia. *Human Remains & Violence* **2**(1): 58–74.

Shalev Greene, K. and Collie, C.J.R. (2021). *People Who Go Missing Abroad: An Examination of Patterns and Investigative Challenges*: International Crime Coordination Centre https://www.newswise.com/pdf_docs/163309295234815_Missing Abroad Report final.pdf.

Tae-Ung, B. (2021). Asia and Pacific. In: *Global Report on Missing Persons 2021* (ed. A. Kleiser), 84–98. The Hague: ICMP.

The American Association for the Advancement of Science (2019) Location-based data in crisis situations – principles and guidelines. https://www.aaas.org/sites/default/files/2019-04/VGI%20Principles%20and%20Guidelines_FINAL%20%28002%29.pdf (accessed 11 October 2021).

Tuller, H. and Salado Puerto, M. (2017). Large-scale forensic investigations into the missing: challenges and considerations. *Forensic Science International* **279**: 219–228.
UN Committee on Enforced Disappearances (2019) Guiding principles for the search for disappeared persons, UN Doc CED/C/7 (May 8, 2019).
UNAMI and OHCHR (2018) Unearthing atrocities: mass graves in territory formerly controlled by ISIL – Report (November 6, 2018). https://www.ohchr.org/Documents/Countries/IQ/UNAMI_Report_on_Mass_Graves4Nov2018_EN.pdf (accessed 11 October 2021).
UNCHR (2005) Report of the independent expert to update the set of principles to combat impunity (Orentlicher principles), February 18, 2005, UN Doc. E/CN.4/2005/102.
UNGA (2006) Basic principles and guidelines on the right to a remedy and reparation for victims of gross violations of international human rights law and serious violations of international humanitarian law (Resolution adopted on March 21, 2006) UN Doc A/RES/60/147.
UNGA (2020) Human rights standards and possible steps towards the respectful and lawful handling of mass graves (October 12, 2020) UN Doc A/75/384.
UNHRC (1982) CCPR General Comment No. 6: Article 6 (Right to Life) (April 30, 1982).
UNHRC (2014) CCPR general comment 31: the nature of the legal obligation imposed on states parties to the covenant (May 26, 2004).
UNSC (1994) Final Report of the United Nations Commission of Experts established pursuant to Security Council Resolution 780 (1992) Annex X Mass graves (December 28, 1994) UN Doc S/1994/674/Add/2 (Vol. V).
UNSC (2019) Resolution 2475 (June 11, 2019) UN Doc S/RES/2474.
Van Schaack, B. (2019). Innovations in international criminal law documentation methodologies and institutions. *SSRN Electronic Journal.* doi: 10.2139/ssrn.3329102.
Wright, R. and Hanson, I. (2016). Forensic archaeology under the auspices of large organizations. In: *Handbook of Forensic Anthropology and Archaeology* (eds. S. Blau and D. Ubelaker), 607–621. London: Routledge.
Yale University (2021) Cambodian genocide program. https://gsp.yale.edu/case-studies/cambodian-genocide-program (accessed 11 October 2021).

CHAPTER 12

Respect for the dead under international law and Islamic law in armed conflicts

Ahmed Al-Dawoody and Alexandra Ortiz Signoret

Legal Advisory Service on IHL, International Committee of the Red Cross (ICRC), Geneva, Switzerland

12.1 Introduction

Many civilizations and religions regard death as a transitional period, bridging one stage of life with another. Religions, traditions, and cultural practices have influenced throughout history the ways in which dead bodies are managed both in times of armed conflicts and in times of peace, and they continue to do so. Under Islamic law, as in many cultures and religions, management of dead bodies is the object of specific rules that aim at ensuring the dignity and respect of the dead as well as the feelings of loved ones who are still alive. Bearing in mind that almost two-thirds of armed conflicts are taking place now in Muslim contexts, this chapter discusses the respect for the dead under both international law, in particular international humanitarian law (IHL), and Islamic law. It mainly focuses on the context of armed conflicts in general and, in some cases, in the Muslim contexts in particular. It analyzes the main obligations under IHL and Islamic law of parties to armed conflicts regarding the protection of the dead such as the obligation to search for, collect, and evacuate the dead without adverse distinction; the identification and recording of the information regarding the dead; the respect for the dead and treating them with dignity; the disposal of the dead with respect; the respect for gravesites; and obligations related to the return of human remains and personal effects.

The chapter also addresses a number of challenges facing humanitarian forensics in Muslim contexts such as exhumations, quick burial, and autopsy. The main objectives of this chapter are twofold: first, to give an overview of IHL and

Anthropology of Violent Death: Theoretical Foundations for Forensic Humanitarian Action, First Edition. Edited by Roberto C. Parra and Douglas H. Ubelaker.

Islamic law positions on these specific obligations and challenges, and second, to provide some advice or insights into how forensic specialists can deal with these challenges.

12.2 The Legal Framework

Before delving into obligations and humanitarian challenges, we will give a brief background about the legal framework regulating the management of the dead in armed conflict. IHL, which applies in armed conflict situations and seeks, for humanitarian reasons, to limit the effects of armed conflict and to protect persons who are not or are no longer participating in the hostilities and to restrict the means and methods of warfare,[1] contains a number of rules regarding the management of the dead. Such rules are established in the Four Geneva Conventions of 1949 (GCs) and in their Additional Protocols of 1977 (API and APII) as well as in customary IHL rules.[2] IHL rules regarding the dead seek to ensure respect for basic humanitarian considerations toward the dead and their families.

International law contains additional rules relevant for the subject at hand, in particular from international human rights law (IHRL). International and regional human rights treaties very rarely expressly refer to respect for the dead or to their dignified treatment as in the traditional approach to IHRL; only subjects having a human quality possess human rights, and such human quality ends with death.[3] Only the 2006 International Convention for the Protection of All Persons from Enforced Disappearance (ICPPED) contains some specific provisions regarding the management of the dead in cases of alleged or suspected enforced disappearance.[4] The guiding principles for the search for disappeared persons adopted by the Committee on Enforced Disappearances (CED) in April 2019, as a soft-law instrument, also has some references in this respect.[5] Universal and regional human rights law treaties are also relevant as UN Treaty Bodies and regional courts have determined that States must fulfill some obligations vis-à-vis the treatment of the dead in order to respect rights such as the right to private and family life, the right to an effective remedy, and the prohibition against cruel, inhuman, or degrading treatment, especially toward the surviving relatives.[6]

International criminal law (ICL), which defines the crimes that entail international criminal responsibility for individuals who have committed, ordered, or assisted in the commission of such crimes, also contains some relevant rules regarding the treatment of the dead.[7]

Several international and regional resolutions refer to the management of the dead in armed conflicts. For example, since 2003, every two years, the United

Nations General Assembly (UNGA) has adopted the resolution "Missing Persons," which, for instance, calls upon States that are parties to an armed conflict to provide families of missing persons with all relevant information that they have on their fate and whereabouts or, if they are dead, the circumstances and cause of their death.[8] The United Nations Security Council (UNSC) adopted in 2019 the first-ever resolution on missing persons in armed conflicts, which also refers to the dead and "[u]rges parties to armed conflict to search for and recover the dead as a result of armed conflict, identify them, including by recording all available information and mapping the location of burial sites, to respect the remains of the dead, including by respecting and properly maintaining their graves, and to return them, whenever possible, to their relatives, consistent with applicable obligations under international humanitarian law and human rights law."[9] At the regional level, for instance, the General Assembly of the Organization of American States (OAS) refers to the dead in its biennial resolution entitled "Promotion and protection of Human Rights."[10]

Finally, this chapter shows that Islamic law, a legal system that emerged in the seventh century and is one of the three major legal systems practiced today, covers most of the questions and addresses most of the humanitarian challenges discussed in this chapter. The Islamic rules regulating the management of the dead in the context of armed conflict are based mainly on the precedents set in the earliest Islamic battle of Badr in March 624 and Uḥud in March 625. These precedents set by the Prophet Muhammad constitute a part of the Sunnah (tradition), the second source of the primary sources of Islamic law. Additionally, Muslim jurists have developed Islamic legal rulings and fatwas (non-binding legal opinions) regulating new cases that have confronted them throughout Islamic history. It is important to note that fatwas are not binding judgments and that it is left to the Muslim individuals or the Islamic courts to abide by a given fatwa or not. This is of course in addition to the modern national legislations based on Islamic law. IHL and Islamic law provide rules that aim at maintaining respect for the dead in armed conflict. The comparative approach between these legal systems used below shows that Islamic law can be invoked to influence the behavior of parties to armed conflict in a manner that will enhance respect for the dead in Muslim contexts.

12.3 Search for, Collect, and Evacuate the Dead without Adverse Distinction

Under IHL, both in international armed conflicts (IACs) and in non-international armed conflicts (NIACs), "[w]henever circumstances permit, and particularly after an engagement, each party to an armed conflict must, without delay, take all possible measures to search for, collect and evacuate the dead without adverse distinction."[11] Fulfilling this obligation is a precondition to comply with other obligations vis-à-vis the dead related to their identification, decent burial, and return to their home country or to their families.[12] It is also one of the first steps to prevent people from going missing.[13] This is an obligation of means as in some circumstances, it might be extremely difficult to collect the dead.[14] It includes allowing humanitarian organizations to perform this task, and the civilian population can be asked to provide support.[15] Parties to the armed conflict shall endeavor to conclude agreements on arrangements for teams to search for and collect the dead from the battlefield areas.[16] This rule applies to all the dead in connection with the armed conflict regardless of which party they belong to and regardless of whether or not they have taken a direct part in hostilities.[17] National practice also supports this view.[18] For instance, Cameroon's Instructor's Manual states that military commanders must ensure that the dead are searched for and evacuated.[19] In the same vein, Chad's Instructor's Manual states that "the parties to the conflict must take the measures needed to trace and collect the dead."[20]

Under IHRL, in cases of alleged or suspected enforced disappearance, States parties to the ICPPED have to search for disappeared persons and, in the event of death, to locate and return their remains and to cooperate with each other to this end as well as to exhume, identify, and return their remains.[21] Although no express mention is made to the collection of the dead, this obligation is implied as it constitutes a prerequisite to the fulfillment of other obligations such as the obligation to return the remains.[22] The *Guiding Principles for the Search for Disappeared Persons* indicate that the search should respect the right to participation of "victims, their legal representatives, counsel or any person authorized by them, and any person, association, or organization with a legitimate interest have the right to take part in the search" and that such right "should be protected and guaranteed at all stages of the search process."[23] This principle regarding the search under IHRL is very important as increasingly, families of disappeared persons seek to be involved actively in the search.

Early Islamic sources reflect a longstanding practice of parties to conflict accounting for dead bodies, sometimes in great detail. Ḥadīth (reported sayings, deeds, and tacit approvals of Prophet Muhammad) collection and *Sīrah* (biographies of Prophet Muhammad) literature indicate that during the Prophet's lifetime on the battlefield, women provided among other things the humanitarian acts and services given by health care personnel and aid societies in contemporary armed conflicts. Apart from the fact – which is documented in many reports – that some women fought in the battlefield at that time, their roles mainly included, as explained by Nusaybah, daughter of al-Ḥārith al-Anṣariyyah – a Ḥadīth narrator and a jurist known by her nickname as Umm 'Aṭiyyah, (d. 643) – treating the injured, looking after the sick, preparing food,[24] and, in the words of al-Rubī', daughter of Mi'wwidh bin 'Afrā' (d. 665), "repatriating the injured and dead bodies back to al-Madinah."[25]

The quotation of the words of al-Rubī' showing that women took part in the evacuation of the mortal remains of Muslim bodies and the documentation of fatalities in every military engagement, particularly in the *Sīrah*, makes an important point. It shows that the search for and collection of dead bodies are essential actions that must be taken to ensure respect for the dignity of human bodies and to inform the families about the death of their loved ones. For example, after the cessation of hostilities in the battle of Uḥud, Prophet Muhammad asked his companions to search for Sa'd ibn al-Rabī' (d. 625) to find out if he is among the fatalities or if he is still alive. In the same battle, Prophet Muhammad searched for the body of his uncle Ḥamzah (d. 625) after the cessation of fighting.[26] The search for and collection of the dead during the Prophet's lifetime is documented in the available *Sīrah* literature because, first, it was much easier during this period compared to later periods in Islamic history since the size of the Muslim army and consequently its fatalities and casualties at the time were much smaller. Second, historians wanted to document everything that was reported about the life of the Prophet. The significance of documenting the Prophet's sayings, actions, and tacit approvals, which all constitute the Sunnah (tradition) of the Prophet, is that it acts as the second source of Islamic legislation after the Qur'ān.

For both Muslim and non-Muslim enemies, there is a duty to collect and bury dead bodies of the adverse party, and returning dead bodies of the adverse party finds precedence in early Islamic history (see Ibn Isḥāq 2000, vol. 3, p. 123 f.; Guillaume 1955, pp. 450–460; Ibn 'Alī ibn Ḥajar al-'Asqalānī n.d., vol. 6, p. 283; ḥadīth number 1715 in Ibn 'Isā al-Tirmidhī n.d., vol. 4, p. 214; Abū al-Wafā 2006, p. 297). If, for any reason, the adverse party does not bury its dead, then it becomes the obligation of the Muslims to do so. The Andalusian jurist Ibn Ḥazm (d. 1064) justifies this obligation by arguing that if Muslims do not bury the dead bodies of their enemy in this case, the bodies will decompose or will be eaten by beasts or birds, which will be tantamount to mutilation, prohibited under Islamic law (Ibn Ḥazm, above note 3, vol. 5, p. 117). Ḥadīth collections and *Sīrah* literature show that Muslims buried the dead bodies of their enemy in the battle of Badr in March 624 in a collective grave in a place known as al-Qalīb and in other places until there was not a single dead body left unburied (see ḥadīth number 26404 in Ibn Ḥanbal, above note 3, vol. 6, p. 276; Ibn Jarīr al-Ṭabarī, n.d., vol. 2, p. 37; Al-Zuḥaylī, above note 6, vol. 7, p. 445 f.; Ibn Muḥammad ibn Ḥabīb al-Māwardī 1985, vol. 1, p. 57; 'A. Ibn Ḥazm, above note 3, vol. 1, p. 124). Moreover, Ya'lā ibn Murrah reported: "I travelled with the Prophet (peace be upon him) on more than one occasion, and I did not see him leave a human corpse behind; whenever he came across one, he ordered its burial, without asking whether the person was a Muslim or an unbeliever" ('Ibn 'Umar Al-Dāraqutnī 2004, vol. 5, p. 204).

12.4 Identification and Recording of Information on the Dead

In IACs and NIACs, under IHL, parties to the conflict must record all available information prior to their disposal and mark the location of the graves, with a view to identifying and accounting for the dead.[27] This obligation is not only a means of preserving the dignity of the dead[28] but also allows their families to know their fate and whereabouts and to start the mourning process, as an identified person is one missing person less (Petrig 2009, p. 351–352). It facilitates the issuance of a death certificate, which is most of the time necessary for relatives to start legal and administrative procedures regarding, for instance, pensions and succession rights.[29] Finally, the identification should take place as soon as possible because it becomes more difficult with time, and it can avoid future exhumations, which can be controversial and more difficult to perform, costlier, in some cases potentially contrary to IHL obligations, and with a stronger psychological impact for the relatives (Sassòli 2019, para. 8.278). The identification of the dead is an obligation of conduct, rather than one of result; it requires parties to take all measures to identify the deceased, with due diligence.[30]

In IACs, the GCs establish that prior to the disposal of the dead, parties to the conflict must carry out a careful examination of the body, preferably a medical examination, to confirm the death, establish identity, and produce a report.[31] All possible measures must be taken to establish the identity of the dead by using a holistic approach for the identification and using a wide range of methods available to ensure its scientific reliability.[32] If nothing else is possible, parties to the conflict must at least take all possible measures to maximize the chances of future identification.[33]

Under IHRL, Article 15 ICPPED refers to the obligation of States to cooperate with each other regarding the identification of the dead in cases of enforced disappearance. The *Guiding Principles for the Search for Disappeared Persons* establish that "[i]f the disappeared person is found dead, the search may be considered as completed when the person has been fully identified in accordance with international standards and handed over to his or her family members or relatives in a dignified manner."[34] In the case *Satabayeva v. Russia* concerning enforced disappearance in Chechnya, the ECtHR noted that a number of essential steps regarding the investigation were not taken such as taking meaningful measures for the bodies' conclusive identification.[35] In the case of *González et al. v. Mexico,* the IACtHR stated that the objective of an autopsy is "[. . .] at the very least, to gather information to identify the dead person, and the hour, date, cause and form of death."[36]

The Islamic law of armed conflict was based on certain texts – scriptural, historical, and legal – which addressed primarily a seventh-century war context in which: (i) the conflicting parties in some cases knew the enemy combatants by name partly because of their tribal affiliations and (ii) the extent of destruction and causalities was very limited, on account of their primitive weaponry and the custom of conducting hostilities away from populated areas.

The identification of the dead was the first and obvious obligation in the process of respecting the dead bodies of heroes/martyrs whose heroism and sacrifices ensured that Islam survived and reached later generations of Muslims until the present. Therefore, these accounts are still being studied until now to commemorate the heroism and sacrifices of the early Muslim martyrs. Furthermore, Islamic rulings at that time were driven by practical concerns. Respecting the mortal remains of the deceased necessitated decently burying them in order to, first, prevent their bodies from being preyed upon by wild animals and, second, to allow their families and loved ones to visit their graves. Third, the identification of the dead ensures that additional rules triggered by the recognition of someone being dead can be implemented, such as the right of the spouse to remarry, paying off debts, and the distribution of inheritance in accordance with Islamic law. Such concerns remain relevant today.

In Muslim contexts, there is still a popular tendency to reject autopsy because it will disfigure, and hence desecrate, the dead body. This practice can hinder the identification of the dead (Al-Dawoody 2011). Autopsy, or post-mortem examination, means the dissection of dead bodies for educational, scientific, or legal purposes, that is, determining the cause of death. This practice was not unknown in Islamic history. Born in today's Iran in 854, Abū Bakr Muḥammad ibn Zakariyyah al-Rāzī, known in the West as Rhazes (d. 925), and Al-Ḥusayn ibn 'Abd Allah ibn Sīnā, known in the West as Avicenna, born in today's Uzbekistan and died in today's Iran in 1037 used to perform autopsy for educational purposes. But the Syrian born and educated 'Alī ibn Abī al-Ḥazm ibn al-Nafīs (d. 1288), later the director of the Nāṣirī Hospital in Cairo, known as the first to describe the pulmonary circulation of the blood, did not perform autopsy for educational purposes because he was of the opinion that it is impermissible under Islamic law (see Mohammed and Kharoshah 2014, p. 81).

At present, autopsy is practiced in Muslim countries by specialists in the department of forensics based either in the Ministry of Justice or in the Ministry of Health. Nevertheless, unless autopsy is performed in the case of a court order because there is a suspicion that death is due to a criminal action and the family themselves are interested to know the cause of death, there is still a popular tendency in Muslim societies to reject autopsy because it will disfigure, and hence desecrate, the dead body. The Arabic word *tashrīḥ*, used for anatomy/autopsy, culturally and psychologically indicates in the mind of Arabic speakers cutting the bodies into pieces or at least cutting the corpse open in a cruel way. In addition to that, the psychological and emotional rejection of autopsy is due to the delay of the burial of the dead (Sheikh 1998). Since the issue of an autopsy is not treated in the Islamic scriptures or classical legal literature, the current Islamic legal deliberations on the issue by many muftis basically reflects a sort of deliberation between the principle of the respect for dead bodies, on one hand, and the legal imperatives of identifying the cause of death in case of suspicion of criminal action and the scientific and educational benefits of autopsy, on the other. Based on the principle of *maṣlaḥah* (public interest) and the Islamic legal maxims *al-ḍarūrāt tubīḥ al-maḥẓūrāt* (necessity overrides the prohibition) and *iktiyār akhaf al-ḍararayn* (choice of the lesser of two evils), most Muslim jurists and major Islamic law and fatwā councils in many Muslim countries such as Egypt, Saudi Arabia, Jordan, and Palestine permit autopsy both for criminal investigations and for scientific and educational benefits. The example of dissecting a dead mother's womb to rescue the fetus given by classical Muslim jurists is borrowed here by contemporary muftis to allow an autopsy.[37]

In order to accommodate the religious beliefs of both Jews and Muslims who object to a post-mortem examination and delayed burials on religious grounds in the UK, the government allows for an alternative examination method, magnetic resonance imaging (MRI) scan of the bodies, that replaces the traditional invasive post-mortem examination.[38] This is a good alternative because it also expedites the burial process, and therefore, in this case, no grounds for objection to a post-mortem examination exists. The main problem with the MRI scan is that its cost is high, specifically in cases where there are large numbers of dead bodies, such as in cases of armed conflicts. Although the current Islamic position on autopsy and the modern scientific achievements can help minimize the popular objection to post-mortem examinations in Muslim contexts, it is still necessary to raise awareness in Muslim societies about the advancement in forensic science and to correct misconceptions that post-mortem examination is cruel mutilation of dead bodies (Mohammed and Kharoshah 2014, note 80, p. 80).

12.5 Respecting the Dead and Dignified Treatment

As we have seen, IHL contains obligations for parties to the armed conflict to respect individuals and to protect their dignity not only during their lifetime but also once they have passed away through specific rules regarding the protection of the dead.[39] As indicated in the 2016 Commentary to GCI, "[t]he underlying purpose of the provisions relating to the dead [. . .] is to preserve the dignity of the dead."[40] Article 34(1) of API explicitly states that the dead shall be respected. In addition, it has been argued that the respect of the dead is inherent in Article 3 Common to the GCs.[41] Rule 115 of the CIHL Study also refers to the respect of the dead as it states that the "dead must be disposed of in a respectful manner and their graves respected and properly maintained." Some national legislations provide for the explicit obligation to take all necessary measures to ensure respect for the dead.[42]

The obligation of humane treatment must guide the actions of parties to armed conflicts,[43] but we may ask ourselves if this obligation also expands to the treatment of the dead and what it would mean toward them. The ICRC's 2016 commentary to GCI mentions that common Article 3 to the GCs prohibits the mutilation of dead bodies as it constitutes an outrage upon personal dignity[44] and recalls that the ICTY in the Tadic case stated that "the victim of an "inhumane act", [. . .], need not necessarily be a living member of humanity [. . .]"[45] and that the prohibition of committing outrages upon personal dignity, including humiliating and degrading treatment, may include acts or omissions committed against the dead according to the ICC Elements of Crimes.[46] Indeed, the ICC Elements of Crimes states that "[f]or this crime, 'persons' can include dead persons."[47] Thus, we may conclude that the obligation of humane treatment under IHL can cover the dead for certain aspects such as the prohibition of outrages upon personal dignity, in particular humiliating and degrading treatment. Some of the acts that can be considered as outrages upon personal dignity against the dead include the mutilation of dead bodies, taking body parts as trophies and exposing a corpse to public display and denigration.[48]

Mutilation of dead bodies is prohibited in IHL in IACs and NIACs.[49] Although Article 3 Common to the GCs expressly prohibits mutilation, this prohibition "applies only to the living and does not extend to the mutilation of corpses" but is covered by the prohibition of outrages upon personal dignity under Article 3 Common to the GCs and can amount under the Statute of the ICC to the war crime of committing outrages upon personal dignity, in particular humiliating or degrading treatment.[50] Courts have also sentenced persons for mistreatment of dead bodies, including for their mutilation or for cannibalism,[51] and the prohibition of mutilating dead bodies is reflected in several legislations.[52]

Parties to the conflict must take all possible measures to prevent the dead from being despoiled in IACs and in NIACs.[53] This obligation is an application of the prohibition of pillage[54] and facilitates future identification of the dead as in some cases the objects found on the body are key to this end (e.g., watch, ring, keys, etc.).[55] In addition, to avoid despoiling the dead, parties to the conflict must also take all possible measures to prevent others from doing so.[56] The violation of this obligation can amount to a war crime,[57] and national laws in several States also prohibit this conduct.[58]

The obligation of humane treatment can be interpreted as including the obligation to protect the dead from being exposed to public curiosity.[59] In IACs, Article 13 of GCIII and Article 27 of GCIV expressly state that prisoners of war and civilian internees "must at all times be protected [...] against public curiosity."[60] Although the GCs do not expressly forbid the exposure of dead bodies to public curiosity in IACs, the Commentary to Article 34 of API clearly states that this obligation "[. . .] consists of preventing the remains from being despoiled and from being exposed to public curiosity, by placing them in an appropriate place before burial or cremation."[61]

Under IHRL, the ECtHR has constantly stated that the prohibition of ill-treatment from Article 3 of the ECHR does not apply in a context of disrespect for dead bodies;[62] it has assessed a violation of such Article by evaluating whether the suffering of the relatives caused by the treatment of the dead body could be considered as inhumane or degrading treatment toward the surviving relatives and not on the basis of a right belonging to the deceased.[63] The IACtHR has found a violation of Article 5 of the ACHR regarding the right to mental and moral integrity due to the additional suffering that the next of kin have endured as a consequence of the subsequent acts or omissions of the authorities regarding the treatment of the dead.[64]

In sum, IHL provides for the respect and humane treatment of the dead by parties to the conflict in IACs and NIACs, which includes in particular the prohibition of committing outrages upon personal dignity, the prohibition of mutilation, the obligation to prevent the dead from being despoiled, and the obligation to protect them from public curiosity. Such obligations concern all the dead in connection with the armed conflict. Under traditional interpretations of IHRL, only the living have human rights, but regional courts of human rights have imposed certain obligations to the State regarding the respect of the dead through the rights of their living relatives, in particular, the right to not be subject to torture and cruel and inhuman or degrading treatment or punishment.

In Islam, human dignity is a right given by God to all humankind who are referred to in the Qur'ān as God's representatives on earth. Whether they are dead or alive, the dignity and respect required includes that of the human body, created by God in the perfect shape.[65] In a ḥadīth narrated by his wife 'Āishah (d. 678), Prophet Muhammad (d. 632) said: "breaking the bones of a dead person is equivalent to breaking it when the person is alive."[66] This ḥadīth underlies the fundamental principle of respecting dead bodies under Islamic law,[67] and in one sense, any crime committed against a dead body remains punishable in the same way as it was when the person was alive.

Therefore, in the same line of protecting the human body as part of the respect for human dignity, under the Islamic law of armed conflict, mutilation of an enemy body is strictly prohibited. Mutilation of enemy bodies as a sign of revenge was recorded in fighting between the Arabs, and a practice of carrying out the severed heads of enemy military leaders was reported as a practice in the wars between the Romans and the Persians.[68] In the battle of Uḥud in March 625, many bodies of the dead Muslims were brutally mutilated including the body of Prophet Muhammad's uncle Ḥamzah ibn ʻAbd al-Muṭṭalib. Prophet Muhammad and other Muslims vowed to revenge on their enemies by mutilating their bodies in future military engagements, and when the Qur'ānic text 16, pp. 126–127, was revealed, Prophet Muhammad prohibited mutilation. Among Prophet Muhammad's instructions regulating the use of force during armed conflicts was: "Do not loot, do not be treacherous and do not mutilate."[69] Affirming the brutality of mutilation, Prophet Muhammad prohibited mutilation even if it was the body of a rabid dog.[70] Similarly, the first caliph Abū Bakr (d. 634) sent written instruction to his governor in Hadramaut, Yemen, which reads: "Beware of mutilation, because it is a sin and a disgusting act."[71]

12.6 Respectful Disposal of the Dead

Under IHL in IACs and NIACs, "the dead must be disposed of in a respectful manner and their graves respected and properly maintained."[72] This means that parties must respect the human remains, the burial place, and the burial ceremony and that they must abstain from conducting offensive acts toward the dead.[73] This obligation should be considered to apply to all persons that die in connection with an armed conflict including, for example, the dead of the adverse party, the dead of the side of the party in question, as well as civilians.[74]

In IACs, respectful disposal of the dead also means that parties to the conflict must ensure that the dead are buried[75] Burial must be the general rule, and cremation the exception;[76] as cremation is irreversible, it renders the identification of the deceased impossible, and it can be easier to hide violations of the law.[77] Cremation is acceptable only "for imperative reasons of hygiene" and "for motives based on the religion of the deceased."[78] Regarding the first exception, the threshold to meet this requirement is high, requiring "imperative" reasons of hygiene; as it has been scientifically proven that the dead rarely spread diseases especially if they died from trauma, as it is mostly the case in armed conflicts, this exception rarely applies.[79] Regarding the second exception, parties to the armed conflict should take into account sufficient factors to determine the person's religion to know if this would militate for cremation of the body, and the decision should be based on the individual's wishes, but burial should be favored if the religion cannot be ascertained or if the person is found to be agnostic or an atheist or if there are doubts.[80] Based on this, this exception will apply only in limited cases. A third exception exists that is not mentioned explicitly in the GC, which is the wish of the deceased formulated explicitly and freely before death to be cremated, even if it is not for religious reasons.[81]

Parties to the armed conflict have the obligation to bury the dead in individual graves or to cremate them individually as far as circumstances permit in IACs.[82] When burial in collective graves is unavoidable, parties to the conflict should respect certain requirements as an absolute minimum to ensure the dignified treatment of the dead and to do their utmost to ensure that subsequent exhumation and identification of every individual will be possible and that each deceased is treated with respect.[83]

In IACs, the GCs specify that the dead must be honorably interred, if possible, according to the rites of their religion.[84] This is not an absolute obligation as it might not be possible in some circumstances to perform the ceremony as required by the deceased's religion, for instance, if parties cannot establish the religion or if the necessary elements to perform the rites, such as the religious figure or a component of the ceremony, are not available.[85] Determining the religion of the deceased might be difficult if he/she did not express it before death as States are multicultural, and a person's religion should not be assumed without sufficient factors to reach a conclusion.[86]

In IHRL, there are no treaty provisions regarding final disposal of the dead, except concerning the return of human remains to their families for cases of enforced disappearance.[87] Nevertheless, both the ECtHR and the IACtHR have referred to the importance of allowing the families of the deceased to bury the dead in a proper manner according to their traditions and religion.[88] According to the IACtHR, some actions such as burying the dead at the place where they were found without the consent of the next of kin[89] and throwing them into a river to ensure that they cannot be found and identified[90] are incompatible with the respectful disposal of a body. The IACtHR has also recalled the importance of burying the dead according to their religious beliefs. In the case of the *Río Negro Massacres v. Guatemala*, it stated that the impossibility of burying the dead and performing the funeral rites according to their religious beliefs increased the suffering and anguish of the next of kin especially due to the importance of the farewell rites for the dead in the Mayan culture and the sacred nature they attribute to their cemeteries.[91] In the case *Physicians for Human Rights v Commander of IDF Forces in the Gaza Strip*, the Israeli High Court of Justice recalled that the duty of the authorities was "to ensure a dignified burial for the bodies."[92] In order to ensure such dignified burial, authorities "must speak with the local authorities [. . .] and find dignified ways to carry out this duty."[93]

In sum, under IHL, respectful disposal of the dead includes favoring burial over cremation, which must remain exceptional, favoring burial in individual graves over collective graves, burying the dead, if possible, according to the rites of the religion to which they belonged, and grouping the graves according to nationality if possible.[94] Although those requirements are only specified for IACs, it is likely that some of these requirements also apply in NIACs on the basis of national law.[95] IHRL has also reaffirmed the importance for families and communities to bury the dead in a proper manner according to their traditions and religion.

Under Islamic law, the burial of the dead is a *farḍ kifāyah* (collective obligation) in the Muslim community, which consists of: (i) *ghusl*, ritual washing of dead bodies; (ii) *kafan*, shrouding with pieces of cloth; and (iii) *salat al-janāzah*, funeral prayer. Islamic law has developed detailed regulations regarding the disposal of the dead bodies of Muslims and, importantly for the concern of this chapter, made a separate body of rules for the disposal of the body of those who died in armed conflict, the *shuhadā'*, singular *shahīd* (martyr). Muslim jurists agree that the following three rules should be observed exclusively in the case of martyrs: first, there should be no ritual washing for the body of the martyr. This majority understanding has been the norm and practice throughout Islamic history until today, despite the fact that there are a host of divergent opinions among the jurists in all of these three rules basically because of conflicting reports attributed to Prophet Muhammed. Second, there should be no shrouding of the martyrs, and they should be buried in the same clothes in which they were killed.[96] Third, no funeral prayer should be performed on the body of the martyrs.[97]

In Islamic law and Muslim cultures, burying the dead in the ground is regarded as the correct way of respecting dead bodies, while *ḥarq* (cremation) is strictly prohibited because, unlike in some cultures, it is considered a violation of the dignity of the human body.[98] It is worth mentioning here that during the Ebola crisis, the current Mufti of Egypt, Dr. Shawki Allam, issued fatwa number 3246 on May 14, 2015, permitting the cremation of dead bodies of Ebola victims and then *burying them in graves* after that if specialized experts confirm that cremation is the required method to stop the spread of the Ebola virus disease. In other words, other people would die as a result of the spread of infection if the dead bodies of Ebola victims are not cremated, and therefore, the Mufti of Egypt grounded his fatwa on the protection of life (*hifẓ al-nafs*): the first of the five ultimate objectives of Islamic law.[99] The current Mufti of Egypt also grounded his fatwa on a number of Islamic legal maxims pertaining to the cases of harm and necessity such as: "harm must be removed," "necessity lifts prohibitions/makes the unlawful lawful," and "necessity is measured according to its proportion."[100]

The rule in Islamic law is that every dead body should be buried in an individual grave.[101] However, in cases of necessity, collective graves are permissible. Beyond the issue of individual graves is the issue of separating the graves of different categories. Male and female dead bodies should be buried in separate graves, and if necessity dictates otherwise, then classical Muslim jurists add that a barrier of dust should be placed between the bodies.[102] Classical Muslim jurists agree that Muslims and non-Muslims should be buried in separate graves.[103] They have, however, deliberated various specific cases in this regard. For example, in case the religious identity of a number of dead bodies cannot be identified, then conflicting opinions are given by the jurists. The majority opine that they are to be buried in special graves, not in the Muslims' graves or the non-Muslims'. However, one minority argues that they are to be buried in the Muslims' graves, and another minority thinks they should be buried in the non-Muslims' graves.[104] Despite this difference of opinion, jurists agree that if a body of a dead child was found and her/his religious identity cannot be identified, then the body should be buried in Muslim graves.[105] The practice of separate Muslim and non-Muslim graves is still observed in Muslim countries, and it would be advisable to observe this practice in cases of armed conflicts if the religious identity of dead bodies can be identified. If this practice is no longer observed in certain Muslim contexts, then the issue of separating the graves should not be raised by international organizations in times of armed conflicts.

Understandably, Islamic law, cultural, and traditional practices play a major role in most of the issues related to the management of the dead. In Muslim as well as some other non-Muslim cultures, there is a tendency to quickly bury the dead, which in some cases hinders the work of forensic specialists working in Muslim contexts. This is mainly because, first, the relatives and neighbors want to prevent the body from starting to emit the odor of death, especially in some countries where temperatures are high and there are not enough fridges to keep the dead bodies in cool temperatures or where electricity blackout occurs often and without warning, let alone in villages and remote places in the desert without electricity. So quick burial in these situations is motivated by the desire to respect the dead bodies. Second, the extended relatives and neighbors want to shorten the pain of the members of the family and their loved ones by burying the dead body and save the family from a state of fear and anxiety that the body of the deceased might decay and start to give the odor of death, which is understandably painful for the family.

The principle of respect for dead bodies has surfaced in the above discussion, and different manifestations of this respect exist in different cultures and periods, however. In normal situations, based on reports attributed to Prophet Muhammed – to use Islamic legal terminology – it is *mustaḥab*, preferred, to bury the dead bodies quickly (see ḥadīth number 1252 in al-Bukhārī 1987, above note 6, vol. 1, p. 442; ‘A. Ibn Ḥazm, above note 3, vol. 5, p. 154; Al-Nawawī, above note 3, vol. 5, p. 230; Al-Khatīb al-Shirbīnī n.d., vol. 1, p. 340); that is, it is not *farḍ/wājib* (compulsory). However, no specific indications of how quickly burial should be is given in these reports. But in cases of *al-maṭ‘ūn* (a plague-ridden person), *al-maflūj* (a hemiplegic person), and *al-masbūt* (a comatose person), some jurists advocate that it is preferred that Muslims wait for *yaūm wa laylah* (a day and a night) until the death of persons in such cases is confirmed (see Al-'Asqalānī n.d. above note 12, vol. 3, p. 184; 'Abd al-Raḥman ibn 'Abd al-Raḥīm al-Mubarkāfūrī n.d., vol. 4, p. 82). The reason behind waiting in these three cases is simply that there is a possibility that they are not dead yet. They may be in a coma, and therefore, the premodern Muslim jurists preferred that the burial should be delayed until death is confirmed. But if there is a suspicion that death is due to criminal action, then burial is to be postponed until the body is examined.[106] Few jurists added that waiting for relatives of the deceased is one of the reasons for postponing burial of the dead body, unless the body will decay (see Al-Ra'ūūf al-Mināwī 1937, vol. 3, p. 310). These discussions about the timeframe do not change if the dead body is unclaimed or unidentified: the same rationale of respecting a human dead body applies. The humanitarian concern of respecting dead bodies will prompt Muslims to quickly bury unclaimed or unidentified bodies.

Therefore, for forensic specialists to be given enough time to undertake their job, providing fridges to protect dead bodies is necessary in addition to engaging community and religious leaders and local authorities in convincing the public and relatives of the dead about the fact that giving forensic specialists enough time to examine the bodies is important for establishing the identity of the dead bodies. Otherwise, families of the dead risk being in pain for the rest of their lives for being unable to identify and visit the grave of their loved ones.

12.7 Gravesites and Other Locations of Mortal Remains

IHL provides for specific obligations regarding gravesites and other locations of mortal remains.[107] Although graves are not defined in the GCs, the notion should be understood broadly as they also refer to "other locations of the remains of persons,"[108] which shows that they include cemeteries, informal burial places, temporal and permanent graves, individual and collective graves, and monuments containing human remains.[109] This broad understanding ensures that different traditions and religions are covered by IHL. Parties to the armed conflict must ensure respect for the graves, including by taking positive measures such as adopting relevant legislation and security measures to protect them.[110]

In IACs and NIACs, the graves must be respected and properly maintained.[111] The location of graves must also be marked with a view to the identification of the dead, and the GCs require that graves be grouped according to the nationality of the deceased if possible.[112] The objective is to ensure the respect of the dead and their honorable inhumation by avoiding speedy unorganized burials, to ensure that the graves are grouped and marked in a way that facilitates future exhumation, the possibility for the home country to honor its dead and/or exhume them for their return and for the families to be able to visit them.[113]

There are different Islamic rulings,[114] regional, cultural, and traditional practices throughout the Muslim world regarding building of graves and marking of graves with the names of the deceased. For example, in some countries graves are built over the ground and marked with the name/s of the deceased and date of death in order to identify the different bodies, which is permissible in Islamic law according to fatwā number 4341 given by the current Grand Mufti of Egypt on March 7, 2018.[115] Nonetheless, in other Muslim countries, bodies are buried under the ground without the names of the deceased, but obviously the gravesites and other locations of mortal remains in which they are buried are marked. Such differences should be respected in the respective regions by the concerned international organizations if services are provided in this context of armed conflicts in the Muslim world. However, if such traditional practices will hinder humanitarian assistance to victims, mainly management of dead bodies by forensic specialists in this context, then engaging with community and religious leaders and explaining the risks and the danger such practices may cause can help gain their support for the work of international organizations.

12.8 Exhumations

IHL seeks to balance the obligation to respect the dead and their graves and the need to exhume the bodies in certain circumstances by allowing exhumations only in limited cases.[116] In IACs, they are permitted only in three cases.[117] First, they are allowed when parties to the conflict conclude agreements to facilitate the return of the remains of the deceased and of personal effects to the home country upon its request or, unless that country objects, upon the request of the next of kin.[118] Second, in the absence of such agreements, if the home country of the deceased is not willing to arrange at its expense for the maintenance of gravesites, the party in whose territory the gravesites are situated may offer to facilitate the return of the remains of the deceased to the home country.[119] If the offer is not accepted, it may adopt the arrangements laid down in its own laws relating to cemeteries and graves, which might require exhumation.[120] Third, exhumations can take place in cases of "overriding public necessity,"[121] which include medical reasons or criminal investigation needs but could also include the implementation of obligations related to the treatment of the dead.[122]

Although there is no specific provision regarding exhumations in NIACs, under customary IHL, there are many rules regarding the protection of the dead that are applicable both in IACs and in NIACs and that may require exhumations for their implementation. For instance, the obligation to account for the dead requires to identify them, which might entail exhumation if the dead was not identified prior burial.[123] In addition, the dead must be disposed of in a respectful manner and their graves respected and properly maintained, which might involve that the dead are exhumed to place them in a permanent burial place.[124]

Under IHRL, the procedural obligation to investigate cases of suspicious deaths may require that the authorities take forensic measures, including exhumations to perform autopsies.[125] The ECtHR considers as an important step in an investigation of suspicious death the exhumation of bodies for their conclusive identification.[126] The IACtHR has also established that "[i]n cases of grave human rights violations, [. . .] the exhumation and identification of the deceased victims forms part of the State's obligation to investigate."[127] It has also recognized as a form of reparation "[. . .] the search, exhumation and identification of those who disappeared and those presumably executed."[128]

Under Islamic law, respect of dead bodies entails not exhuming their graves, and therefore, classical Muslim jurists agree on the prohibition of exhuming graves without necessity.[129] There is a precedent in the battle of Uḥud in 625 of exhuming one of the dead bodies who were buried in a collective grave to be transferred to an individual grave in Medina, close to his family.[130] Shaykh Makhlūf, the Grand Mufti of Egypt from January 5, 1946, to May 7, 1950, and from March 1952 to December 1954, gave a fatwā permitting the transfer of the mortal remains of "the last Ottoman sultan, 'Abd Al-Majīd, and his wife, who were embalmed and buried in France, to be buried in Egypt."[131]

Other examples of exhuming graves were also deliberated for (i) religious purposes (or what is described in Islamic parlance as the rights of God), (ii) civil liability cases (rights of humans), or even (iii) public interest considerations.

Examples of exhuming mortal remains for religious purposes include: if a dead body is buried without the ritual washing, or shrouding, or the funeral prayer. The jurists agree that there is no need for exhuming the mortal remains to perform the funeral prayer because it can be performed at the grave without exhuming the body. Similarly, they tend to reject exhumation if the body was buried without shrouding because they argue that the grave already satisfies the purpose of covering the body, while they tend to accept exhuming the dead body if it was buried without the ritual washing.[132]

Examples of exhuming mortal remains for civil liability cases include: if gold,[133] money, or valuable belongings are buried with the dead bodies, if the deceased swallowed a piece of jewelry before death, or if the body is buried in a usurped land and the land owner asks for the removal of the grave from his/her land. In all of these examples, the jurists support the exhumation of the graves[134] because after death, the possession of all such items accompanying the dead body is to be legally transferred to the heirs of the dead according to their prescribed shares under Islamic law. Hence, loose personal items, belongings, and valuables found with the dead bodies during armed conflicts should be handed to their next of kin. Likewise, the right of the living, in this case the owner of the usurped land upon which the grave is built, overrides the respect of dead bodies.

Examples of exhuming mortal remains for the purpose of public interest include: exhuming graves for building public roads[135] or if the graves were hit by floods or leaks.[136] Public interest considerations here constitute legitimate grounds for exhumation of graves.

Therefore, the issue of the exhumation of human remains as deliberated in Islamic legal tradition reflects not only the Islamic religious, legal, and ethical dimensions but also the cultural and contextual dimensions of the seventh and eighth centuries. As shown, exhumation of human remains is permissible in some cases and prohibited in others. On one hand, the prohibition in some of these cases is based solely or mainly on the jurists' discretion of what constitutes disrespect for human dignity. On the other hand, the permissibility is based in some cases on the jurists' discretion of what constitutes the public interest of the Muslim community. This explains the different rulings developed by the jurists and the various practices adopted in the Muslim societies accordingly.

12.9 Return of Human Remains and Personal Effects of the Dead

Under IHL in IACs, parties to the conflict must endeavor to facilitate the return of the remains of the deceased upon request of the party to which they belong or upon the request of their next of kin,[137] and they must return their personal effects.[138] The return of the human remains to their families has been considered as "a basic humanitarian goal" for different reasons.[139] Some families may mistrust the death certificate issued by the other party; others may need the remains to accept the death of their loved one and begin the mourning process (Sassòli 2019, para. 8.281, and Baranowska 2017, p. 714). Besides, many religions and cultures require the performance of certain rituals with the dead body to permit it to transcend to the afterlife and to find peace.[140] In sum, there seems to be "[. . .] a universal human need to bury one's dead" (Baranowska 2017, p. 714) and to perform our own ritual to give a final rest to our dead.

In IACs, parties to the conflict may either inter the dead honorably themselves or return them to their home country for burial or cremation.[141] According to the 2016 Commentary to GCI, the return of the mortal remains should be favored because it facilitates the mourning process of the deceased's relatives and because it allows them to ensure that the final disposal of the dead is carried out in accordance with their religious beliefs and customs.[142] The request for the return can come from the home country or from the next of kin but the home country has the possibility to oppose to such request in certain circumstances (Petrig 2009, pp. 353–354).[143] However, IHRL has strongly reinforced the rights of the family of the deceased through, for instance, the right to family and private life. Thus, it seems that today, it will be difficult for a State to oppose to the request of family members to have the remains of their loved ones returned to them.

While in IACs, the return of the dead is envisaged to the home country, in classic NIACs, the dead will be most likely in his/her own country, which means that the return should be interpreted as the return to his/her relatives.[144] In NIACs, there are no treaty provisions and no customary rule regarding the return of human remains to their families, but there is a growing trend toward recognition of the obligation of parties to a conflict to facilitate the return of remains to their families upon their request, as it is in keeping with the requirement of respect for family life and the right of families to know the fate and whereabouts of their relatives, which apply in both types of conflicts.[145]

Under IHRL, Article 15 and Article 24(3) of the ICPPED establish that State parties to the Convention shall return the remains of disappeared persons and shall cooperate with each other and afford one another the greatest measure of mutual assistance to return the remains to their families. Although the ICPPED specifically refers to cases of enforced disappearance, those articles represent an important step toward the recognition of a right of families to have the remains of their loved ones returned to them. The ECtHR has established the violation of the right to family life in some cases concerning the refusal of the State to return the human remains to their relatives[146] and cases concerning an excessive delay in the return of a body.[147] In the cases *Maskhadova and Others v. Russia* and *Sabanchiyeva and Others v. Russia*, the ECtHR concluded that there was a violation of the right to private and family life due to the State's refusal to return the human remains of the Chechen insurgents to their relatives.[148] The IACtHR has recalled the importance for the relatives to receive the body of their forcibly disappeared loved one to allow them to bury him/her according to their beliefs and to grieve based on the right of family members to not be subject to cruel, inhuman, and degrading treatment in cases such as *García and Family Members v. Guatemala*.[149]

As documented in the earliest Islamic sources, Muslims observed the practice of returning the dead bodies of the Muslim soldiers from the battlefield to their families.[150] Otherwise, when it is impossible to return bodies from the battlefield to their families, then burying dead bodies in collective graves will be permitted in this case of necessity. Likewise, returning dead bodies to the adverse party finds precedence in early Islamic history. At the Battle of the Trench in 627 where Muslims numbered less than one third of the coalition of their enemy attackers,

Nawfal ibn ‘Abd Allah ibn al-Mughīrah died when he attempted to jump the trench with his horse, which Muslims dug around Medina to prevent the Meccans' attack. When the Meccans offered payment for receiving the body of Nawfal, Prophet Muhammed gave them the body and refused their offer.[151]

Regarding personal effects of the deceased, parties to the conflict must return them to the party to which they belong or to their next of kin in IACs.[152] The objective of this rule is to give back to families objects that are important to them or that have a sentimental value.[153] The GCs establish that the return should be done through the National Information Bureaus,[154] which then transmits them to the Central Tracing Agency or the Protecting Power, which finally transmits them to the families. The articles should be sent in sealed packets, accompanied by statements giving all particulars necessary for the identification of the deceased owners as well as by a complete list of the contents.[155] They should also be sent as soon as possible given the importance they may have for the family not only for administrative and legal reasons[156] but also for sentimental reasons. Article 34(2–3) API states that agreements should be concluded to facilitate the return and establishes a particular procedure in case no agreement is concluded. "Personal effects" shall be interpreted broadly and include one half of a double identity disc, last wills, other documents of importance to the next of kin, money, and all articles of an intrinsic or sentimental value, which are found on the dead, as well as other unidentified articles.[157] Regarding what is meant by "other documents of importance," it has been interpreted that this object must be of documentary nature and may even include an "electronic matter that provides information or evidence,"[158] and it must be important or useful to the relatives, which excludes documents of a military value.[159] As the "intrinsic or sentimental value" of an object is relative and depends on the culture and personal criteria, it is important to return all possible objects and to let the family of the dead decide if they want to keep the object or not.[160]

In NIACs, there are no treaty provisions and no customary rules regarding the return of personal effects to their families. Nevertheless, arguments have been made that under IHRL, the State must return personal effects of the dead to their relatives when there is no legitimate aim to retain them based on the right to property established for instance in Article 17 UDHR and Article 1 of the first AP to the ECHR.[161] In addition, this issue is normally regulated under national law.[162]

As was the norm in international relations at the time, classical Islamic law provides that the property of a defeated non-Muslim enemy becomes war booty. The classical Islamic rules on war booty are largely based on the scriptural sources, the Qur'ān 8:41 and the Sunnah, and regulated in detail in the Islamic legal compendia. In brief, one fifth of the booty is to be distributed to certain beneficiaries,[163] and the rest is to be distributed to the army. Some Ḥanafī and Shāfi‘ī jurists give the ruler the freedom to return to the defeated adversary their property. The general and strict rule is that the ruler is the one in charge of distributing the booty,[164] and therefore, it is prohibited for Muslims to take anything from the booty before it is given to them by the ruler; otherwise, this constitutes an act of looting, which is a major sin/crime in the Qur'ān 3:161.[165] The Second Caliph, 'Umar ibn al-Khaṭṭāb (r. 634–644), sent written instructions to his officials that reads: "Do not steal from the booty, do not betray; do not kill a child; and fear God in the farmers."[166] In conflicts between Muslims or what can be classified as NIAC, according to classical Islamic law, money and weapons confiscated from armed rebels – both living and dead – must be returned to them after the cessation of hostilities.[167] In other words, it is prohibited for both adversary parties to take war booty in inter-Muslim fighting. If respected, this specific ruling in inter-Muslim fighting can protect personal valuables. This is particularly if one or both parties of armed conflict use Islamic law as their source of reference.

12.10 Conclusion

IHL provides a comprehensive set of obligations to parties to the conflict regarding the protection of the dead in armed conflicts. The rules for IACs are substantially more detailed and developed than for NIACs as it is often the case. Nevertheless, most of the broad obligations are customary law applicable to both types of situations. In summary, IHL contains rules regarding parties to the conflict's obligations to search for, collect and evacuate the dead, to ensure that they are treated with respect, to take measures to identify them and to record relevant information to this end, to dispose them honorably, to respect their graves, and to return them to their relatives. Such rules seek to directly ensure the respect of the dead and their dignified treatment, in addition to ensuring respect and protection to their families. Thus, IHL recognizes that parties have the obligation to treat the dead with respect, independently of their relatives' rights. This recognition comes from the most fundamental and basic human belief in most cultures, societies, and religions that the dead should be respected and honored: human dignity should be preserved, even after death.

Contrary to IHL, IHRL contains extremely few treaty provisions specifically relating to the treatment of the dead. Nevertheless, through UN bodies' and regional Courts' jurisprudence, IHRL has complemented IHL obligations regarding the dead by interpreting some rights of their relatives as requiring that a specific conduct is followed toward the dead. Such obligations have notably been developed through the obligation to respect the right to life and the procedural obligation of investigation that comes with it as well as from the right to family life and the prohibition of ill-treatment against relatives of the deceased person.

IHRL has also strengthened the place and the role of families regarding their deceased loved ones.

In order to ensure that the obligations regarding the treatment of the dead are respected, the authorities need to adopt relevant domestic measures including policies, laws, regulations, protocols, and other practical measures to ensure the respect and protection of the dead and their families in accordance with international law.[168]

The specific legal issues and contemporary challenges discussed in this chapter under international law and Islamic law lead to the following conclusions: first, although the two legal systems have different sources, emerged in two different eras and, therefore, address primarily different conflict contexts, they both attempt to protect the dignity and respect of the dead. Second, the two legal systems can complement each other at the present time to achieve the protection of the dead in the context of armed conflicts in the Muslim contexts. That is because Islamic law provisions have strongly shaped the practice of the management of dead bodies in Muslim majority states. Third, Islamic rules are still being revisited, sought after by the average Muslims. and deliberated by both local and international Islamic law institutions as well as by Islamic law experts. Muslims are self-motivated to abide by Islamic law, and hence, if Muslim scholars disseminate Islamic law of armed conflict among Muslims, it could have a big influence on ensuring the dignity and respect for the dead. Fourth, in the same vein, if forensics specialists working in Muslim societies familiarize themselves with the Islamic law positions on the issues and challenges they are confronted within the Muslim contexts, they can better communicate their humanitarian and scientific messages. In cases where cultural practices constitute challenges to the forensic specialists' work, then engaging with Islamic institutions, scholars, and community leader becomes inevitable in order to address the challenges if such communal practices may change. Fifth, the legal, technical, and specialized forensic expertise that institutions such as the ICRC have developed are indispensable for achieving the protection of dead bodies in contemporary armed conflicts in Muslims contexts.

Notes

1. ICRC (2004).
2. For more detail on the rules of customary international humanitarian law identified by the ICRC, see: Henckaerts and Doswald-Beck 2005, Rules 112–116. Hereafter: ICRC, CIHL Study.
3. See for instance ECtHR, *Akpinar and Altun v. Turkey*, no. 56760/00, February 27, 2007, para. 82.
4. ICPPED, Art. 15, 17(3)(g), 18(1)(g), and 24(3).

5. CED, "Guiding principles for the search for disappeared persons," adopted by the Committee at its 16th session, April 8–18, 2019, preambular para. 3.
6. ICRC (2020).
7. With reference to the war crime of outrages upon personal dignity, the 2000 ICC Elements of Crimes specifies that Article 8(2)(b)(xxi) and (c)(ii) of the 1998 ICC Statute also applies to dead persons. See ICC Statute, Footnote 57 relating to Article 8(2)(c)(ii).
8. UNGA Res. 57/207, "Missing Persons," UN Doc. A/RES/57/207, February 14, 2003 and UNGA, Res. 75/184, "Missing Persons," UN Doc. A/RES/75/184, December 16, 2020, para. 7.
9. UNSC, Res. 2474, June 11, 2019, para. 8.
10. OAS, General Assembly Res. AG/RES 2961 (L-O/20), "Promotion and Protection of Human Rights," October 20–21, 2020.
11. ICRC, CIHL Study, Rule 112. See also GCI, Art. 15(1); GC II, Art. 18(1); GCIV, Art. 16(2); API, Art. 17(2) and 33(4); APII, Art. 8.
12. ICRC, CIHL Study, explanation to Rule 112 and Gavshon 2015, pp. 279–280.
13. ICRC, *Commentary on the First Geneva Convention: Convention (I) for the Amelioration of the Condition of the Wounded and Sick in Armed Forces in the Field, 2nd edition*, 2016, Art. 15, paras. 1508 and 1510. Hereafter: ICRC, *Commentary on the First Geneva Convention*, 2016.
14. ICRC, *Commentary on the First Geneva Convention*, 2016, Art. 15, para. 1509 and ICRC, CIHL Study, explanation to Rule 112.
15. API, Art. 17(2); ICRC, *Commentary on the First Geneva Convention, 2016*, Art. 15, para. 1509; and ICRC, CIHL Study, explanation to Rule 112.
16. API, Art. 33(4) and ICRC, CIHL Study, explanation to Rule 112.
17. ICRC, CIHL Study explanation to Rule 112.
18. ICRC, CIHL Study, explanation to Rule 112 and related practice.
19. Cameroon, *Droit International Humanitaire et droit de la guerre, Manuel de l'instructeur en vigueur dans les Forces Armées*, Présidence de le République, Ministère de la Défense, Etat-major des Armées, Troisième division, Edition 1992. See ICRC, CIHL Study, explanation to Rule 112 and related practice.
20. Chad, Droit international humanitaire, Manuel de l'instructeur en vigueur dans les forces armées et de sécurité, Ministère de la Défense, Présidence de la République, Etat-major des Armées, 2006, p. 52. See ICRC, CIHL Study, explanation to Rule 112 and related practice.
21. ICPPED, Art. 15 and Art. 23(3).
22. ECtHR, *Benzer and Others v. Turkey*, no. 23502/06, November 12, 2013. See also Last Rights, "The Dead, the Missing and the Bereaved at Europe's International Borders, Proposal for a Statement of the International legal obligations of States," May 2017, p. 2.
23. CED, "Guiding principles for the search for disappeared persons," adopted in the Committee 16th session, April 8–18, 2019, Principle 5.
24. See ḥadīth number 1812 in Ibn al-Ḥajjāj al-Qushayrī (n.d.), vol. 3, p. 1447; ḥadīth number 1065 in Ibn Ḥanbal (n.d.), above note 3, vol. 5, p. 84; ḥadīth number 33650 in Ibn Muḥammad ibn Abī Shaybah (1998), vol. 6, p. 537.
25. See ḥadīth number 2727 in Ibn Ismā'īl al-Bukhārī (1987), vol. 3, p. 1056; Al-Zuḥaylī (2010), vol. 7, p. 437.
26. See Al-Zuḥaylī (2010), above note 6, vol. 7, p. 448.

27. GCI, Art. 16–17; GCII, Art. 19–20; GCIII, Art. 120–122; GCIV, Art. 129–131; API, Art. 33(2)(b) and 33(4); ICRC, CIHL Study, Rule 116. See also ICRC, *Commentary on the First Geneva Convention*, 2016, Art. 17, para. 1672.
28. GCI, Art. 16–17; GCII, Art. 19–20; GCIII, Art. 120–122; GCIV, Art. 129–131; API, Art. 33(2)(b) and 33(4); ICRC, CIHL Study, Rule 116. See also ICRC, *Commentary on the First Geneva Convention*, 2016, Art. 17, para. 1634.
29. *Ibid.*
30. ICRC, *Commentary on the First Geneva Convention*, 2016, Art. 17, para. 1664 and ICRC, CIHL Study, explanation to Rule 116. See also Sassòli and Tougas (2002, p. 731).
31. GCI, Art. 17(1); GCII, Art. 20(1); GCIII, Art. 120(3). For civilian internees, deaths must be certified by a doctor and a death certificate made out, showing the cause of death and the conditions under which it occurred: see GCIV, Art. 129(2). See also ICRC, CIHL Study, Rule 116; and ICRC, *Commentary on the First Geneva Convention*, 2016, Art. 17, para. 1672.
32. GCI, Art. 17(1); GCII, Art. 20(1); GCIII, Art. 120(3). For civilian internees, deaths must be certified by a doctor and a death certificate made out, showing the cause of death and the conditions under which it occurred: see GCIV, Art. 129(2). See also ICRC, CIHL Study, Rule 116; and ICRC, *Commentary on the First Geneva Convention*, 2016, Art. 17, para. 1661.
33. GCI, Art. 17(1); GCII, Art. 20(1); GCIII, Art. 120(3). For civilian internees, deaths must be certified by a doctor and a death certificate made out, showing the cause of death and the conditions under which it occurred: see GCIV, Art. 129(2). See also ICRC, CIHL Study, Rule 116; and ICRC, *Commentary on the First Geneva Convention*, 2016, Art. 17, para. 1673; ICRC, *Operational Best Practices Regarding the Management of Human Remains*, para. 3.2.
34. CED, "Guiding principles for the search for disappeared persons," adopted in the Committee 16th session, April 8–18, 2019, Principle 5 para. 3.
35. ECtHR, *Satabayeva v. Russia*, No. 21486/06, November 29, 2009, para. 126,
36. IACtHR, *González et al. ("Cotton Field") v. Mexico*, November 16, 2009, para. 310.
37. See http://fatwa.islamweb.net/fatwa/index.php?page=showfatwa&Option=FatwaId&lang=A&Id=56064
38. See https://www.telegraph.co.uk/news/religion/5195466/Muslims-and-Jews-to-be-allowed-to-have-different-post-mortems.html; https://www.manchestereveningnews.co.uk/news/greater-manchester-news/body-scans-instead-of-post-mortems-955338
39. ICRC, *Commentary on the First Geneva Convention*, 2016, Art. 17, para. 1634.
40. ICRC, *Commentary on the First Geneva Convention*, 2016, Art. 17, para. 1634.
41. Colombia, Council of State, Case No. 9276, Statement of the Prosecutor, Concepto del Procurador Primero Delegado, August 19, 1994. See also ICRC, CIHL Study, Rule 113, explanation and State practice.
42. See for instance Italy, *Law of War Decree* (1938 amended in 1992), Art. 94 states: "[c]ommanders shall take all necessary measures to ensure respect for the bodies of enemy dead on the battlefield."
43. GC I–IV, Art. 3(1); GCI, Art. 12; GCII, Art. 12; GCIII, Art. 13; GCIV, Arts. 5 and 27; API, Arts. 10 and 75; APII, Arts. 4, 5, and 7; ICRC, CIHL Study, Rule 87.
44. ICRC, *Commentary on the First Geneva Convention, 2016*, Common Art. 3, para. 611.
45. ICTY, Tadić Trial Judgment, 1997, para. 748.

46. ICRC, *Commentary on the First Geneva Convention, 2016*, Common Art. 3, para. 668. See ICC Statute, Footnote 57 relating to Article 8(2)(c)(ii) and UN Human Rights Council, Advisory Committee, Fourth Session, January 25–29, 2010, Study on best practices on the issue of missing persons, UN Doc.A/HRC/AC/4/CRP.2/Rev.1, January 25, 2010, paras. 66–71.
47. ICC Statute, Footnote 57 relating to Article 8(2)(c)(ii).
48. ICRC, *Commentary on the First Geneva Convention*, 2016, Art. 3, footnote 541.
49. GC I–IV, Art. 3(1)(c); AP II, Art. 4(2)(e); ICRC, CIHL Study, Rule 113; ICC Statute, Footnote 57 relating to Article 8(2)(c)(ii)).
50. ICRC, *Commentary on the First Geneva Convention, 2016*, Art. 3, para. 611 and 668; ICC Statute, Footnote 57 relating to Article 8(2)(c)(ii).
51. Petrig (2009), p. 350; ICRC, CIHL Study, Rule 113, interpretation.
52. See Australia, *War Crimes Act*, 1945, Section 3(xxxiv) and (xxxv); Australia, *ICC (Consequential Amendments) Act*, 2002, Schedule 1, paras. 268.58(2) and 268.74(2) and Ethiopia, *Criminal Code*, 2004, Art. 275.
53. ICRC, CIHL Study, Rule 113; GCI, Art. 15(1); GCII, Art. 18 (1); GCIV, Art. 16(2); API, Art. 34(1); APII, Art. 8(2).
54. ICRC, CIHL Study, explanation to Rule 113.
55. Gaggioli (2018), p. 187.
56. Pictet (1952).
57. See US Military Tribunal at Nuremberg, *Pohl case*, Judgment, November 3, 1947, which said that "Robbing the dead, even without the added offence of killing, is and always has been a crime. And when it is organized and planned and carried out on a hundred-million-mark scale, it becomes an aggravated crime, and anyone who takes part in it is a criminal."
58. ICRC, CIHL Study, explanation to Rule 113. See for instance Albania, *Military Penal Code*, 1995, Art. 91–93; Algeria, *Code of Military Justice*, 1971, Art. 287; Chad, *Code of Military Justice*, 1962, Art. 62.
59. Petrig (2009), Sandoz, Swinarski and Zimmermann (eds.), *Commentary on the Additional Protocols of 1977*, Art. 34, para. 1307.
60. GCIII, Art. 13 and GCIV, Art. 27.
61. ICRC, Sandoz, Swinarski and Zimmermann (eds), *Commentary on the Additional Protocols of 1977*, Art. 34, para. 1307.
62. ECtHR, *Akpinar and Altun v. Turkey*, no. 56760/00, February 27, 2007, para. 82.
63. See ECtHR, *Akpinar and Altun v. Turkey*, no. 56760/00, February 27, 2007; ECtHR, *Sabanchiyeva and Others v. Russia*, no. 38450/05, June 6, 2013; and ECtHR, *Akkum and Others v. Turkey*, no. 21894/93, June 24, 2005. See also Last Rights, "The Dead, the Missing and the Bereaved at Europe's International Borders, Proposal for a Statement of the International legal obligations of States," May 2017, p. 5.
64. E.g. IACtHR, *Case of the 19 Merchants v. Colombia*, Judgment, July 5, 2004, para. 210.
65. Qur'ān: 95:4. This and other Qur'ānic texts 20:55; 77:25–26 make it clear that dead bodies are to be buried.
66. See ḥadīth number 24783 in Ibn Ḥanbal (n.d.), vol. 6, p. 105; ḥadīth number 2307 in Ibn al-Ash'ath Abū Dāwūd (n.d.), vol. 3, p. 212; Ibn Aḥmad ibn Sa'īd ibn Ḥazm (n.d.), vol. 5, p. 166, vol. 11, p. 40; Ibn Sharaf al-Nawawī (1997), vol. 5, p. 263; http://www.alifta.net/Fatawa/fatawaDetails.aspx?languagename=en&BookID=7&View=Page&PageNo=1&PageID=3094.
67. Aman Andrabi (2018), p. 114.

68. See Ibn al-Ḥassan al-Shaybānī (1997), vol. 1, p. 79.
69. M. ibn Anas, *Al-Muwaṭṭa'*, above note 34, vol. 2, p. 448.
70. See Ibn Aḥmad ibn Abī Sahl al-Sarakhsī (n.d.), vol. 9, pp. 135, 196, vol. 10, pp. 129, 131, vol. 16, p. 145, vol. 26, p. 175.
71. Quoted in 'A. Ṣaqr, above note 2, p. 57.
72. ICRC, CIHL Study, Rule 115. See also GCI, Art. 17; GCII, Art. 20; GCIII, Art. 120; GCIV, Art. 130; API, Art. 34(1) and (2); APII, Art. 8.
73. ICRC, *Commentary on the First Geneva Convention*, 2016, Art. 17, para. 1684.
74. ICRC, *Commentary on the First Geneva Convention*, 2016, Art. 17, para. 1655.
75. GCI, Art. 17(1–2); GC II, Art. 20(2); GC III, Art. 120(5); GCIV, Art. 130(2).
76. GCI, Art. 17(1–2); GC II, Art. 20(2); GC III, Art. 120(5); GCIV, Art. 130(2). See also ICRC, CIHL Study, explanation to Rule 115 and ICRC, *Commentary on the First Geneva Convention*, 2016, Art. 17, para. 1647.
77. ICRC, *Commentary on the First Geneva Convention*, 2016, Art. 17, paras., 1675–1676.
78. Art. 17(2); GC II, Art. 20(2); GCIII, Art. 120(5); GCIV, Art. 130(2); and ICRC, CIHL Study, explanation to Rule 115.
79. ICRC, *Commentary on the First Geneva Convention*, 2016, Art. 17, para. 1678.
80. ICRC, *Commentary on the First Geneva Convention*, 2016, Art. 17, para. 1678.
81. ICRC, *Commentary on the First Geneva Convention*, 2016, Art. 17, para. 1680.
82. GCI, Art. 17(1); GCII, Art. 20(1); GCIII, Art. 120(5); GC IV, Art. 130(2). ICRC, *Commentary on the First Geneva Convention*, 2016, Art. 17, para. 1648.
83. GCI, Art. 17(1); GCII, Art. 20(1); GCIII, Art. 120(5); GC IV, Art. 130(2). ICRC, *Commentary on the First Geneva Convention*, 2016, Art. 17, para. 1651.
84. GCI, Art. 17(3); GCIII, Art. 120(4); GCIV, Art. 130(1); and ICRC, CIHL Study, explanation to Rule 115.
85. ICRC, *Commentary on the First Geneva Convention*, 2016, Art. 17, para. 1686.
86. ICRC, *Commentary on the First Geneva Convention*, 2016, Art. 17, para 1679.
87. ICPPED, Art. 15 and Art. 24(3).
88. See for instance IACtHR, *Río Negro Massacres v. Guatemala,* September 4, 2012, paras. 156–158.
89. IACtHR, *Juan Humberto Sánchez v. Honduras,* Judgment June 7, 2003, para. 102.
90. IACtHR, *Bámaca-Velásquez v. Guatemala,* Judgment November 5, 2000, para. 174.
91. IACtHR, *Río Negro Massacres v. Guatemala,* September 4, 2012, paras. 156–158.
92. Israel, High Court of Justice, *Physicians for Human Rights v. Commander of IDF Forces in the Gaza Strip,* Judgment, May 30, 2004, para. 27, available at: https://versa.cardozo.yu.edu/sites/default/files/upload/opinions/Physicians%20for%20Human%20Rights%20v.%20IDF%20Commander%20in%20Gaza.pdf.
93. *Ibid.*
94. GCI, Art. 17; GCII, Art. 20; GCIII, Art. 120; GCIV, Art. 130; and ICRC, CIHL Study, explanation to Rule 115.
95. ICRC, CIHL Study, Rule 115.
96. Al-'Umarī, above note 23, pp. 259–275.
97. Al-'Umarī, above note 23, pp. 276–289.
98. See, for example, fatwa number 1896 issued by Dar al-Ifta of Egypt on June 26, 2001: https://www.dar-alifta.org/Foreign/ViewArticle.aspx?ID=8348&CategoryID=1; fatwa number 17513 issued by the General Presidency of Scholarly Research and Ifta in the Kingdom of Saudi Arabia: http://www.alifta.net/Search/ResultDetails.aspx?languagename=ar&lang=ar&view=result&fatwaNum=&FatwaNumID=&ID=12862&searchSco

pe=3&SearchScopeLevels1=&SearchScopeLevels2=&highLight=1&SearchType=exact&SearchMoesar=false&bookID=&LeftVal=0&RightVal=0&simple=&SearchCriteria=allwords&PagePath=&siteSection=1&searchkeyword=2161732161772171300322161722161712161710322161672171322171332171362161702171 37#firstKeyWordFound; fatwa number 87734 issued by the Assembly of Muslim Jurists of America's Resident Fatwa Committee: https://www.amjaonline.org/fatwa/en/87734/the-rights-of-the-muslims-who-die-with-covid-19-on-the-muslim-community; fatwa issued by the Islamic High Council of Australia: http://www.darulfatwa.org.au/ar/%D8%AD%D9%83%D9%85-%D8%A5%D8%AD%D8%B1%D8%A7%D9%82-%D8%AC%D8%AB%D9%85%D8%A7%D9%86-%D8%A7%D9%84%D9%85%D8%B3%D9%84%D9%85/.

99. http://www.dar-alifta.gov.eg/ar/ViewFatwa.aspx?sec=fatwa&ID=13425.

100. http://www.elnabaa.net/632207.

101. Ibn Muḥammad ibn Aḥmad ibn al-Ikhwah (n.d.), p. 106; 'A. Ibn al-Saḥaybānī, above note 35, p. 218; fatwā number 4263 given by the current Grand Mufti of Egypt on January 24, 2018, available at: http://www.dar-alifta.gov.eg/ar/ViewFatwa.aspx?ID=14229&LangID=1.

102. M. Ibn al-Ikhwah, above note 38, p. 106. See also 'A. Ibn al-Saḥaybānī, above note 35, p. 223.

103. M. Ibn al-Ikhwah, above note 38, p. 106. See also 'A. Ibn al-Saḥaybānī, above note 35, p. 231.

104. M. Ibn al-Ikhwah, above note 38, p. 106. See also 'A. Ibn al-Saḥaybānī, above note 35, p. 229.

105. M. Ibn al-Ikhwah, above note 38, p. 106. See also 'A. Ibn al-Saḥaybānī, above note 35, p. 236.

106. See fatwā number 66120 issued by the Fatwā Centre affiliated to the Qatari Ministry of Endowments (Awqaf) and Religious Affairs, available at: http://fatwa.islamweb.net/fatwa/index.php?page=showfatwa&Option=FatwaId&Id=66120.

107. GCI, Art. 17(3); GCIII, Art. 120(4); GCIV, Art. 130(1); API, Art. 34(1); and ICRC, CIHL Study, Rule 115.

108. API, Art. 34(2); Petrig (2009) p. 344.

109. ICRC, *Commentary on the First Geneva Convention*, 2016, Art. 17, para. 1687.

110. ICRC, *Commentary on the First Geneva Convention*, 2016, Art. 17, para. 1689.

111. GCI, Art. 17; GCII, Art. 20; GCIII Art. 120; GCIV, Art. 130; API, Art. 34(1–3); and ICRC, CIHL Study, Rule 115.

112. GCI, Art. 17(3); GCII, Art. 20(2); GCIII, Art. 120(4); GCIV, Art. 130(1 and 3); API, Art. 34(1–3); and ICRC, CIHL Study, Rules 115 and 116.

113. ICRC, *Commentary on the First Geneva Convention*, 2016, Art. 17, paras. 1692, 1695, and 1696. See also Anna Petrig, "The war dead and their gravesites," IRRC, vol. 91, No. 874, 2009, p. 346.

114. See, for example, 'A. Ibn al-Saḥaybānī, above note 35, pp. 147–212.

115. http://www.dar-alifta.gov.eg/ar/ViewFatwa.aspx?ID=14347&LangID=1.

116. GCI, Art. 17(3); GCIII, Art. 120(6); and API Art. 34(4). See ICRC, Sandoz, Swinarski and Zimmermann (eds.), *Commentary on the Additional Protocols of 1977*, Art. 34, p. 377, paras. 1354–1362 and Petrig (2009), p. 360.

117. API, Art. 34(4). See ICRC, Sandoz, Swinarski and Zimmermann (eds.), *Commentary on the Additional Protocols of 1977*, Art. 34, p. 377, paras. 1354–1362.

118. *Ibid.*

119. *Ibid.*
120. *Ibid.*
121. *Ibid.*
122. API, Art. 34(4). See ICRC, Sandoz, Swinarski and Zimmermann (eds.), *Commentary on the Additional Protocols of 1977*, Art. 34, , p. 377, paras. 1354–1362. See also ICRC, CIHL Study, explanation to Rule 116; and Petrig (2009), p. 361.
123. ICRC, CIHL Study, explanation to Rule 116.
124. *Ibid.*
125. Last Rights, "The Dead, the Missing and the Bereaved at Europe's International Borders, Proposal for a Statement of the International legal obligations of States," May 2017, p. 11.
126. ECtHR, *Satabayeva v. Russia*, no. 21486/06, November 29, 2009, para. 126.
127. IACtHR, *Río Negro Massacre v. Guatemala*, September 4, 2012, para 217.
128. IACtHR, *Río Negro Massacre v. Guatemala*, September 4, 2012, paras 217 and 268.
129. See Kuwaiti Ministry of Awqaf and Islamic Affairs, above note 51, vol. 40, p. 25.
130. See Ibn al-Ḥussein ibn 'Ali al-Bayhaqī (1994), vol. 4, p. 58; Ibn al-Saḥaybānī:above note 35, p. 494.
131. *Ibid.*
132. Al-Ghazālī (1997), vol. 2, p. 390; Ibn al-Ikhwah, above note 38, p. 106. It is worth adding here that the jurists Ashhab and Saḥnūn from the Māliki school of law prohibit performing the funeral prayer at the grave, see 'A. Ibn al-Saḥaybānī, above note 35, p. 350.
133. See ḥadīth number 3088 in Abū Dāwūd, above note 3, vol. 3, p. 181.
134. See, for example, M. al-Ghazālī, above note 74, vol. 2, p. 390; Ḥ. Shurunbulālī, *Kitāb nūr al-Iḍāḥ*, above note 75, p. 98; M. Ibn al-Ikhwah, above note 38, p. 106.
135. 'A. Ibn al-Saḥaybānī, above note 35, p. 492.
136. 'A. Ibn al-Saḥaybānī, above note 35, p. 493.
137. GCI, Art. 17(3); GCIII, Art. 120(6); GCIV, Article 130(2); API, Article 34(2–3); and ICRC, CIHL Study, Rule 114.
138. GCI, Art. 16(4); GCII, Art. 19(3); GCIII, Art. 122(9); GCIV, Art. 139; AP I, Art. 34(2); and ICRC, CIHL Study, Rule 114.
139. ICRC, *Commentary on the First Geneva Convention*, 2016, Art. 17, para. 1645. See also Gavshon (2015).
140. *Ibid.*
141. ICRC, *Commentary on the First Geneva Convention*, 2016, Art. 17, para. 1644.
142. ICRC, *Commentary on the First Geneva Convention*, 2016, Art. 17, para. 1645.
143. Sandoz Y, Swinarski C, and Zimmermann B. (eds.), *Commentary on the Additional Protocols of 1977*, Art. 34, paras. 1345–1346.
144. In some NIACs today, the dead find themselves in countries to which they are not nationals (e.g. cases for foreign fighters).
145. ICRC, CIHL Study, explanation to Rule 114.
146. EctHR, *Maskhadova and Others v. Russia*, No. 18071/05, June 6, 2013.
147. ECtHR, *Girard v. France*, No. 22590/04, June 30, 2011.
148. EctHR, *Maskhadova and Others v. Russia*, No. 18071/05, June 6, 2013 and EctHR, *Sabanchiyeva and Others v. Russia*, No. 38450/05, June 6, 2013.
149. IACtHR, *García and Family Members v. Guatemala*, November 29, 2012.
150. See ḥadīth number 2727 in Ibn Ismā'īl al-Bukhārī (1987), vol. 3, p. 1056; Al-Zuḥaylī (2010), vol. 7, p. 437.

151. See Ibn Isḥāq (2000), vol. 3, p. 123 f.; Guillaume (1955), 450–460; Ibn 'Alī ibn Ḥajar al-'Asqalānī (n.d.), vol. 6, p. 283; ḥadīth number 1715 in Ibn 'Isā al-Tirmidhī (n.d.), vol. 4, p. 214; Al-Wafā (2006), p. 297.
152. GCI, Art. 16(3); GCII, Art. 19(3); GCIII, Art. 122(9); GCIV, Art. 139; ICRC, CIHL Study, Rule 114.
153. ICRC, *Commentary on the First Geneva Convention*, 2016, Art. 16, para. 1618.
154. GCI, Art. 16(3); GCII, Art. 19(3); GCIII, Art. 122(9); GCIV, Art. 139; ICRC, CIHL Study, Rule 114. See also ICRC, *Commentary on the First Geneva Convention*, 2016, Art. 16, para. 1616.
155. GCI, Art. 16(4).
156. ICRC, *Commentary on the First Geneva Convention*, 2016, Art. 16, para. 1612.
157. GCI, Art. 16(3); GCII, Art. 19(3); GCIII, Art. 122(9); GCIV, Art. 139; ICRC, CIHL Study, explanation to Rule 114.
158. See Concise Oxford English Dictionary (2011), p. 1202 and ICRC, *Commentary on the First Geneva Convention*, 2016, Art. 16, para. 1623.
159. ICRC, *Commentary on the First Geneva Convention*, 2016, Art. 16, para. 1623.
160. ICRC, *Commentary on the First Geneva Convention*, 2016, Art. 16, para 1625.
161. ECtHR, *Vasilescu v. Romania*, No. 27053/95, May 22, 1998, Reports of Judgments and Decisions 1998-III, paras. 44–55. See also Last Rights, "The Dead, the Missing and the Bereaved at Europe's International Borders, Proposal for a Statement of the International legal obligations of States," May 2017, pp. 10–11.
162. ICRC, CIHL Study, explanation to Rule 114 and State practice. See for instance procedure by Coroners Court in Australia available at: http://www.coroners.justice.nsw.gov.au/Pages/what_happens_process/first_steps/personal_belongings.aspx
163. Qur'ān 8:41.
164. W. al-Zuḥaylī, above note 6, vol. 7, p. 614.
165. See, for example, Ibn Ibrāhīm al-Anṣārī (n.d.), p. 48; Ibn al-Ḥasan al-Shaybānī (n.d.), vol. 4, pp. 1206, 1208, 1239; Ibn Idrīs al-Shāfi'ī (1973), vol. 4, pp. 251, 262, vol. 7, pp. 336, 345.
166. The instructions of the Second Caliph 'Umar ibn al-Khaṭṭāb to his soldiers to "fear God in the farmers" means beware of deliberately targeting non-combatant farmers because this will incur the punishment of God. Ibn Aḥmad ibn Muḥammad ibn Rushd (n.d.), vol. 1, p. 281; Ibn Aḥmad ibn Qudāmah (1984), vol. 9, p. 251; Peters (1996), p. 35.
167. See Al-Dawoody (2011), p. 164; Ibn al-Ḥasan al-Shaybānī (1975), p. 229; Ibn Qudāmah, above note 20, vol. 9, p. 11; Al-Qādir (2005), vol. I, p. 119; Abou El Fadl (2006), p. 238.
168. On the importance of national implementation of IHL regarding missing persons see Londoño and Signoret (2017). See also OAS, General Assembly Res. AG/RES 2961 (L-O/20), "Promotion and Protection of Human Rights," October 20–21, 2020.

References

Abou El Fadl, K. (2006). *Rebellion and Violence in Islamic Law*, paperback e. Cambridge: Cambridge University Press.

Abū al-Wafā, A. (2006). *Al-Naẓariyyah al-'Āmmah lil-Qānūn al-Dawlī al-Insānī fī al-Qānūn al-Dawlī wa fī al-Sharī'ah al-Islāmiyyah*. Cairo: Dār al-Nahḍah al-'Arabiyyah.

Al-Dawoody, A. (2011). *The Islamic Law of War: Justifications and Regulations.* Palgrave Series in Islamic Theology, Law, and History, Vol. **2**. New York: Palgrave Macmillan.
Al-Dīn 'Abd Allah ibn Aḥmad ibn Qudāmah, M. (1984). *Al-Mughnī: Fī Fiqh al-Imām Aḥmad Ibn Ḥanbal al-Shaybānī.* Beirut: Dār al-Fikr.
Al-Ghazālī, M. (1997). In: *Al-Waṣīṭ fī al-Madhhab* (eds. A. Maḥmūd Ibrāhīm and M. Muḥammad Tāmir). Cairo: Dār al-Salām.
Al-Khatīb al-Shirbīnī, M. (n.d.). *Mughnī al-Muḥtāj ilā Ma'rifah Ma'ānī Alfāẓ al-Minhāj.* Beirut: Dār al-Fikr.
Al-Ra'ūūf al-Minawī, A. (1937). *Fayḍ al-Qadīr Sharḥ al-Jāmi' al-Ṣaghīr.* Cairo: Al-Maktabah al-Tujāriyyah al-Kubrā.
Al-Wafā, A. (2006). *Al-Naẓariyyah al-'Āmmah lil-Qānūn al-Dawlī al-Insānī fī al-Qānūn al-Dawlī wa fī al-Sharī'ah al-Islāmiyyah.* Cairo: Dār al-Nahḍah al-'Arabiyyah.
Al-Zuḥaylī, W. (2010). *Mawsū'ah al-Fiqh al-Islāmī wa al-Qaḍāyā al-Mu'āṣirah.* Damascus: Dār al-Fikr.
Aman Andrabi, A. (2018). Medical ethics within the Islamic tradition and the specific issues in the modern scientific era. *International Journal of Multidisciplinary Research and Development* **5**(2).
Baranowska, G. (2017). Advances and progress in the obligation to return the remains of missing and forcibly disappeared persons. *International Review of the Red Cross* **99**(905).
Gaggioli, G. (2018). International humanitarian law: The legal framework for humanitarian forensic action. *Forensic Science International* **282**: 187.
Gavshon, D. (2015). The dead. In: *The 1949 Geneva Conventions: A Commentary*, 1 e. Oxford: Oxford University Press.
Guillaume, A. (trans.) (1955). *The Life of Muhammad: A Translation of Isḥāq's Sīrat Rasūl Allāh.* Oxford: Oxford University Press.
Henckaerts, J.-M. and Doswald-Beck, L. (eds.) (2005). *Customary International Humanitarian Law. Vol. I: Rules.* Cambridge: Cambridge University Press. https://www.icrc.org/customary-ihl/eng/docs/v1 (accessed 2022).
Ibn 'Abd al-Raḥīm al-Mubarkāfūrī, A. (n.d.). *Tuḥfah al-Aḥwadhī bi-Sharḥ Jāmi' al-Tirmidhī.* Beirut: Dār al-Kutub al-'Ilmiyyah.
Ibn 'Umar Al-Dāraqutnī, A. (2004). In: *Sunan al-Dāraqutnī* (eds. S.'a. al-Arna'ūṭ, Ḥassan, '.A. al-Mun'im Shalabī, and S.'i. al-Laḥām). Beirut: Mu'assasah al-Risālah.
Ibn Aḥmad ibn Abī Sahl al-Sarakhsī, M. (n.d.). *Kitāb al-Mabsūt.* Beirut: Dār al-Ma'rifah.
Ibn Aḥmad ibn Muḥammad ibn Rushd, M. (n.d.). *Bidāyah al-Mujtahid wa Nihāyah al-Muqtaṣid.* Beirut: Dār al-Fikr.
Ibn Aḥmad ibn Sa'īd ibn Ḥazm, A. (n.d.). In: *Al-Muhallā* (ed. Committee of the Revival of Arabic Heritage). Dār al-Āfāq al-Jadīdah: Beirut.
Ibn al-Ash'ath Abū Dāwūd, S. (n.d.). In: *Sunan Abī Dāwūd* (ed. Muḥammad Muḥyī al-Dīn 'Abd al-Ḥamīd). Beirut: Dār al-Fikr.
Ibn al-Ḥajjāj al-Qushayrī, M. (n.d.). In: *Ṣaḥīḥ Muslim* (ed. Muḥammad Fū'ād 'Abd al-Bāqī). Beirut: Dār Iḥyā' al-Turāth al-'Arabī.
Ibn al-Ḥasan al-Shaybānī, M. (n.d.). In: *Al-Siyar al-Kabīr* (ed. Ṣalāḥ al-Dīn al-Munjid). Cairo: Ma'had al-Makhṭūṭāt.
Ibn al-Ḥassan al-Shaybānī, M. (1975). In: *Al-Siyar* (ed. M. Khadduri). Beirut: Al-Dār al-Muttaḥidah.
Ibn al-Ḥassan al-Shaybānī, M. (1997). In: *Sharḥ Kitāb al-Siyar al-Kabīr* (commentary by Muḥammad ibn Aḥmad al-Sarakhsī (ed. Abī Abdullah Muḥammad Ḥassan Muḥammad Hassan Ismā'il al-Shafi'ī). Beirut: Dār al-Kutub al-'Ilmiyyah.

Ibn al-Ḥussein ibn 'Ali al-Bayhaqī, A. (1994). In: *Sunan al-Bayhaqī al-Kubrā* (ed. Muḥammad 'Abd al-Qādir 'Aṭṭā). Mecca: Dār al-Bāz.

Ibn 'Alī ibn Ḥajar al-'Asqalānī, A. (n.d.). In: *Fatḥ al-Bārī Sharhḥ Ṣaḥīḥ al-Bukhārī* (ed. Muḥib al-Dīn al-Khaṭīb). Beirut: Dār al-Ma'rifah.

Ibn Ḥanbal, A. (n.d.). *Musnad al-Imām Aḥmad Ibn Ḥanbal.* Cairo: Mu'assasah Qurṭubah.

Ibn Idrīs al-Shāfi'ī, M. (1973). *Al-Umm*, 2 e. Beirut: Dār al-Ma'rifah.

Ibn 'Isā al-Tirmidhī, M. (n.d.). In: *Al-Jāmi' al-Ṣaḥīh Sunan al-Tirmidhī* (eds. A. Muḥammad Shākir et al.). Beirut: Dār Iḥyā' al-Turāth al-'Arabī.

Ibn Isḥāq, M. (2000). In: *Al-Sīrah al-Nabawiyyah* (ed. 'Abd al-Malik ibn Hishām), annotated by Fu'ād ibn 'Alī Ḥāfiẓ. Beirut: Dār al-Kutub al-'Ilmiyyah.

Ibn Ismā'īl al-Bukhārī, M. (1987). In: *Al-Jāmi' al-Ṣaḥīḥ al-Mukhtaṣar* (ed. Muṣṭafā Dīb al-Baghā), 3 e. Damascus/Beirut: Dār ibn Kathīr.

Ibn Jarīr al-Ṭabarī, M. (n.d.). *Tarīkh al-Ṭabarī.* Beirut: Dār al-Kutub al-'Ilmiyyah.

Ibn Muḥammad ibn Abī Shaybah, A. (1998). In: *Al-Kitāb al-Muṣannaf fī al-Aḥādīth wa al-Āthār* (ed. Kamāl Yūsuf al-Ḥūt). Riyadh: Maktabah al-Rushd.

Ibn Muḥammad ibn Aḥmad ibn al-Ikhwah, M.eds. M. Maḥmūd Sha'bān and Ṣ. Aḥmad 'Isā al-Muṭī'ī *M'ālim al-Qurbah fī Ṭalab al-Ḥisbah.* Cairo: Al-Hay'ah al-'Āmmah lil-Kitāb.

Ibn Muḥammad ibn Ḥabīb al-Māwardī, A. (1985). *Kitāb al-Aḥkām al-Sulṭāniyyah wa al-Wilāyāt al-Dīniyyah.* Beirut: Dār al-Kutub al-'Ilmiyyah.

Ibn Sharaf al-Nawawī, M. (1997). *Al-Majmū'*. Beirut: Dār al-Fikr.

Ibrāhīm al-Anṣārī, I. (n.d.). In: *Al-Radd 'alā Siyar al-Awzā'ī* (ed. Abū al-Wafā al-Afghānī). Beirut: Dār al-Kutub al-'Ilmiyyah.

ICRC (2004). What is international humanitarian law? Advisory Service Factsheet, Geneva, ICRC, p. 1. https://www.icrc.org/eng/assets/files/other/what_is_ihl.pdf

ICRC (2020). Humanity after life: Respecting and protecting the dead. Advisory Services Fact-sheet, *ICRC*, Geneva, p. 4. https://www.icrc.org/en/document/humanity-after-life-respect-and-protection-dead

Londoño, X. and Signoret, A.O. (2017). Implementing international law: An avenue for preventing disappearances, resolving cases of missing persons and addressing the needs of their families. *IRRC* **99**(2): 551–552.

Mohammed, M. and Kharoshah, M.A. (2014). Autopsy in Islam and current practice in Arab Muslim countries. *Journal of Forensic and Legal Medicine.* **23**: 80–83.

Oxford University (2011). *Concise Oxford English Dictionary*, 12 e. Oxford: Oxford University Press.

Peters, R. (1996). *Jihad in Classical and Modern Islam.* Markus Wiener: Princeton, NJ.

Petrig, A. (2009). The war dead and their gravesites. *International Review of the Red Cross* **91**: 874.

Jean Pictet (ed.) *The Geneva Conventions of 12 August 1949: Commentary, Vol. I (Geneva Convention for the Amelioration of the Condition of the Wounded and Sick in Armed Forces in the Field)*, 1952, para. 152

Sassòli, M. (2019). In: *International Humanitarian Law, Rules, Controversies, and Solutions to Problems Arising in Warfare* (eds. A. Clapham, P. Gaeta, and M. Sassòli). Cheltenham/Northampton: Edward Elgar Publishing.

Sassòli, M. and Tougas, M.-L. (2002). The ICRC and the missing. *International Review of the Red Cross* **84**(848).

Sheikh, A. (1998). Death and dying—a muslim perspective. *Journal of the Royal Society of Medicine.* **91**(3): 138–140. doi: 10.1177/014107689809100307.

CHAPTER 13

Unmaking forgotten mass graves and honorable burials: engaging with the Spanish civil war legacy[1]

Francisco Ferrándiz

Institute for Language, Literature and Anthropology (ILLA), Center for Human and Social Sciences (CCHS), Spanish National Research Council (CSIC)

13.1 Overture

This chapter is based on a 20-year-long ethnography of mass grave exhumations in contemporary Spain and deals with the tortuous, painful, much-disputed, and incomplete unmaking of a concrete and massive militaristic inscription of Spain, which related to its last internal war (1936–1939) and subsequent dictatorship (1939–1975).[2] To understand the intricacy of this process and its historical roots, it first dissects the formation of a *funerary apartheid* in the country since the end of the war,[3] where the dictatorial regime increasingly forced the corpses of the winners and losers to inhabit two quite dissimilar *spaces of death* (Taussig 1987), as necropolitics became a salient feature in the architecture of national sovereignty (Mbembe 2003; Verdery 1999).

Second, it analyzes the shocking impact on the social fabric of the mass grave exhumations of Republican civilians that started in the year 2000, as part of a broader social movement, challenging the impunity of Francoist crimes. Franco's forgotten victims, in the form of unburied wounded skeletons, started posing uncomfortable questions about the scope and depth of Franco's legacy and the enduring impunity machine still covering it up decades after his death. This bottom-up process, initially driven by the grandchildren of those defeated in the war, defied public institutions and the judicial system's capacity to respond, and provoked surprising aftereffects that have brought to light profound contradictions in Spain's relationship with its Civil War past.

Anthropology of Violent Death: Theoretical Foundations for Forensic Humanitarian Action, First Edition. Edited by Roberto C. Parra and Douglas H. Ubelaker.

Third, as one crucial consequence, the chapter traces how these politically charged twenty-first-century disinterments came to intersect with Spain's most prominent Francoist stronghold, the Valley of the Fallen (recently renamed as Valley of Cuelgamuros in the 20/2022 Democratic Memory Law), and started to threaten both its patrimonial integrity, the status of its huge Civil War cemetery, and, very importantly, the dictator's resting place behind the monument's main altar. The disturbing finding that Republican civilians executed in the war could also be found in its subterranean crypts, ignited a debate over the monument's *status*. The pressure to remove Franco's body from El Valle has unsettled the war-derived funerary hierarchy established during Francoism, especially the priority accorded to burial sites of other prominent generals participating in the 1936 coup d'état, whom public opinion growingly perceives as perpetrators of crimes against humanity (Ferrándiz 2014, pp. 205–259, 2022; Garibian 2016).

This demilitarization process does not mean that Spain departs in any significant way from broader transnational processes where largely patriarchal military logics, technologies, and imaginaries increasingly seep into other non-military dimensions of social life, right into the most intimate spaces of experience, creating tenacious reverberations and resisting undoing (Enloe 2007; Lutz 2001). In fact, rolling back militarization by dismantling war-derived cartographies of death using forensic protocols, challenging military burial arrangements, or degrading statues of generals necessarily involves a certain level of remilitarizing by other means. I call this mirroring and deeply embodied memorial backfiring *phantom militarism*.

As argued throughout the chapter, this reflective militarism infiltrates the political memorial cultures accompanying the historical memory process, inevitably drenched by the warmongering traces, logics, and narratives unveiled in forensic grave disclosure based on crime scenes (Crossland 2002; Dziuban 2017; Iturriaga 2022; Renshaw 2011) – which mostly highlight modalities of perpetration, obscuring alternate narratives of those executed – or in the professional military careers and historically proven cruelty of rebel leaders under critical public scrutiny (Cazorla 2014; Preston 1993).

These ghostly resonances of the multiple manifestations of a specific military apparatus are not just spectral or metaphorical yet socially determinant forces. They are also grounded in concrete forms of materiality, be they injured skeletons, grandiose monuments, or authoritative statues. (González-Ruibal 2016; Gordon 1997; Kwon 2008; Labanyi 2002; Winter 1995). It is the resilience or fragility of this phantom militarism in the long term that marks the success or failure of a demilitarization process.

13.2 On Funerary Militarism

The Spanish Civil War, originating in a military rebellion against the democratically elected Republican government on July 18, 1936, lasted for almost three years, leaving around 500 000 Spaniards dead. Around 300 000 were killed in combat, and up to 200 000 civilians were executed. These figures are only estimates, as there is still disagreement over casualties among historians, certain regions are understudied, and many data are still missing or difficult to access. As for the massive execution of civilians during the conflict, contemporary historiography places the numbers at around 55 000 killed in the Republican-controlled zone and as many as 150 000 in the rebel Nationalist zone during the war and the repression of the early postwar years (Ferrándiz 2013; Rodrigo 2008). To this figure, Preston (2012, p. 17) adds a further 20 000 executions after the war, not counting those who died from hunger and disease while trapped in a dense network of jails and concentration camps.

The killing sprees in the Republican and Nationalist zones were dramatic but differed significantly in numbers and scale. For Juliá, "in the rebellious zone, repression and death had to do with the building of a new power; in the loyalist [to the Republic], repression and death were related to the collapse of any power" (1999, pp. 25–26). The main instigator and leader of the military uprising until his death in a plane crash in June 1937, General Emilio Mola, openly referred to the insurgents' plan in a meeting with Municipal Mayors in Navarra right after the coup: "It is crucial to create an atmosphere of terror . . . We have to establish an overwhelming feeling of dominion eliminating without any scruple or reservation all those who do not think like us. No cowardice is allowed. If we hesitate and do not proceed with the utmost vigor, we will not win. Anybody hiding or protecting a communist or a Popular Front supporter [the left-wing coalition that won the 1936 elections] shall be executed" (Preston 2012, p. 253). Drawing on Mola's instructions and subsequent War Edicts, radio broadcasts by coup leaders, and archival evidence, particularly death certificates and the bureaucratic records of "kangaroo military courts" ***(Consejos de guerra),*** historian Javier Rodrigo also argues that there were "crucial differences between the repressive actions on civilians carried out behind the front lines in Republican and Nationalist zones" (2008, pp. 42–49; see also Casanova, 1999, pp. 159–177). According to Rodrigo, the violence exercised by the Francoists responded to a "well-designed terror investment associated with a profoundly militaristic blood pedagogy, designed to paralyze the opponent during the war and inhibit any political or military response in its aftermath" (2008, p. 95, 73).

After the war ended on April 1, 1939, Franco shifted his attention from open battleground conflict and extensive rearguard killing to other forms of repression and containment of the enemy in jails and concentration camps as well as to trials, purges, forced labor, evictions, expropriation of property, and so on (Gómez Bravo 2017; Preston 1993; Rodrigo 2005). But he also looked to celebration, commemoration, and, very important for the core argument of this chapter, honorable relocation of those who were killed on the nationalist side, both on the frontlines or in the rearguard. During the early postwar years, the State issued abundant funerary legislation specifically affecting the corpses claimed by the dictatorship. Meanwhile, the bodies of the defeated – expelled from the legitimate community of the war dead as "reds," "Marxist hordes," and ultimately "traitors" to their country – continued to accumulate in mass graves and remained outside lawmaking, ignored, and excluded from the triumphant military–political–religious project of a New Spain. The formation of a *funerary apartheid*, establishing asymmetrical connections between territory and necropower, therefore became a cornerstone in the construction of dictatorial sovereign control of the country (Mbembe 2003; Robben 2015).

The first wave of civilian exhumations took place immediately after the war, as part of the mourning for losses on the winning side, national reconstruction, and the organization of the new dictatorial militarized state. Both the military forces and core forensic institutions participated in hundreds of unburials and identifications, and the central government issued formal instructions to prevent spontaneous diggings (Ferrándiz 2014, pp. 145–155; Saqqa 2020; Solé i Barjau 2008, pp. 96–102). In an unparalleled high point in November 1939, José Antonio Primo de Rivera, the founder of *Falange* (Spain's main fascist party), was dramatically paraded for almost 500 km over 10 days as his coffin was carried on the shoulders of his followers from his tomb in Alicante to the Monastery of El Escorial, the most distinguished symbol of the Spanish Monarchy and Empire, where he was reburied in the Basilica above the Royal Pantheon (Box 2009). Many others were reburied with religious and military honors in local cemeteries, occupying visible priority pantheons that can still be seen today. Plaques with the names of those "Fallen for God and Spain" – always presided over by the name of Jose Antonio, "martyr of martyrs" – were placed outside church walls in almost every village in the country, refreshing a centuries-deep alliance between nation, military, and Catholic Church.

As years went by, in parallel with the consolidation of the dictatorship and the honorable relocation of the mass graves of the victors, the country underwent an exhaustive militarization of its public spaces. Monuments to the memory of Francoist war martyrs were inaugurated everywhere. Streets were named after military officials and heroes across Spain. The sites of heroic battles were preserved in ruins, transformed into symbols of resilience and triumph

(Viejo-Rose 2011, pp. 45–104). Roman-style equestrian statues of Franco were placed in prominent locations in Spanish cities. A Triumphal Arch commemorating the military victory was erected in one of Madrid's main gateways. If the three-year fratricidal war had not already generated enough combat, repression, executions, military operations, and long lines of terrorized civilians painfully shuffling into exile, Spain was now thoroughly re-inscribed by a militarized symbolic and political logic. The memorial choreography of the war dead took place within a pervasive official narrative of military victory anchored in the concepts of religious crusade, heroism, and martyrdom – known in Spanish political history as National Catholicism – where the cult to the *fallen* played a predominant role in refashioning the new political body (Aguilar 2000; Box 2009, 2010). Many of these pantheons, plaques, monuments, and other heterogeneous infrastructures are still in their original locations in contemporary Spain, albeit now heavily questioned by sectors on the political left (Rubin 2018, 2020).

In 1959, 20 years after the end of the conflict, a new wave of unburials was to stir the Civil War dead, reinscribing worn-out religious and militaristic notions of martyrdom, sacrifice, and patriotism in the corpses of many war winners and generating further funerary slippage between the death spaces of triumphant and defeated. Over two decades, more than 33 800 bodies, both military and civilian, were dug up from burial locations across Spain and transferred to subterranean crypts in the Valley of the Fallen (Ferrándiz 2022; Olmeda 2009). An early arrival was José Antonio Primo de Rivera, transferred from the Monastery of El Escorial and ceremoniously placed before the main altar. For 15 years, he presided over the monument on his own, as the side crypts were filled with thousands of bodies of diverse origin. It was an honor he was to share as of November 1975, when, after a heavily militarized state funeral, the Valley became the burial place of Franco himself, who was placed behind the main altar, creating a politically charged funerary axis with Primo de Rivera. The fact that both men had died on November 20, albeit 49 years apart, consolidated a powerful commemorative date for the victors. The arrival of the dictator's remains in *El Valle* unequivocally sealed the monument as Spain's chief Francoist stronghold. Although most were brought during the 1960s, bodies from all over the country continued to arrive in the Valley until 1983.

Meanwhile the vast majority of mass graves containing Republican loyalists – which continued to grow in the postwar as a result of a repression that lasted well beyond the limits of the formal conflict – remained abandoned in miscellaneous locations outside cemeteries (at times right outside the wall) or in "second-class" civil sections of formal burial grounds. This topography of death was initially the result of a funerary punishment meted out in addition to the killing of people who were thus expelled not only from the legitimate community of the living by means of summary executions but also from the community of the dead by inappropriate or dishonorable burial. These undignified graves, outside conventional funerary spaces and ignored by postwar reburial laws, carried an admonitory message to potential political dissidents. As decades passed, some of these unprotected mass graves slid progressively into public secrecy, while others simply vanished. In cemeteries, bones frequently ended up in mixed ossuaries during refurbishments and relocations. Meanwhile, an unknown number of outdoor mass graves have been destroyed under Spain's infrastructure modernization and real-estate development, which entailed freeways, high-speed trains, urban and rural development, and general landscape transformation.

Oral testimonies from elderly people suggest that a small number of graves were furtively opened by relatives during the war itself and the subsequent dictatorship, and the bodies clandestinely reburied in family pantheons in cemeteries. After Franco's death in 1975, relatives conducted many exhumations with little institutional or technical support and limited media attention, within the framework of the emerging political cultures accompanying the transition to democracy. These local unburials – some followed by massive reburials in municipal cemeteries – gave those defeated in the war a crucial glimpse of public visibility after decades of erasure affecting both the executed and the survivors and initiated the process of acknowledgment and commemoration of their decades-long suffering and marginalization (Aguilar 2017; Aguilar and Ferrándiz 2015; de Kerangat 2017; Mateo and de Kerangat 2020).

13.3 Franco's Militarist Imprint Under Siege

In his 1969 Christmas speech, approaching death, Franco reassured supporters that his militaristic legacy was *atado y bien atado* ("sewn up, all sewn up") with the recent designation by Parliament of Prince Juan Carlos de Borbón as his successor. A new monarchy was to emerge from his glorious military victory and dictatorial regime. There was at least some truth to this. His dictum is still recalled in public debates whenever a progressive initiative is successfully blocked or resisted by his political heirs. It is a fact that Spain is still struggling to get fully rid of the conspicuous traces of a dictatorial militarism dating back to the 1930s and that certain conservative forces that originated and flourished during Francoism remain strong in democratic guise, particularly in the political and legal arenas as well as in powerful sectors of the Catholic Church. Paradoxically, the armed forces, heavily reformed during the tenure of Socialist president Felipe González (1982–1996), are credited by international observers like Pablo de Greiff, UN's Special Rapporteur on the Promotion of Truth, Justice, Reparation, and Guarantees of Non-recurrence, with a more professional and politically neutral role, except for some vanishing – though tenacious – nostalgic right-wing pockets (2014, pp. 5–7).

To cut a complex debate short, in Spain's transition to democracy (1975–1982), the dominant driving force was that of reconciliation, and the crimes committed by the rebellious army and paramilitaries during the War, and later during Francoism, were purposefully "thrown into oblivion" for the sake of peaceful coexistence, as Santos Juliá, a highly influential Socialist historian, has put it (2003; Ferrándiz 2008). An Amnesty Law passed in 1977 secured impunity for Francoist crimes. Despite these major concessions by the descendants of the defeated, a failed military coup in 1981 – during which the Parliament was taken by Civil Guards during the investiture of Prime Minister Calvo Sotelo and the city of Valencia, occupied by tanks, was declared in a state of emergency – sent shivers down the collective spine, reminding the country that the army remained vigilant and ready to restore order if necessary. As years went by, Spain's transition, deemed exemplary across the world, was thoroughly studied by political scientists and even became a model to export (Aguilar 2000; Bermeo 1997; Encarnación 2012; Gunther 1992).

Yet troubling turn-of-the-century events – when the grandchildren of those defeated in the war began to revisit the repression of civilians by Franco's army and paramilitary – threatened to destabilize these consensually sanitized perceptions of the Civil War, dictatorship, and transition to democracy (Labrador 2017; Sánchez León and Izquierdo 2017). In October 2000, sociologist and journalist Emilio Silva opened the latest chapter in Spain's Civil War unburials when he promoted the exhumation of a Republican mass grave in Priaranza del Bierzo (León) containing the body of his grandfather and 12 others. Led by forensic doctors and archeologists who were acquainted with the internationally approved technical manuals for the search of disappeared persons available at the time, like the Minnesota Protocol, it set off a dizzying wave of excavations and reburials, increasingly linked to the global expansion of human rights protocols to promote truth, justice, and reparation for victims (Ferrándiz 2014; Ferrándiz and Robben 2015; Moreno 2021; Silva and Macías 2003; Wagner 2008) (Figure 13.1).

A political and media storm regarding the proper handling of these anachronistic and highly disturbing bodies struck Spain in the following years, with international repercussions. The political right wing, in good part heir of the dictatorship's political elites, loudly resisted this emergent process, arguing that reconciliation from the painful conflict had been satisfactorily achieved during the transition to democracy and looking back amounted to the unnecessary opening of old wounds. Despite such staunch opposition, exhumations multiplied in the following years, mostly promoted by the grandchildren and later the great-grandchildren of executed Republicans, originating what Rojas-Perez has defined as a new and alternative "necro-governmentality of postconflict," altering "the wartime relationship between the geography of violence and the geography of memory" (2017, p. 259).

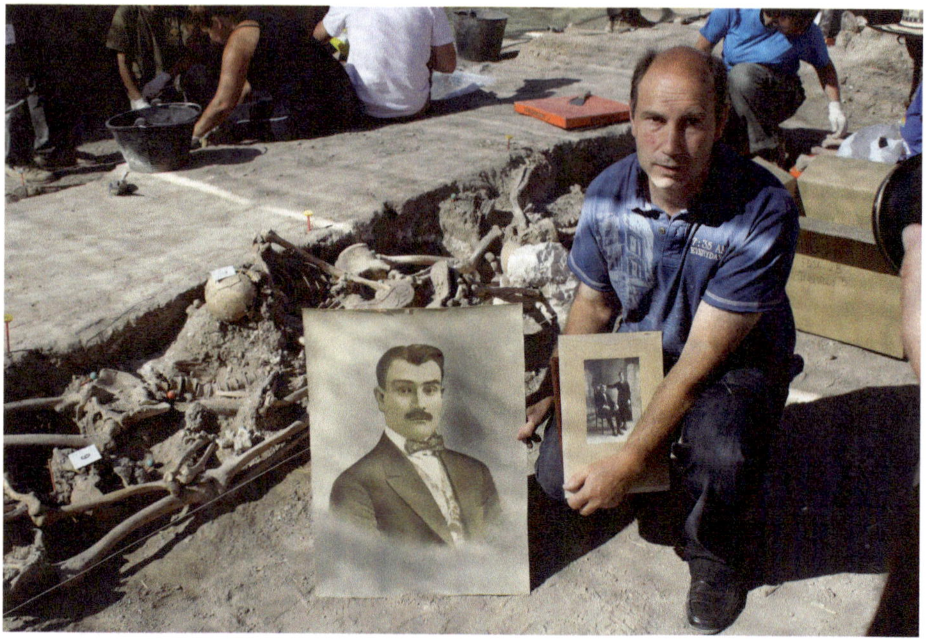

Figure 13.1 Exhumation of 45 Republican civilians executed by rebel militias in the rear guard in the early stages of the war. Milagros (Burgos), July 18, 2009. Source: Francisco Ferrándiz.

The main developments in Spain since the Priaranza unburial can be summarized as follows: the passing in 2007 of a Memory Law to "recognize and increase rights and establish measures in favor of those who suffered persecution and violence during the Civil War and the Dictatorship" (BOE 2007) by a Socialist government after heated debates in Parliament and more generally in the public sphere; the unsuccessful attempt in 2008 by Judge Baltasar Garzón – internationally renowned for issuing an arrest warrant against Chilean dictator Augusto Pinochet for genocide, international terrorism, torture, and forced disappearances in 1998 (Golob 2002) – to connect the Spanish case with international human rights law by reframing Francoist repression as crimes against humanity (Ferrándiz 2014, pp. 205–259); the judicial testimony of victims of Francoism in the Supreme Court during Garzón's trial for malfeasance; the development of memorial institutions in some of Spain's Autonomous Communities, with uneven scope and results; a second lawsuit filed in 2010 by a number of Spanish associations for the recovery of historical memory and victims in Argentina regarding crimes against humanity committed during the Civil War and Francoism, under international law (known as *Querella Argentina*); the 2011 appointment by the government of a Commission of Experts, in which I participated, to decide on the fate of Francisco Franco's tomb and the controversial monument housing it;

the uneven drafting of regional memory policies in certain parts of Spain, affecting the exhumation of mass graves, the recognition of the suffering of diverse types of victims, the removal of physical traces of apology to Francoism, and the memorialization of anti-Francoist resistance, among other controversial topics (Basque Country, Andalusia, Catalonia, Navarra, and others); and the creation in 2020 of a State Secretariat for Democratic Memory in the central government.

In the 2005–2011 period, José Luis Rodríguez Zapatero's Socialist government funneled more than 20 million euros of state public funding to support exhumations and other commemorative activities related to rescuing the memory of the war's defeated, although a tiny part was also assigned to projects pursuing the promotion of the "other" memory, as some authors refer now to the memory of the Francoist winners (Salas 2006; García Alonso 2018). During this period, unburials and reburials, documentaries, commemorative monuments, local research on repression, conferences, and acts of tribute proliferated, as other traces of the Francoist regime started to be called into question. The online initiative "Hunt a Fascist Monument," launched by one major memorial association, *Foro por la Memoria*, is a good example.[4] But when the right-wing Partido Popular (PP) came to power in December 2011, state funding for exhumations and related Civil War memorial activities ceased completely. Spain's 2011–2018 conservative prime minister, Mariano Rajoy, publicly stated his disdain for the Memory Law and soon stated his intention to starve it to death economically. In all, since 2000, more than 950 mass graves have been opened and over 11 000 bodies have been unearthed (Francisco Etxeberria, personal conversation, January 2022).

Whatever the political leanings of the party in power, the Spanish case became increasingly entangled with transnational human rights processes, a connection promoted by many sectors of the associative movement and skillfully dodged by successive governments. In 2014, two UN reports (by the Working Group on Enforced and Involuntary Disappearances and the Special Rapporteur on the Promotion of Truth, Justice, Reparation, and Guarantees of Non-recurrence) admonished the Spanish State for refusing to frame these unburials and the bigger issue of crimes against humanity committed during the war and the dictatorship – within international human rights legislation and transitional justice frameworks. They demanded that the State acknowledge these crimes as *forced disappearances*, assuming the responsibility to investigate all of them (de Greiff 2014). A new Law of Democratic Memory, responding to some of the demands of the memory associations and the UN rapporteurs, was sent to parliament for debate in late 2021. The new Law was passed on October 2022. amidst controversy.

The history of the bullet-riddled bodies now retrieved began with denunciations, arrests, jails, military trials, tortures and mistreatment, executions, and hasty mass grave burials several decades ago. All of these repressive techniques are to be understood as instruments of a generalized political terror that was an integral part of Franco's military strategy: to sow fear and eliminate dissidence as his troops took control of the country. Thus, the memory work around mass graves and the exhumation and reburial of the executed skeletons raises the highest stakes, as it necessarily unmakes a systematic form of military sovereign domination that included the intentionally offensive placement of executed cadavers in unnamed ditches.

This process of reclamation required the bodies' relocation within a legitimate funerary and memorial cartography. Yet initially, for many families and memorial associations, it was not easy to know how to deal with the unexpected homecoming of 60- or 70-year-old skeletons inscribed with decades-old repressive violence, in a context of full media visibility and in a highly politicized and confrontational social environment. None of the available funerary arrangements provided either by the Church – Spain's main provider in this respect, albeit one strongly rejected by many associations due to its complicity with the dictatorship and the very crimes unearthed – or by the funeral homes' service charts could properly accommodate, as a general principle, these unsettling corpses rescued *in extremis* from oblivion and destruction.[5]

Most activists and relatives involved in the internally diverse and troubled memorial social movement agree that unburials and reburials make sense only if those executed during the war and postwar and later abandoned and mistreated by the nation for decades are somehow "dignified" in the process. Yet there are crucial disagreements on how to proceed – technically, politically, and symbolically – with the undoing and relocation of this stigmatized space of death (Ferrándiz 2014, pp. 191–203). Early initiatives to commemorate and resignify mass graves without unburials or public exposure of the bones were soon sidelined by the success of a body-centric *forensic turn* in the memory-recovery associative field after 2000, as technical exhumations accumulated, archeologists, and forensic doctors operating under the umbrella of transnational human rights discourses and practices become crucial interpreters of the Civil War and postwar repression, and the executed skeletons took center stage in memorial public displays, debates, and the media, including the new digital media (Dziuban 2017; Ferrándiz 2016; Ferrándiz and Baer 2008) (Figure 13.2).

Ironically, due to the 1977 Amnesty Law and the statute of limitations in Spanish criminal law (20 years), in the absence of the kind of legal framework for the exhumations that exists in countries like Argentina or Bosnia (Robben 2015; Wagner 2008), forensic interventions are carried out in an *as if* mode, creating the legal fiction that some justice is being done. That is, although in many cases, forensic doctors write internationally approvable scientific reports on the exhumations, they have no legal value as of today – though they could be legally reactivated as evidence if in the future there were some sort of trial of Francoist crimes. The epistemological status of the evidence documented at

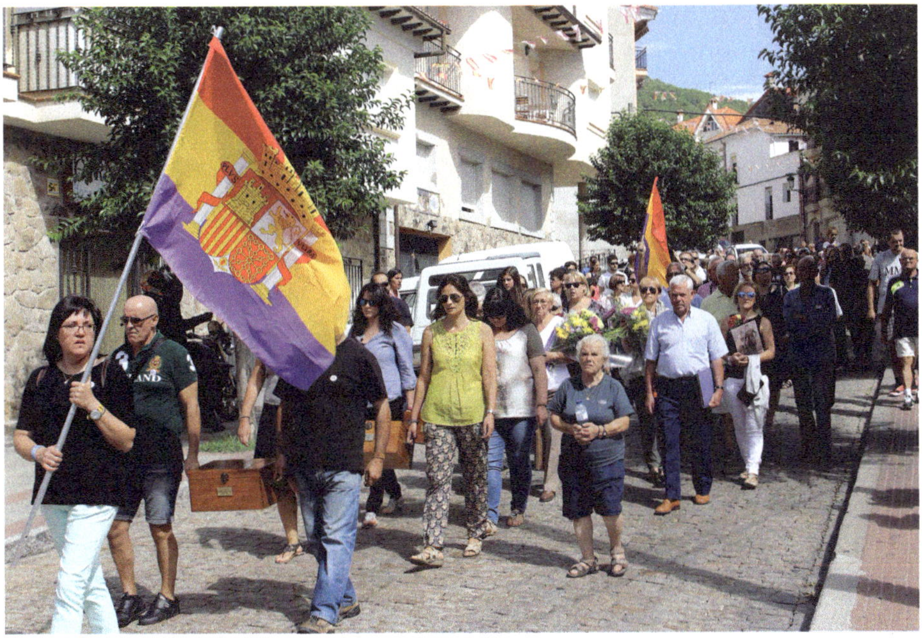

Figure 13.2 Parading through the streets of Gavilanes (Ávila) during the reburial ceremony of three people exhumed from a mass grave, as they are brought to the local cemetery, September 12, 2015. Source: Francisco Ferrándiz.

excavations and in laboratories is therefore scientific, but not, as things stand, judicial (Crossland 2013). That they have no current legal status does not detract from their social and symbolic efficacy for relatives, as they provide powerful scientific evidence that there were large-scale, thus undermining revisionist approaches to the war and the dictatorship.

In this eye-catching *bare bones* forensic scenography, wounded human remains; *premortem, perimortem,* and *postmortem* violence traces; *coups de grâce*; calibers; ammunition shells; tying ropes and wires; blindfolds; quicklime; and personal objects came to express the *ground zero* of Franco's militaristic repression, often overshadowing other alternative narratives of the past (Anstett and Dreyfus 2015; Crossland and Joyce 2015; Davis 2017; Dziuban 2017; Ferrándiz 2013; Ferrándiz and Robben 2015; Rosenblatt 2015; Weizman 2012). Transmission of this forensic connection to the past occurs in diverse ways: in the "mobile seminars" where experts give attendees their interpretation of the day's scientific progress at the exhumations (Bevernage and Colaert 2014); in PowerPoint presentations that have become an integral part of the return ceremonies; or in the flow of scientific data to different types of non-official archives, either personal, familial, or managed by memorial associations

(Aragüete-Toribio 2017), to name some relevant ones. In this authoritative evidence-driven interpretative framework where forensic medicine becomes the crucial memory science, and *crime-scene* – in its *crimes against humanity* version – logics, and esthetics develop into a salient access point to the violent past in public space, the violent repression inscribed in the executed civilians lying in the graves necessarily colors the memorial culture that attempts to dismantle it (Ferrándiz 2021; Hacking 1996; Keenan and Weizman 2012).

13.4 Unmaking the *Generalissimo's* Burial

A 2003 exhumation of a mass grave in the province of Ávila turned the Valley of Cuelgamuros into a very uncomfortable hotspot, directly connected to the emerging unburial process. When technicians attempted to exhume the grave, they were unable to find more than a few broken, scattered bones, suggesting that a previous, and rather careless, excavation had already taken place. Fausto Canales was the driving force behind this 2003 exhumation, when searching for his father and six fellow residents from the village of Pajares de Adaja, all members of the local Socialist party, killed in 1936 by *Falange* paramilitary. A retired engineer, he undertook private investigations after the exhumation fiasco, following evidence that the bodies had been moved to the Valley in 1959. The case was particularly striking because it was the first documented example that a Republican mass grave had been raided without the relatives' knowledge during Francoism to help fill up the Valley's crypts. Many local officers had been under pressure to contribute bodies to the Francoist monument and saw this as an opportunity to erase awkward evidence pointing to the embarrassing killing of neighbors during the war (Olmeda 2009). The discovery was a bombshell, bringing Fausto Canales media attention both at home and abroad, and transforming him into a symbol of courage and resilience for historical memory recovery associations, ranging from ephemeral local clusters of relatives of victims to full-fledged legally constituted organizations with national implantation. Yet this was only part of a broader and equally striking public revelation – that the Valley's crypts actually hosted more than 33 000 Civil War bodies, around 12 000 of them *unknowns*, an indeterminate number of which were executed Republican civilians removed from mass graves, as well as Republican soldiers transplanted from military cemeteries (Figure 13.3).

As research provided more information on the genealogy and magnitude of the crypts, memorial activists, initially spearheaded by Canales, started filing legal injunctions for their relatives' immediate exhumation from the Valley, and return to their families. For more than a decade, these lawsuits languished in religious, bureaucratic, political, and legal labyrinths and are threatened by

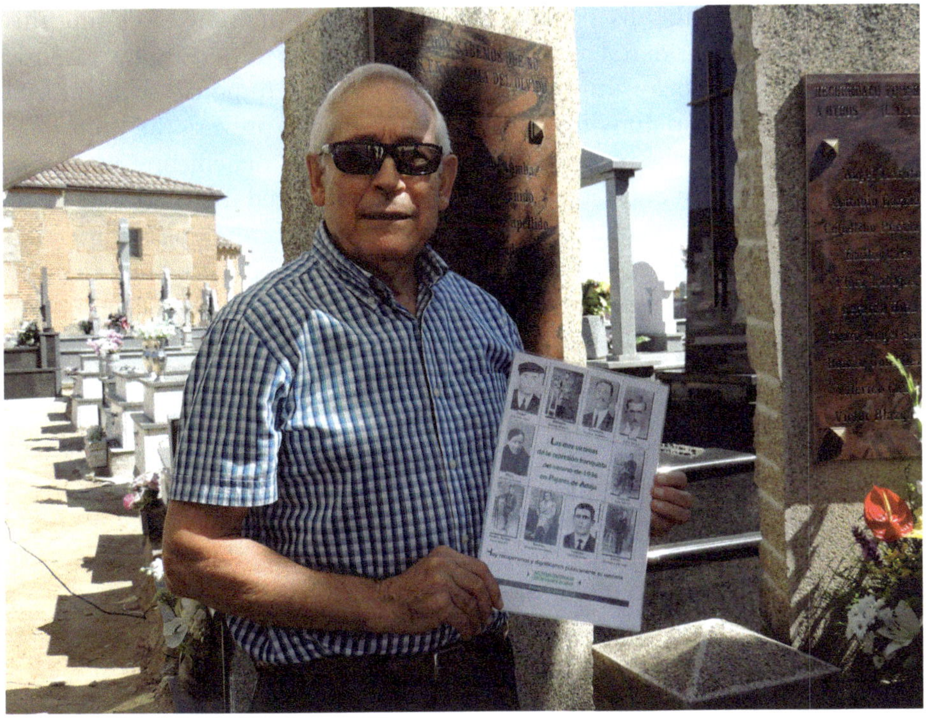

Figure 13.3 Fausto Canales pins a home-made print-out with the faces of all the Republican civilians from Pajares de Adaja (Ávila) executed in 1936, during a commemorative act in his village's cemetry. Seven of them were exhumed from a mass grave in Aldeaseca (Ávila) and transferred to the Valley of the Fallen in 1959. Source: Francisco Ferrándiz.

counter-litigation for funerary profanation by the main association defending the Francoist essence of the Valley (Ferrándiz 2014, pp. 261–303). A firm legal ruling of 2016 authorizing the disinterment of anarchist brothers Manuel and Antonio Ramiro Lapeña from the town of Calatayud, executed in 1936 and transferred to the monument in 1959, initially hailed as historic, met with "Kafkaesque" judicial, political, and technical obstacles, in the words of Manuel's granddaughter (Ejerique 2016). With the creation of the State Secretariat for Democratic Memory in 2020, these demands found the political support they had lacked for years, and the necessary technical provisions for the potential unburials were set in motion, led by the prestigious forensic doctor Francisco Etxeberria (who was already present in the Priaranza exhumation in 2000). This involved the development of a sophisticated and very detailed forensic plan to meet all Spain's legal, technical, funerary, and ethical regulations as well as the high standards put forward in the internationally validated forensic protocols used in the search for the disappeared. In late 2022, at the time of closing this text, what has been considered by some experts as Spain's most complex forensic operative ever is stuck, awaiting a legal resolution in response to a judicial demand by an extreme-right wing association designed to prevent the unburials.

Keepers of the monument's most hidden secrets, the Benedictine monks in charge of the monument and the cult of the dead transferred there since its inauguration by Franco in 1959, reacted quickly to preempt any attempt at unmaking the crypts. First, they argued that their own census might be wrong and that the actual number of bodies was probably double the number on file. Second, they conveyed to the press the impossibility of any kind of exhumation or individualized identification of remains, claiming that the leaks and seepage the monument had suffered over the decades had affected the crypts where the corpses were buried to such an extent that the ossuary had dissolved into the rock, making one body indistinguishable from another. An anonymous declaration by Valley sources states verbatim: "The remains were used to fill the internal chambers of the crypts and are now part of the building's structure. Damp has done the rest." It reads as a euphemism for the radical melting of biographical and political identities into one complex, contradictory, and indissoluble collective corpse, architecturally consolidated in the cement of the monument's underground vaults (Junquera 2008). This powerful religious allegory would express, according to these sources, the definitive embrace of the *two Spains* under the welcoming arms of the huge cross: a truly devastating prospect for those opposed to preservation of the monument's *status quo*, who are eager to open and clarify this subterranean cemetery.

Let's rewind a few decades for a better understanding of why relatives of Republican victims are so disturbed by these developments regarding the monument they see as the staunchest and most extravagant stronghold of Francoism – in Canales' words (personal conversation), a "cavern of horror" unconceivable in a democratic State. The Valley of Cuelgamuros is Spain's most conspicuous militarist–religious compound. The monument was visualized by Franco during the war to host the bodies of the victors, creating a permanent religious cult to commemorate their martyrdom and sacrifice, as suggested in the foundational decree signed by Franco in April 1, 1940:

> The magnitude of our Crusade, the heroic sacrifices that victory entails, and the transcendence of this epopee for the future of Spain cannot be perpetuated by the unassuming memorials commonly used in towns and villages to commemorate the outstanding deeds of our History and the glorious episodes of its sons.
>
> The stones erected must be endowed with the splendor of ancient monuments, defying time and oblivion, and must constitute a place of meditation and rest where future generations can pay a tribute of admiration to those who left them a better Spain (published in BOE April 2, 1940; translated by the author).

Parts of the monument imitate the imperial style created by the architect Juan de Herrera and canonized in the nearby Monastery of El Escorial, built by Philip II in the sixteenth century, which currently houses the Royal Pantheon. Just 13 km apart, these two architectural power structures are joined by an umbilical cord connecting different imperial utopias. Indeed, Franco always sought to recast his military victory as a continuation of the Crusades and the Spanish Empire. To this day, both monuments are included on an "Imperial Route" in tourist itineraries. Christianity's tallest cross soars 150 m above the Valley site, hewn into the granite hill. The subterranean Basilica is packed with a blend of Catholic and militaristic symbols, sealing a decades-long alliance (Casanova 2011). Welcoming visitors at the entrance are two huge angels holding downward-pointing swords, made out of melted bronze cannons from the Civil War. The six side chapels in the central nave are dedicated to Virgins, each representing a different military force. The impressive tiled dome reviews Spain's history as a Catholic country, featuring representations of the Nation's martyrs. One section alludes directly to the Civil War and its share of martyrs, where Francoist and Falangist flags are on full display (Figure 13.4).

Just before its formal inauguration on April 1, 1959, on the 20th anniversary of Franco's military victory, one of the first bodies to be transferred to the monument,

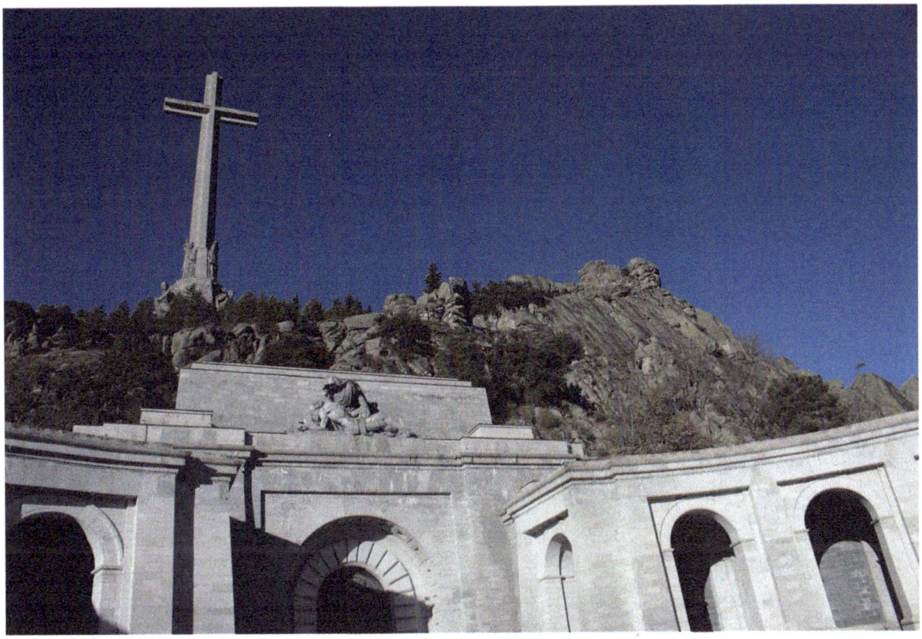

Figure 13.4 Digital memory. Use of mobile devices to record resources to be used in the social media in a commemorative act in Calera y Chozas (Ávila), February 10, 2013. Source: Francisco Ferrándiz.

as we have seen, was that of fascist leader Primo de Rivera, reexhumed from the Monastery of El Escorial and placed before the Basilica's main altar. The next few years saw a large-scale funerary parade of Civil War dead, with thousands of bodies – ranging from senior military officers to rank-and-file and civilians killed in the war – brought to the monument from different parts of Spain. In 1969, all of the 3185 soldiers believed to be resting in the military cemetery of Griñón, a town close to Madrid, were transferred to the Valley (Olmeda 2009, pp. 281–284).

But the Valley's militaristic profile was particularly sharpened in 1975. Although it is unclear how the decision to bury the *Generalissimo* in the monument was reached, or if he had even agreed to it, on November 23, he was brought to the pantheon, after a two-day vigil in the Royal Palace (Alija Fernández 2016). Buried in full dress uniform right behind the altar, he was set in a heroic axis with Primo de Rivera's tomb. For decades, the Valley became the main site of militaristic nostalgia for bygone times on their shared death date of November 20. Although their numbers faded over time, groups of Francoist supporters and *Falange* members staged celebratory rituals, including military parades from Madrid to the Valley, Roman salutes, and the singing of fascist anthems by the tombstones. In their outdated homilies, the Benedictines still pray daily for the "unity of Spain" and the blood shed by Civil War martyrs. While Jose Antonio's tomb has lost prominence with time, Franco's grave – and more specifically his bodily remains – have increasingly become the ultimate bastion of his regime's protracted but decaying sovereignty (Yurchak 2015).

In 2011, the Socialist government appointed a Commission of 12 experts to propose alternatives to "democratize" and "resignify" the monument, stripping it of its explicit militaristic and pre-democratic tone (BOE 2011). As a result of my ongoing research on mass graves and long-standing relationship with memorial associations, I was a member of this body, to which the political right and their associated media were openly hostile in view of their position that Valley is already a place of reconciliation. The Commission's plenary sessions were held in the Prime Minister's compound in Moncloa and was subdivided into three sections dealing with the legal status of the monument; the preservation or removal of its symbolic elements; and finally, the provision of ideas, in which I participated, to resolve the ongoing contradictions and tensions emanating from both the privileged burial sites in the Basilica and the huge underground cemetery.

In our Crypt Subcommission, we established that any transformation of the monument required radical elimination of the Francoist funerary hierarchy dominating the Valley, as this was the keystone of the broader funerary apartheid being dismantled in State-wide exhumations since 2000. First, we argued, if the monument was truly to the Civil War dead, Franco had to be exhumed and handed over to his family for private burial. Next, Primo de Rivera should be moved to a side crypt, away from his privileged burial site. Finally, the cemetery should change its status from a pseudo-religious character into a special public cemetery under the full oversight of the State. This would facilitate exhumations like the ones demanded by the relatives of the Republicans surreptitiously buried there.

The Commission's three most conservative members signed a private vote against Franco's exhumation from the Valley, warning of the social alarm that this would create in Spain and arguing that no such proposal existed anywhere else in Europe. Furthermore, as both leaders were buried on holy ground (in the Basilica), any removal had to abide by the 1979 agreement between the State and Vatican, involving permission from the Pope and therefore tricky and delicate international diplomacy. In the extreme case that the unburial eventually occurred, the operation should be performed as befit a Head of State.[6] Since then, the inviolability of Franco's tomb become a major red line for a political right which shrinks away from claiming explicit ties with his military regime but actively resists every effort to dismantle its legacy. Yet for the first time since his death, Franco's tomb had come under siege, as the very possibility of his removal entered public debate and periodically gave rise to bold media headlines.

Yet the circle was definitely closing in on Franco's resting place as his iron-fist militarist inscription of the country progressively comes apart and the fallout spreads from the mass grave exhumations of Republicans that started in 2000. This directly affected other senior members of his military entourage, with a rise in public consciousness of their role as the perpetrators of crimes against humanity and sight increasingly restored to the blind eye that political elites agreed to turn to the atrocities of Francoism during the transition to democracy. Late 2016 saw removal of the remains of Generals Emilio Mola – the true mastermind of the 1936 military rebellion – and José Sanjurjo – a recidivist putschist who had already made a previous attempt to overthrow the Republican government in 1932. Both killed in plane crashes during the war, they were reunited in the same mausoleum during the dictatorship and have now been exhumed from a crypt located below the Monument to the Fallen – now an exhibition center – in downtown Pamplona and returned to their relatives, amidst heavy controversy.

Although Mola's disinterment on October 24 was more discreet, the conditions imposed by Sanjurjo's relatives and the Church for disinterring his body on November 16, following tense negotiations and legal skirmishes with the City Council, were strict: the exhumation was to be carried out by religious and municipal personnel – thus excluding any forensic handling; it had to be registered by a notary, and no pictures were to be taken, much less reach the public domain. In a press release, Sanjurjo's family expressed their "profound pain for the substance of the case, the form and purpose of the exhumation" (La Gaceta 2016). This major development in conservative Pamplona seemed unthinkable until 2015, when the City Council changed political hands and a

Basque pro-independence mayor came to power for the first time (Martínez Magdalena 2017). As part of the same process, 900 km away, the tomb of another top Francoist commander in a famous Basilica in Seville, General Gonzalo Queipo del Llano, was removed on early November 2012–2022, just a few days after the passing of the new Democratic Memory Law. General Queipo del Llano is known for his cruelty and incendiary radio broadcasts during the war, in which he openly called for indiscriminate rapes and killings and had the ultimate responsibility for the ruthless wave of repression in Andalucía that resulted in the execution of thousands of civilians, including the well-known poet Federico García Lorca on August 18, 1936 (Espinosa 2000; Gibson 2005, pp. 174–175).

In July 2018, soon after the Socialist party won the general election, petitions that it should abide by its own proposal regarding Franco's unburial were not long in coming. A powerful example was the opinion piece in *El País* by prestigious writer and journalist Manuel Vicent, who urged the new President Pedro Sánchez to act swiftly on this matter. "If the new Socialist government needs a symbolic action with a high moral impact, this is it," wrote Vicent, adding, "At this stage, it would be truly scandalous for the reverential fear inspired by the dictator's remains until now to continue, as if his grave were a concrete pot containing a nuclear fuel rod capable of releasing an uncontrolled radioactive load. Be bold, Prime Minister" (2018). And so it happened. Barely two weeks after he was sworn in, Sánchez announced that he was mandating Franco's exhumation from the Valley, as the 2011 report recommended.

Whereas for the Socialist government and the political Left, the exhumation was seen as an act of justice to the victims and a necessary step to dismantle the main stronghold and monumental expression of Francoism, the status of the Valley and the inviolability of Franco's tomb became a major red line for the political Right. But it was the extreme Right that took up the fight, spearheaded by Franco's family, the Francisco Franco National Foundation (FFNF) and, with less public visibility, the Association for the Defence of the Valley. To cut a long story short, on September 13, 2018, the Royal Decree to exhume Franco was adopted by Parliament. A few days later, Franco's family rejected the exhumation and pointed, if worse came to worst, to Madrid's Cathedral (right beside the Royal Palace) as the final resting place for the body, requesting military honors and a state funeral for the reburial. The government rejected any such honors but was caught off-guard by the decision to relocate Franco's body in the cathedral and resorted to the Vatican for help in preventing this move (Franco was buried in sacred land in the Valley's Basilica). A report commissioned by the government declared the Cathedral an unsuitable place due to public security concerns. Meanwhile, in coordination with Franco's family, the prior of the Benedictines order in the Valley refused to acknowledge the State's authority and repeatedly vowed to keep Franco's body in the Valley.

Finally, in the midst of rising tension and confusion, the Supreme Court ruled in the government's favor on September 24, 2019, with reference both to the unburial and to the final destination of the body of the dictator, a crypt in the Mingorrubio cemetery, where Franco's wife, Carmen Polo, was buried. The process of exhuming and transferring the body finally took place on October 24, 16 months after Sanchez's announcement. The exhumation conveyed a strong political statement: Spain is no longer a comfort zone for dictators who so bluntly violated basic human rights. The choreographed exhumation, another political thriller carefully designed by top officials, was imposed on the family by the government, who decided to have full control over both the protocol and the information flow. No images of the exhumation in the Valley's Basilica were allowed, and the state provided a single audio–visual signal broadcast by Spain's national TV and rebroadcast live nationally and internationally. It made for great expectation and entertainment, as the country ground to a halt to watch such a historical moment. The TV spectacle left in the Spanish public conflicting senses of relief, indifference, or outrage, depending on political leanings and whether Franco was considered villain, relic from the past, or moral hero whose tomb had been shamefully desecrated.

13.5 Military disassemblage

Unmaking militaristic legacies is a daunting, lengthy, multileveled, incomplete, shadowy, and often frustrating task, in Spain or elsewhere (Figure 13.5). Franco, who fought and won a scorched-earth war and led an iron-fisted 36-year-long dictatorship, is still deeply ingrained in Spanish institutional, political, symbolic, and emotional landscapes. After 40 years of democracy, opening abandoned mass graves, relocating generals, erasing the names of perpetrators from street maps, removing statues of a dictator, or dismantling politico–religious cults paying homage to a tyrant or his most prominent comrades still suffuses Spanish society with a surprising uneasiness. When the transition was hailed as a neat example of a clean democratization, none of this belated "warped mourning" process could even have been imagined (Etkind 2013).

Yet this is the juncture at which Spain currently stands, caught up in an intense debate about the Civil War, the protracted dictatorship that followed it, and the scope and depth of its legacy of militarism. Opening the mass graves of the defeated and the increasing social and political pressure on the General's burial sites and monuments are proving decisive tools in the historical, political, and emotional unlearning of Francoism, and yet they are also testimony to the endurance of its foundations and the historical and political depth of its terror machinery, deeply suffusing the memorial process as a lingering militaristic phantom.

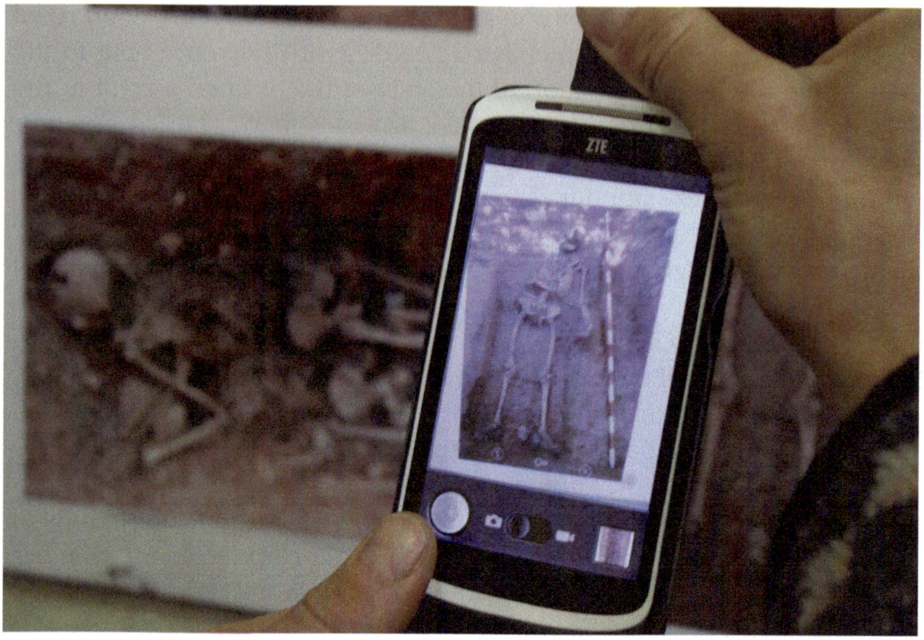

Figure 13.5 The Valley of the Fallen. Front view. Source: Francisco Ferrándiz.

This demilitarization of Spanish society through exhumation practices and the questioning and removal of other Francoist traces or bodies is forcing the country to travel to the depths of the physical wounds inscribed on the executed corpses and to decipher and unmake the military honors invested in the burial arrangements of perpetrators. So too this process must critically decipher the corpses' afterlives, from deep emotions to cyberspace (Figure 13.5), from artistic proposals to judicial resolutions, from fleeting biological traces to impregnable monuments, from political laws to grassroots commemorations, from statues to street-name signs, and from local dynamics within families or villages to transnational processes.

Above all, after more than 20 years of hectic hereafter, the exhumed bodies of those defeated in the Civil War have become crucial actors in the final dismantling of a political corpse that, though decaying, is still influential. The tensions, fissures, and backlash provoked by their uncontrollable flooding into civil society, the judicial system, political agendas, media circuits, emotional regimes, and the country's historical consciousness are bound to extinguish the agonic breath of a vanishing military regime, which in many senses has outlived its formal conclusion and is only now starting to lose its claim to impunity. Far from a necrophilic anecdote, the comeback of the executed Republicans is not just part of the history of Spain, but the history of humankind, increasingly claiming a significant slot in the universal catalog of complicities between totalitarian militarism and extensive human right violations.

Notes

1. This paper is a revised and abridged version of the paper "Unburials, Generals and Phantom Militarism: Engaging with the Spanish Civil War Legacy" published in 2019 in *Current Anthropology* 60(S19): S62–S76, copyright by The Wenner-Gren Foundation for Anthropological Research (DOI: 10.1086/701057). It is a result of Research Project PID2019-104418RB-I00 financed by the Spanish Ministry of Economy and Competitiveness.
2. The Webpage of the nationally-funded research team I have been leading since 2007 can be visited at http://www.politicasdelamemoria.org/en/ (accessed January 26, 2022).
3. I take the notion of *funerary apartheid* from Emilio Silvia, who translated in these terms my earlier notion of the two differential *spaces of death* during a public debate in the Universidad Complutense in Madrid.
4. See http://www.foroporlamemoria.info/simbolos_franquistas.php?id_prov=2 (accessed January 26, 2022).
5. On the development of funerary arrangements for exhumed bodies, see Ferrándiz 2018.
6. See the final report by the Commission of Experts at http://digital.csic.es/bitstream/10261/85710/1/INFORME%20COMISION%20EXPERTOS%20VALLE%20CAIDOS%20PDF.pdf (accessed January 26, 2022).

References

Aguilar, P. (2000). *Memory and Amnesia: The Role of the Spanish Civil War in the Transition to Democracy*. Oxford: Berghahn Books.

Aguilar, P. (2017). Unwilling to forget: Local memory initiatives in post-Franco Spain. *South European Society and Politics* **22**(4): 405–426.

Aguilar, P. and Ferrándiz, F. (2015). Memory, media and spectacle: *Interviú's* portrayal of Civil War exhumations in the early years of Spanish democracy. *Journal of Spanish Cultural Studies* **17**(1): 1–25.

Alija Fernández, R.A. (2016). El inextricable camino entre el lecho de muerte y la lucha contra la impunidad: Los casos de Franco y Pinochet. In: *La muerte del Verdugo. Reflexiones interdisciplinarias sobre el cadáver de los criminales en masa* (ed. S. Garibian), 101–121. Buenos Aires: Miño y Dávila.

Anstett, É. and Dreyfus, J.M. (eds.) (2015). *Human remains and Identification: Mass Violence, Genocide and the 'Forensic Turn'*. Manchester: Manchester University Press.

Aragüete-Toribio, Z. (2017). *Producing History in Spanish Civil War Exhumations*. New York: Palgrave Macmillan.

Bermeo, N. (1997). Myths of moderation: Confrontation and crisis during democratic transition. *Comparative Politics* **29**(3): 305–322.

Bevernage, B. and Colaert, L. (2014). History from the grave? Politics of time in Spain mass grave exhumations. *Memory Studies* **7**(4): 440–456.

Boletín Oficial del Estado (BOE) (1940). Decreto de 1 de abril de 1940 disponiendo se alcen Basílica, Monasterio y Cuartel de Juventudes, en la finca situada en las vertientes de la Sierra de Guadarrama (El Escorial), conocida por Cuelga-muros, para perpetuar la memoria de los caídos en nuestra Gloriosa Cruzada, 2240. Madrid: Presidencia del Gobierno.

Boletín Oficial del Estado (BOE) (2007). LEY 52/2007, de 26 de diciembre, por la que se reconocen y amplían derechos y se establecen medidas en favor de quienes padecieron persecución o violencia durante la Guerra civil y la dictadura, 5341053416–5341053453. Madrid: Presidencia del Gobierno. https://www.boe.es/boe/dias/2007/12/27/pdfs/A53410-53416.pdf (accessed January 26, 2022).

Boletín Oficial del Estado (BOE) (2011). Orden PRE/1396/2011 por la que se publica el Acuerdo del Consejo de Ministros por el que se crea la Comisión de Expertos para el furuto del Valle de los Caídos, 53148–53153. Madrid: Presidencia del Gobierno. https://www.boe.es/boe/dias/2011/05/28/pdfs/BOE-A-2011-9320.pdf (accessed January 26, 2022).

Box, Z. (2009). Rituales funerarios. Culto a los caídos y política en la España franquista: A propósito de los traslados de José Antonio Primo de Rivera. In: *Políticas de la muerte. Usos y abusos del ritual fúnebre en la Europa del siglo XX* (eds. J. Casquete and R. Cruz), 265–298. Madrid: Catarata.

Box, Z. (2010). *España: Año Cero*. Madrid: Alianza.

Casanova, J. (1999). Rebelión y revolución. In: *Víctimas de la Guerra Civil* (ed. S. Juliá), 57–177. Madrid: Temas de Hoy.

Casanova, J. (2011 [2001]). *La iglesia de Franco*. Barcelona: Crítica.

Cazorla, A. (2014). *Franco: The Biography of the Myth*. London: Routledge.

Crossland, Z. (2002). Violent spaces: Conflict over the reappearance of Argentina's disappeared. In: *Matériel Culture: The Archaeology of Twentieth-Century Conflict* (eds. J. Schofield, W.G. Johnson, and C.M. Beck), 114–131. London: Routledge.

Crossland, Z. (2013). Evidential regimes of forensic archaeology. *Annual Review of Anthropology* **42**: 121–137.

Crossland, Z. and Joyce, R.A. (eds.) (2015). *Disturbing Bodies: Perspectives on Forensic Anthropology*. Santa Fe, NM: SAR Press.

Davis, E.A. (2017). Time machines. In: *Unfinished: The Anthropology of Becoming* (eds. J. Biehl and P. Locke), 217–242. Durham: Duke University Press.

De Greiff, P. (2014). *Report of the Special Rapporteur on the Promotion of Truth, Justice, Reparation and Guarantees of Non-recurrence. Mission to Spain*. New York: United Nations.

De Kerangat, Z. (2017). Beyond local memories: Exhumations of Francoism's victims as counter-discourse during the Spanish transition to democracy. In: *The Twentieth Century in European Memory: Transcultural Mediation and Reception* (eds. B. Törnquist-Plewa and T. Sindbaek), 104–121. Leiden: Brill.

Dziuban, Z. (2017). Introduction: Forensics in the expanded field. In: *Mapping the 'Forensic Turn'* (ed. Z. Dziuban), 7–35. Vienna: New Academic Press.

Ejerique, R. (2016). Entrevista a Purificación Lapeña. *eldiario.es* (Spain) (15 November). Historical Memory sec. https://www.eldiario.es/sociedad/Nieta-republicanos-Lapena-Valle-Caidos_0_572892959.html (accessed January 26, 2022).

Encarnación, O. (2012). Justice in times of transition: Lessons from the Iberian experience. *International Studies Quarterly* **56**: 179–192.

Enloe, C. (2007). *Globalization and Militarism: Feminists Make the Link*. Lanham, MD: Rowman and Littlefield Publishers.
Espinosa, F. (2000). *La Justicia de Queipo*. Barcelona: Crítica.
Etkind, A. (2013). *Warped Mourning: Stories of the Undead in the Land of the Unburied*. Stanford, CA: Stanford University Press.
Ferrándiz, F. (2008). Cries and whispers: Exhuming and narrating defeat in Spain today. *Journal of Spanish Cultural Studies* **9**(2): 177–192.
Ferrándiz, F. (2013). Exhuming the defeated: Civil War mass graves in 21st-century Spain. *American Ethnologist* **40**(1): 38–54.
Ferrándiz, F. (2014). *El pasado bajo tierra: exhumaciones contemporáneas de la Guerra Civil*. Barcelona: Anthropos.
Ferrándiz, F. (2016). From tear to pixel: Political correctness and digital emotions in the exhumation of mass graves from the Civil War. In: *Engaging the Emotions in Spanish Culture and History* (eds. L.E. Delgado, P. Fernández, and J. Labanyi), 242–261. Nashville, TN: Vanderbilt University Press.
Ferrándiz, F. (2018). Death on the move: Pantheons and reburials in Spanish Civil War exhumations. In: *A Companion to the Anthropology of Death* (ed. A.C.G.M. Robben), 189–204. Hoboken, NJ: Wiley-Blackwell.
Ferrándiz, F. (2021). Mass graves as crime scenes: Forensic operatives and scenographies in contemporary Spain. In: *Geographies of Perpetration. Re-Signifying Cultural Narratives of Mass Violence* (eds. B. Jirku and V. Sánchez-Biosca), 149–169. Berlin: Peter Lang.
Ferrándiz, F. (2022). Francisco Franco is back: The contested reemergence of a fascist moral exemplar. *Comparative Studies in Society and History* **64**(1): 208–237.
Ferrándiz, F. and Baer, A. (2008). Digital memory: The visual recording of mass grave exhumations in contemporary Spain. *Forum: Qualitative. Social Research* **9**(3): art. 35. http://www.qualitative-research.net/index.php/fqs/article/view/1152 (accessed January 26, 2022).
Ferrándiz, F. and Robben, A.C.G.M. (2015). *Necropolitics: Mass Graves and Exhumations in the Age of Human Rights*. Philadelphia, PA: University of Pennsylvania Press.
García Alonso, M. (2018). "¿Qué es lo que quieren ahora si nosotros ya les habíamos perdonado?" Resistencias y transformaciones de la memoria de los vencedores de la Guerra Civil española. In: *El pasado como testimonio: Memoria de la Resistencia y resistencias de la memoria* (eds. M. Mastrángelo and M. Cardina). Special Issue, *EOLLES Identités et Cultures*, Vol. **9**. https://gric.univ-lehavre.fr/IMG/pdf/maria_garcia_alonso-2.pdf.
Garibian, S. (dir.) (2016). *La muerte del Verdugo: reflexiones interdisciplinarias sobre el cadaver de los criminales en masa*. Buenos Aires: Miño y Dávila.
Gibson, I. (2005). *El asesinato de García Lorca*. Madrid: Punto de Lectura.
Golob, S. (2002). "Forced to be free": Globalized justice, pacted democracy, and the Pinochet case. *Democratization* **9**(2): 21–42.
Gómez Bravo, G. (2017). *Geografía humana de la represión franquista: del Golpe a la Guerra de ocupación (1936-1941)*. Madrid: Cátedra.
González-Ruibal, A. (2016). *Volver a las trincheras: una arqueología de la Guerra Civil española*. Madrid: Alianza Editorial.
Gordon, A. (1997). *Ghostly Matters: Haunting and the Sociological Imagination*. Minneapolis, MN: University of Minnesota Press.
Gunther, R. (1992). Spain: The very model of a modern elite settlement. In: *Elites and Democratic Consolidation in Latin America and Southern Europe* (eds. J. Higley and R. Gunther), 38–80. Cambridge: Cambridge University Press.

Hacking, I. (1996). Memory sciences, memory politics. In: *Tense Past: Cultural Essays in Trauma and Memory* (eds. P. Antza and M. Lambek), 67–87. New York: Rouledge.

Iturriaga, N. (2022). *Exhuming Violent Histories: Forensics, Memory, and Rewriting Spain's Past.* New York: Columbia University Press.

Juliá, S. (1999). De "guerra contra el invasor" a "guerra fratricida". In: *Víctimas de la Guerra Civil* (ed. S. Juliá), 11–54. Madrid: Temas de Hoy.

Juliá, S. (2003). Echar al olvido. Memoria y amnistía en la transición. *Claves de Razón Práctica* **129**: 14–25.

Junquera, N. (2008). Juicio a la barbarie. *El País* (Madrid) (14 December). Sunday sec. https://elpais.com/diario/2008/09/14/domingo/1221364353_850215.html (accessed January 26, 2022).

Keenan, T. and Weizman, E. (2012). *Mengele's Skull: The Advent of Forensic Aesthetics.* Berlin: Stenberg.

Kwon, H. (2008). *Ghosts of War in Vietnam.* Cambridge: Cambridge University Press.

La Gaceta (2016). La familia Sanjurjo habla sobre la exhumación del general. *La Gaceta.*

Labanyi, J. (2002). Introduction: Engaging with ghosts; or, theorizing culture in modern Spain. In: *Constructing Identity in Contemporary Spain: Theoretical Debates and Cultural Practice* (ed. J. Labanyi), 1–14. Oxford: Oxford University Press.

Labrador, G. (2017). *Culpables por la literatura. Imaginación política y contracultura en la transición española (1968-1986).* Madrid: Akal.

Lutz, C. (2001). *Homefront: A Military City and the American 20th Century.* Boston, MA: Beacon Press.

Martínez Magdalena, S. (2017). *El Monumento a los caídos como dispositivo sinóptico: tres retóricas etnográficas en la ciudad de Pamplona/Iruñea.* Cuadernos de Etnología y Etnografía de Navarra, 91, Pamplona.

Mateo, L. and de Kerangat, Z. (2020). The limits of remembrance during the Spanish transition: Questioning the "pact of oblivion" through the analysis of a censored film and a mass grave exhumation. *Memory Studies* **13**(6): 1144–1165.

Mbembe, A. (2003). Necropolitics. *Public Culture* **15**(1): 11–40.

Moreno, J. (2021). Etnografía de una ausencia. Los sentidos de la fotografía familiar en la transmission de la memoria traumática. *Disparidades: Revista de. Antropología Social* **76**(2): e023. https://dra.revistas.csic.es/index.php/dra/article/view/909/1104 (accessed January 25, 2022).

Olmeda, F. (2009). *El Valle de los Caídos: una memoria de España.* Barcelona: Península.

Preston, P. (1993). *Franco: A Biography.* New York: Harper Collins.

Preston, P. (2012). *The Spanish Holocaust: Inquisition and Extermination in Twentieth-Century Spain.* London: Harper Press.

Renshaw, L. (2011). *Exhuming Loss: Memory, Materiality and Mass Graves of the Spanish Civil War.* London: Routledge.

Robben, A.C.G.M. (2015). Exhumations, territoriality and necropower in Chile and Argentina. In: *Necropolitics: Mass Graves and Exhumations in the Age of Human Rights* (eds. F. Ferrándiz and A.C.G.M. Robben), 53–75. Philadelphia, PA: University of Pennsylvania Press.

Rodrigo, J. (2005). *Cautivos. Campos de concentración en la España franquista (1936-1947).* Barcelona: Crítica.

Rodrigo, J. (2008). *Hasta la raíz. Violencia durante la Guerra Civil y la dictadura franquista.* Madrid: Alianza.

Rojas-Perez, I. (2017). *Mourning Remains: State Atrocity, Exhumation and Governing the Disappeared in Peru's Postwar Andes*. Stanford, CA: Stanford University Press.
Rosenblatt, A. (2015). *Digging for the Disappeared: Forensic Science After Atrocity*. Stanford, CA: Stanford University Press.
Rubin, J. (2018). How Francisco Franco governs from beyond the grave: An infrastructural approach to memory politics in Contemporary Spain. *American Ethnologist* **45**(2): 1–14.
Rubin, J. (2020). Exhuming death persons: Forensic science and the making of post-fascist publics in Spain. *Cultural Anthropology* **35**(3): 345–373.
Salas, N. (2006). *La otra memoria histórica*. Córdoba: Almuzara.
Sánchez León, P. and Izquierdo, J. (2017). *La guerra que nos han contado y la que no*. Madrid: Postmetrópolis.
Saqqa, M. (2020). Las exhumaciones de los "Caídos por Dios y por España". La gestión de los cuerpos. In: *Luces sobre un pasado deformado. La Guerra Civil ochenta años después* (eds. J.A. Blanco Rodríguez, J.A. Martínez, and Á. Viñas), 503–524. Madrid: Marcial Pons.
Silva, E. and Macías, S. (2003). *Las fosas de Franco*. Madrid: Temas de Hoy.
Solé i Barjau, Q. (2008). *Els morts clandestins: les fosses comunes de la Guerra Civil a Catalunya (1936-1939)*. Barcelona: Afers.
Taussig, M. (1987). *Shamanism, Colonialism and the Wild Man: A Study in Terror and Healing*. Chicago, IL: The University of Chicago Press.
Verdery, K. (1999). *The Political Lives of Death Bodies*. New York: Columbia University Press.
Vicent, M. (2018). De una vez. *El País* (Spain) (10 June). Opinion sec. https://elpais.com/elpais/2018/06/09/opinion/1528551194_758513.html (accessed January 26, 2022).
Viejo-Rose, D. (2011). *Reconstructing Spain: Cultural Heritage and Memory After Civil War*. Brighton: Sussex Academic Press.
Wagner, S. (2008). *To Know Where He Lies: DNA Technology and the Search for Srebrenica's Missing*. Berkeley, CA: University of California Press.
Weizman, E. (2012). *The Least of All Possible Evils: Humanitarian Violence from Arendt to Gaza*. New York: Verso.
Winter, J. (1995). *Sites of Memory, Sites of Mourning: The Great War in European Cultural History*. Cambridge: Cambridge University Press.
Yurchak, A. (2015). Bodies of Lenin: The hidden science of Communist sovereignty. *Representations* **129**: 116–157.

CHAPTER 14

Dealing with bad death in post-conflict societies: forensic devices, burials of exhumed remains, and mourning processes in Peru*

Valérie Robin-Azevedo

Université Paris Cité, Migrations and Society Research Unit (URMIS), Paris, France
Co-director of the research project "Transfunerary: Mass violence and funerary practices in Europe and Latin America."

**Translated by Cadenza Academic Translations.*

14.1 Models for dealing with death: morphologies of "good death" and "bad death"

Human societies often turn to classifications to bring order and meaning to the world around them. Among these, typical ideal models of "good death" and "bad death" feature prominently. Good death, produced by way of the ritual "fabrication" of the deceased at the end of a supposedly fulfilled existence, is often imagined as perfectly framed, in order to bring the inescapability of death under control. In many societies, good death is associated with circumstances in which death, meaning arrival at the end of life, is met with certain practices that mark a farewell and separation from the land of the living, which include the suitable treatment of the body as well as an ideal model of accompanying the souls and the bereaved. This seeks to construct a new, peaceful relationship with the deceased, now invisible in – yet not entirely absent from – the lives of their relatives and the group they belonged to. Good death is also associated with the idea of a successful grieving process, in the sense that it brings about the desired emotional peace and consolation for the bereaved. It is important to note here the difference between grief and mourning (Cordeu et al. 1994). While grief refers to intrapsychic processes, mourning denotes social practices and rituals of

Anthropology of Violent Death: Theoretical Foundations for Forensic Humanitarian Action, First Edition.
Edited by Roberto C. Parra and Douglas H. Ubelaker.

separation of the deceased and the temporary liminality of the bereaved, which accompany more intimate and individual grieving processes. In fact, grief and mourning feed into each other, in a reciprocity that allows the changes caused by the death of an individual member of society to be confronted. Yet it is not always possible to put in place devices aimed at caring for the deceased and preparing the body – devices that may take very different forms depending on the cultural system concerned. I would even go as far as to say that good death is the exception rather than the rule.

Violent, suspect, or disruptive deaths that cannot be dealt with through prescribed social practices and rituals, or in which the treatment of the body is considered inappropriate, turn into bad death. A bad death can refer, therefore, to both the specific circumstances of the death and to the treatment of the body (or its absence) and the ritual practice in general (Panizo and Robin Azevedo 2021). Bad death also evokes the idea of someone who died in painful circumstances and who continues to suffer: a lost soul who cannot rest, a distressed corpse, a "*malmuerto*," who often appears to the living through oneiric or ghostly apparitions to demand unfinished care and rest, echoing an incomplete death. Bad death symbolizes the difficulty humankind experiences in its desire to control the randomness of death. It means the dead cannot be pacified or separated from the land of the living, something granted through the rituals of funeral ceremonies that seek to socialize the dead as "good," as a "*buenmuerto*." Bad death is undoubtedly the product of an act of often multidimensional violence. But while violence is key, it is not enough alone to explain the complex phenomenon of bad death, which relates rather to an incomplete biography. As Baptandier (2001) reminds us, what characterizes the life of a "*malmuerto*" is having been interrupted before its time. This premature death cuts existence off before the time assigned to that life by destiny. It is precisely this "remainder" of life – unused and unresolved but also still active – that produces bad death. Thus, it brings a sense of "incompleteness" linked to an untimely death.

14.2 Contexts of mass violence through the lens of bad death

In contexts of mass violence and its aftermath, the hard and painful process of dealing with ill-treated, incomplete, or absent bodies, as well as the ontological uncertainty related to these deaths, encourages in a paradigmatic way the emergence of bad death, of postponed grief, and of seemingly endless pain. Furthermore, it involves the idea of the debt that the living and survivors owe the dead. In Vietnam, in the years after the wars against France and the United States, bad death was expressed through the ubiquity of "invisible neighbors" associated with the local concept of "unjust death," which condemned the souls of massacred civilians without descendants to posthumous incarceration, trapped in the memory of terror, and condemned to materially relive the agony of a violent death, a grievous death, expressed in accounts of the apparition and laments of ghosts, making claims in the name of the unalienable right of the dead to be freed from the brutal history of death (Kwon 2012). In the Peruvian Andes, in the context of the internal armed conflict at the end of the twentieth century that pitted communist guerrilla fighters of the Shining Path and the Túpac Amaru Revolutionary Movement (Movimiento Revolucionario Túpac Amaru, MRTA) against countersubversive state forces, the notion of bad death was expressed in the Quechua language with the Spanish term "*mala muerte*," to refer to death that was sudden and out of place and to the ensuing state of affliction of the deceased and the bereaved, as a result of extrajudicial killings, massacres, and forced disappearances. The expression "bad luck" is also used to evoke tragic death and wretched luck, as a broader category of tragedy and misfortune whose semantic field includes a combination of events that are negative or destructive of individual and collective existence (Robin Azevedo 2008).

In Latin America, armed conflicts and sociopolitical violence lead to a burgeoning number of bad deaths, especially through the damage inflicted on bodies postmortem, such as the dismembering and mutilation of corpses that create divided, dehumanized, and animalized bodies (Uribe 2018). A corpse being in that state generates horror among the living and prevents the deceased from complying with a widely shared criteria for a good death: to go to the afterlife whole. In addition, the lack of a grave or even the prohibition of burial – a practice known to have been carried out by all violent agents, including counterinsurgents of the national armies – lead to fragmented, dispersed, and abandoned bodies being scattered across local and familial landscapes. These deteriorated bodies have been stained, from the perspective of the living, thus embodying a new extreme form of bad death (Losonczy and Robin Azevedo 2021). Another form of bad death is expressed through the disappeared, whose bodies are unreachable and invisible, having been tossed into rivers or caves, thrown off cliffs, abandoned to the elements, or cremated and concealed in mass graves. Uncertainty about their death, and the persistent hope of one day finding them, make both the ritual tasks of the construction of the deceased and their memory, and the mourning practices and the internal grief work of the bereaved, implausible. For the living, the disappeared cast the piercing and paradoxical figure of an open gap between life and death (Gatti 2014; Panizo 2012). Thus, bad death creates obstacles for grief. While it cannot be claimed that grief is impossible under these circumstances, it is possible to talk of disturbed and prolonged grief, of literally extraordinary grief. Similarly, the hampering of mourning rituals can hinder grieving processes. These deaths may be called "unattended deaths,"[1] as

Laura Panizo described them in relation to forced disappearances perpetrated by the Argentinian military, whereby the absence of a body prevents the death from being confronted in a clear and precise manner. In "unattended death," mourning rituals are obstructed, and no social spaces of "care" are created for the deceased and the bereaved. There is no body that may be venerated, and there are none of the usual practices to support the bereaved (Panizo 2021).

14.3 Transitional justice, the forensic turn, and the "dignified burial": can we reverse bad death?

In the context of the mass production of bad deaths, since the end of the twentieth century, there have been a growing number of campaigns to exhume mass graves, through a framework based on transitional justice and deployed worldwide in countries considered to be post-conflict (Lefranc 2012) or that have seen civil war in the recent or more distant past. This particular moment in recent history reflects the so-called "forensic turn," typical of contemporary societies in the new millennium (Anstett and Dreyfus 2015; Anstett 2020). It can be seen, for example, in Spain (Ferrándiz 2013), Rwanda (Korman 2017), Cambodia (Guillou 2012), Guatemala (Sanford 2003; Duterme 2016, 2017), and Peru. Understood as "reparations" policies for the victims of mass violence, these campaigns consist in locating, exhuming, and identifying the dead and disappeared as well as delivering the recovered "human remains"[2] to relatives. The aims of the international organizations working on these operations are to help "restore dignity" to the deceased and to allow affected families to finally be able to bury their dead and complete what was presumed to be an impeded grieving process. So, the already widely socially accepted idea of allowing the bereaved to finally carry out the "dignified burial" of their loved ones has become widespread. Another underlying idea is that the individual grief of those affected should then be reflected in the collective grief of the Nation, in order to achieve lasting peace, especially in contexts where there was fratricidal conflict. Furthermore, the language of compassion employed in this area highlights the now socially recognized and legitimate place of the victim and the pressing need to alleviate their pain (Fassin and Rechtman 2009). Exhumations thus become central to the "humanitarian reason" extended to the vulnerable by the most powerful, in which appealing to moral sentiments has become an essential and effective part of contemporary politics, fueling discourse and legitimizing practices (Fassin 2011).

However, it is worth questioning whether the act of returning exhumed bodies – or rather, piles of bones, often of incomplete skeletons – within a framework of forensic, legal, and ritual devices subject to certain norms, does in fact allow the wounds of the past to heal as easily as it is claimed, thus reversing the associated bad death. Moreover, which methods are used to do this? Indeed, if forced disappearances can be understood as events that involve the rupture of a previously coherent relationship with the world (see Bensa and Fassin 2002), then the opening of mass graves and the "return" of the disappeared and these poorly buried bodies means, in turn, a new and drastic change in the relationship with death, with corpses or their substitutes, and with the pain of the bereaved. This makes exhumations and subsequent burials difficult to comprehend, at both an individual and a collective level. Exhumations mean that the ontological chaos caused by the status of the "*malmuerto*," the disappeared, the absence of a body, and the uncertainty this absence generates about a presumed death, is compounded by another phase that is equally hard for the relatives and members of the group to which the victim belonged.

Indeed, beyond the demands of those who wait, often for decades, to find traces of the disappeared or to recover the bodies that had to be hurriedly buried in pits, the *extraordinary* appearance of these dead involves a complex process of managing these unexpected reunions, on both a material (in terms of the necessary treatment of the remains) and a symbolic level (in terms of managing the new identity of these remains and the place assigned to them from this point on). Exhumations in fact lead to a reconfiguration of ritual and cultural forms of action – adapted or even reinvented, often in the midst of the urgency created by these new circumstances – and to new, collectively created sociocultural responses to mourning. Thus, it is about reconnecting in a different way and creating new relationships with these beings who now leave behind their liminal status – that "no man's land," related to "bad death," of being neither entirely alive nor dead – to take on the category of deceased, being socially and culturally recognized as such. Based on the example of Peru, this chapter therefore aims to address the circulation of exhumed human remains, the ritual devices that frame them, and the postmortem destination of the deceased found or not, during campaigns to exhume mass graves and burial sites of the period of internal armed conflict.

14.4 From the necropolitics to the necrogovernamentality of the Peruvian state

For the past two decades, in accordance with the recommendations of the Truth and Reconciliation Commission (Comisión de la Verdad y Reconciliación, CVR) – set up in 2001 during the political transition following the authoritarian regime of Alberto Fujimori – exhumations carried out in Peru have concerned burial sites from the period of the internal armed conflict of 1980–2000, between

Marxist guerrillas, comprising the Castroite MRTA and the Maoist communist Shining Path, and the Peruvian state. Unlike its Southern Cone neighbors (Chile, Argentina, Uruguay, and Brazil), armed conflict in Peru did not take place during a military dictatorship but rather in the context of democracy. Nevertheless, constitutional rights were suspended in areas where a state of emergency was declared, and the armed forces sent to these areas took on military and political power. This situation gave rise to a considerable number of abuses (extrajudicial killings, massacres, rapes, etc.) perpetrated by state agents, which were considered by the CVR to be part of a systematic policy to violate the human rights of the civilian population. The continuity of the Peruvian state during the internal armed conflict and the post-conflict period, through an officially democratic regime, also explains – at least in part – the reticence of the state in accepting responsibility for past crimes perpetrated by state agents and in applying reparations policies.

The final report of the CVR (2003, Vol. I, Chap. 1 and Vol. VIII, Conclusions) concludes that around 70 000 people died during this conflict. The CVR holds the MRTA responsible for 1.5% of those killed, and the Shining Path for 53.68%, making the latter group the main perpetrator of deaths during the conflict. State agents (police, armed forces, and paramilitary rural self-defense committees) were thought to be responsible for 37.26% of deaths and disappearances. Peru does not, therefore, reproduce the classic Latin American pattern of state agents as the main perpetrators, although the CVR does state that the armed forces committed crimes against humanity.[3] According to the most recent estimations of the National Register of Disappeared Persons and Burial Sites (Registro Nacional de Personas Desaparecidas y Sitios de Entierro, RENADE) there are more than 21 334 disappeared people. In turn, there are a total of 4934 registered burial sites, 83% of which are in the Andean Department of Ayacucho, the epicenter of the armed conflict (Ministry of Justice and Human Rights 2020). In this regard, it is worth noting that Ayacucho – where I carried out my ethnographic questionnaires – and neighboring departments, which are among the most rural, deprived, and "indigenous" regions of Peru,[4] recorded almost 85% of total deaths and disappearances. Thus, the historically poorest and most marginalized sectors of Peruvian society are also the main group interested in exhumations being carried out.

Exhumations in Peru are coordinated by the Public Prosecutor's Office through the Specialized Forensic Team (*Equipo Forense Especializado*, EFE), part of the Medical Examiner's Office and created in 2003 with the purpose of excavating mass graves from the internal armed conflict and analyzing their contents. Only their personnel, or specialized state-authorized non-governmental organizations (NGOs), are permitted to carry out this kind of investigation, under the direction of an assistant district attorney responsible for initiating a concurrent judicial investigation. Therefore, examination of the exhumed remains must provide the scientific proof needed for the criminal prosecution of those responsible for the extrajudicial killings. However, the enactment of the Law on the Search for Disappeared Persons (2016) with a humanitarian focus, together with the creation of an Office for the Search for Disappeared Persons (2017), within the Ministry of Justice, responsible for enacting the law, sought to disassociate criminal investigations from the return of bodies to relatives. This was in order to speed up the return process that has dragged on for many years, and so that, in cases where there were no remains to be returned, at least information on the fate of those disappeared can be provided.

It is worth noting that the category of "disappeared," used by the Peruvian state, also applies to those whose resting place is known by the family and even to those who were buried in the community cemetery by relatives but for whom there is no legal documentation of death (that is, they do not have a death certificate). Although it is not stipulated by law, state actors use the expression "disappeared with body" as opposed to "disappeared without body." The use of the category "disappeared with body" – a peculiar oxymoron – has been questioned by some human rights organizations, who see this broad definition of the "disappeared" as a way of waiving responsibility for future effective investigation in cases where the fate of those disappeared remains unknown. To date, preference has been given precisely to exhumations of those buried without legal recognition and whose resting place was known by relatives. Most of the victims of forced disappearance at the hands of state agents have disappeared in the classic sense of the term, that is, "disappeared without body." Unlike the Shining Path, who carried out "public" executions and massacres as a warning to others, the armed forces and the police always sought to hide the crimes they committed. Therefore, the corollary of accepting the concept of "disappeared with body" is an overall increase in the number of "disappearances" attributed to the Shining Path, given that many of the killings carried out by this organization were followed by rapid burials that meant relatives could not report the death to the relevant authorities. Even when taking into account the responsibility of the Shining Path for disappearances and kidnappings – particularly of minors who were enrolled in the People's Guerrilla Army (Ejército Guerrillero Popular, EGP), a kind of recruitment that has been underestimated and not precisely identified – the armed forces were certainly the main perpetrators of forced disappearances.

Thus, the way the term "disappeared," with all its ambiguities, has been constructed and used by the state, together with the generic naming of "burial sites" to include both mass graves and the graves where families buried their dead, forms part of a framework of post-conflict "necrogovernmentality" practices related to the "fabrication of corpses" (Rojas-Pérez 2017). Indeed, Rojas-Pérez argues that the state, in an effort to regain a positive role, has used exhumations as reparations policies, returning human remains found to the relatives and thus restoring citizen rights, in contrast to the repressive and destructive capacity of the state's previous "necropolitics" (Ferrándiz and Robben 2015), which involved making citizens disappear during dictatorships or internal armed conflicts.

14.5 Exhumation of mass graves and the reactivation of bad death in the Andes

On February 4, 1984, a group of people affiliated with the Shining Path entered Cceraocro, a small village to the south of the Andean city of Ayacucho, armed with machetes and knives, and carried out a massacre of the unarmed population, leaving the gruesome tally of 17 deaths. A brief vigil was held for the mutilated corpses overnight, after which the local people then buried their dead in an improvised grave, dug close to the place where they had been killed, a few meters from the main square. The survivors then sought refuge in the village of Ocros, located approximately 400 m below Cceraocro. After several months of fierce fighting between the regular army and the guerrilla group, the inhabitants who had not migrated returned to live in the village. The grave, and its dead, had remained intact. The children of two of the victims of the massacre had a cement gravestone put up, with a cross on top bearing the names of their murdered parents. Other relatives put candles and flowers in the space on All Saints' Day, although these were not structured or enduring rituals. With the resumption of agricultural activities, farmers began to plant crops ever closer to the grave, and while they did not encroach on the actual space of the grave, it did sometimes end up being hidden by the fava bean crops grown there. In 2002, when staff from the CVR visited Cceraocro, this grave was included on a list of thousands of mass graves from the Peruvian armed conflict. The Public Prosecutor's Office finally ordered its exhumation in 2011.[5]

Therefore, almost 30 years passed between the bodies being buried and the reappearance of their remains. The "bracketing off" or even the relative "forgetting" of these dead, whose physical presence in the village was a constant reminder of their unfortunate fate, seems to have been necessary in order for daily life to carry on. By way of comparison, in Cambodia, Guillou (2012, p. 216) explains that farmers began to sew rice over graves all over the country, as a sign of the renewal of the life cycle in the wake of the Khmer Rouge regime. In her analysis of the alternation between phases of forgetting and remembering the dead of this period, Guillou proposes the idea of a local memory device of the genocide, which she argues is sometimes "switched on" and sometimes "switched off." During reconstruction phases following mass destruction, it may be necessary to forget the dead. This does not, however, stop the dead from sometimes reappearing in oneiric apparitions. It is common after such an apparition for an altar to be set up for those lost souls to be venerated, for a length of time that varies.[6] In Cceraocro, various inhabitants told me that the dead of the mass grave were still buried and should remain that way, like the violent past they wished to be forgotten and let go. The graves should not be dug up, nor the past awoken. Ricoeur (2004) has described the interest, and even the therapeutic dimension of the figure of forgetting, as long as it is not a "prescribed" forgetting, which would be equivalent to an "abuse of forgetting."

However, in this Andean village, the opening of the grave by the forensic team drastically changed the physical landscape and local memory as well as the relationship with these dead who made a physical reappearance in community life. Indeed, there was an issue with the harmful emissions emanating from the unearthed corpses, especially since it was the inhabitants themselves who opened up the grave and dug until the bodies appeared. Young children were kept away from the graves to protect them from the "wind of the dead" (*alma wayra*), and older children were told off if they got too close to the excavation. Normally, contact with the dead and the vapors that supposedly emanate from their remains during the funeral can cause "bad wind" (*mal viento*). The dead can give rise to *fright*, a nosological category caused by the improper exit of the soul from the body of the living, which must be restored under penalty of sickness or even death.[7] Nevertheless, in the present case, no recent or decomposing body caused the kind of contamination that occurs in the liminal context of ordinary funeral rituals. Furthermore, over the years, contact with the grave, and the presence of the dead who had not been buried in the cemetery, did not seem to have been problematic for the inhabitants. Indeed, I was surprised to see that the groups of children between 8 and 12 years old, who would sometimes accompany me during my trips to Cceraocro, did not hesitate to run around and play on top of the grave.

In a way, the exhumation "reconnected" the local memorial device of the dead. Their appearance reactivated the discourse around misfortune related to the "*malmuertos*" and the pathogenic potential of the unearthed remains. Delacroix (2016, 2021) shares similar accounts from the neighboring department of Apurímac of the dangers associated with mass graves from the armed conflict, from which gases may escape that can cause a range of maladies, even though those graves had not been opened. This also suggests that the relationship inhabitants have with these sites may vary between regions. Contaminated and contaminating, these "*malmuertos*," extracted from the ground, came to contaminate the living (Baptandier 2001). The fear that was sparked in that moment relates to the fact that appropriate rituals could not be carried out for the dead who, in stained clothing, were hurriedly tossed into mass graves. It is crucial that the deceased be dressed in clean or even new clothes for the funeral, in order to prevent the soul from wandering as a result of the "imprints" (blood, sweat, hair, and nails, for example) that remain on the clothing, preventing the deceased from departing as a complete whole to the "next life" (*huk vida*). This is why clothes worn at the time of death are washed or burned in specific rituals. Although it largely refers to an ideal type of "good death," in this case, the process of ritual "fabrication" of the deceased was cut short. The opening of the grave meant skeletons and clothing being raised up to the surface, revealing their incompleteness and their condition as victims of bad death.

People whose bodies have suffered injuries pre- or postmortem, and even those who were not able to be properly buried, run the risk of becoming distressed dead, whose lost souls may return to torment their loved ones. The massacres perpetrated during the war meant that funerals – generally highly codified in the Andes – were held only very rarely. For example, this happened when the Shining Path prevented the burial of those slaughtered in many places in their lamentably infamous "popular trials," which in reality were summary trials accompanied by public executions for cautionary purposes. This did not stop families from burying their murdered relatives when they had the opportunity to do so. For their part, combatants endeavored to make the bodies "disappear" so as to hide the evidence of their crimes. In these cases, the misfortune attributed to these lost souls ought to be seen as the manifestation of a grief that cannot be performed, a suspended grief (Robin Azevedo 2008), since, as Thomas (1980, p. 10) rightly notes, the funeral is a farewell ritual that also allows pain to be codified for the bereaved and their milieu.

Moreover, contamination and the risks involved in opening the grave were not the only cause for discussion and concern among inhabitants. Some assigned new attributes to the earth in the disturbed grave. In fact, various people assured me that after the exhumation of the grave in Cceraocro, some inhabitants had, at night and in secret, retrieved some of this "earth with power" (*kallpayuq allpa*) to later carry out preventive or propitiatory rituals or even witchcraft. Information gathered on this topic is still incomplete, but it seems that ambivalence about the exhumed graves is also due to the fact that they are not only sites contaminated by the impregnation of violated bodies, and therefore dangerous, but also places blessed with a certain kind of sacredness, carriers of a power that should be appropriated and channeled in the best possible way. Once excavation had been completed, the bones were sent to the Medical Examiner's Office in the city of Ayacucho and were returned to the families only a year later, in May 2012. During the autopsies, the identification of the exhumed bodies did not present any technical difficulties. In Cceraocro, the grave had been excavated by the local inhabitants, who had also buried the victims of the massacre. The clothing in which they had been buried helped the process of identifying the remains that were recovered.

Nevertheless, since most graves are clandestine, they contain people whose bodies were hidden and whose identity is still unknown, often having been the victims of extrajudicial killings at the hands of the Peruvian armed forces, who did not wish to leave any trace of their actions. Unlike in Cceraocro, the identification of these exhumed bodies is problematic, and they are sent to the Medical Examiner's Office where a series of tests and procedures are carried out to identify the exhumed remains, using *antemortem*[8] reference cards, visual recognition by the family, and even DNA tests if budget allows.

14.6 The task of identification or the process of rehumanization of ill-treated bodies

Bodies are given to relatives in the morgue, in the presence of a district attorney, once the final forensic examinations have been carried out. However, the return of the exhumed remains requires a final "identification" of them by the family. This identification has sometimes already happened during the exhumation of the grave, if one of the members of the family was present. But the handing over of bodies in the morgue is necessarily preceded by a mandatory process of "visual recognition." Some families dread the violence of this situation, and for some of our interlocutors, this visual confrontation was as unbearable as the exhumation itself. Painful accounts abound: terror on seeing the fleshless remains, feeling faint at the sight of seeing the bones displayed in the cold storage unit, nausea on having to verify the forearm fracture of a childhood accident, the violence of the obligatory forensic photos, and so on. While there is some consensus that exhumation procedures cause emotional suffering in the families concerned, to date, little attention has been paid to the sociocultural impact of the reappearance of the "disappeared" in terms of ontological, ritual, and symbolic disorganization/reorganization. Yet, the violence created by this new contact also stems from the fact that people faced with exhumations lack the recognized sociocultural references to deal with the situation and have to develop new tools with which to confront this kind of experience.

During the opening of mass graves and the subsequent identification of remains by the families in the morgue, the physical relationship established between the living and the remains of the dead is drastically altered, a literally extraordinary change in the normal course of funeral rituals. The general economy of the management of death is disrupted, and there is a change in the relationship with the body and the remains. First, the dead who have emerged from the earth are skeletons. They are no longer the bodies of flesh and bone that are normally buried. In the Andes, there are no double funeral rites (Hertz 1960) or funerary handling of the bones, as happens in Madagascar, for example, in "return of the dead"[9] rituals. Furthermore, in the context of exhumations, the bodies are rarely whole. In addition, the skeletons show signs of the violence that lead to death. Therefore, the unearthed bodies are fragmented, be that as a result of scavenging animals or because they were mutilated at the moment of death – bullet holes in the skull, traces of blows from a machete, broken bones, and so on. Lastly, the bodies are often dressed in scraps of the clothes they were wearing at the time of their violent death; in other words, they hold the injuries suffered by the person at the moment of death: fabrics stained by blood, torn from stab wounds, pierced by bullets.

Once found, the bones and associated objects are handled first by the forensic anthropologists during the exhumation of the mass grave and then by the forensic staff in the morgue. Information on the method of execution and on identity emerges during this process of removal and subsequent laboratory analysis. Therefore, it could be said that the forensic experts literally *work* these bodies, gradually trying to put them back in order. There are at least two ways of doing this. In the case of the disappeared, the process starts with them being officially granted a recovered identity. The disappeared find (again) a place in society and become (again) individualized beings. Given that these violent collective deaths are characterized precisely by the destruction of individuality (Guillou and Vignato 2012, p. 170), forensic experts name them (again). This act of naming is not just a formality; rather, it exercises real performative power over the very nature of the exhumed remains, whose social existence is restored. The disappeared, with their identity restored, exist again, or put another way, they can finally become fully dead and fit into the usual categories that distinguish the living from the deceased. This makes it possible to redraw the boundary between life and death, which up to that point was blurred. The second method is of a material nature. In the course of the examination, the forensic experts reconstruct the skeleton, especially when the bones have been mixed together in mass graves where the bodies were piled up. The dispersed bones are meticulously grouped together in the anatomically recognizable human form of a skeleton that is as whole as possible. Ideally, each bone is in its rightful place, before then being placed in a casket. Forensic staff arrange the skeleton in front of the family and oversee the first phase of administration of the death, despite not being, in theory, responsible for the care of the body in the funeral.[10] As Duterme (2017) shows in the case of Guatemala, forensic anthropologists who exhume bodies and return them to the relatives have become key actors in the conduct of reinterment rites of exhumed victims of the armed internal conflict.

In addition, the bones are often returned to the families in ossuaries. Although the forensic officers assure them that all the bones recovered are in the ossuaries, these containers resemble small "coffins," which, as some relatives point out, are "like a child's coffin." This situation is difficult for the families to accept, who see it as another form of violence that once again denies the identity of the deceased, this time as adults. In the context of the exhumations of those disappeared during the Argentinian military dictatorship, Panizo (2012) finds the same unease among those who receive the remains of their adult disappeared relatives in what look like urns for children. In some cases, when the Peruvian state had not provided funds for the purchase of caskets or urns, and the families could not afford to buy one, bones were returned to them in undignified containers such as plastic bags or tin cans (Office of the Ombudsman 2013; Koc-Menard 2014; Robin Azevedo 2021). With no social recognition and "considered insignificant," these human remains are treated like "disposable waste" (Thomas 1980, p. 100), which makes the fact that they are associated with the person whose remains were found and must be buried again, even more difficult and painful.

Moreover, recovery of the bones does not lead to an obvious or immediate correspondence between the materiality of the remains and who that person was when alive (Panizo 2012). Therefore, a cognitive process is needed to restore meaning to the bones, so that they are not only officially considered to be those of the deceased, as affirmed by the forensic officers, but also *become* the deceased and take on his or her new identity in the eyes of the relatives. It is about the synchronization of these remains with the image of the person at the time of their disappearance. The performance of the ritual process is possible from the moment these elements are recognized as such by those around them. The remains and artifacts of the deceased (bone fragments, clothing, ash, objects found) must be "resignified" if they are to be able to represent the deceased. This phase is crucial for the subsequent burial, with its ritual innovations. It allows the deceased to be suitably venerated and for the cycle of waiting and uncertainty to end, as if finally bringing indefinite temporality to a close.

Many mass graves contain bodies whose identities, at the time of excavation, are unknown, such as in the emblematic case of La Hoyada, an area located close to the Cabitos antisubversive military base, which was the main center of operations of the fight against the Shining Path in the city of Ayacucho and also the most important "*chupadero*"[11] (Gatti 2014) in the country, that is, the main "producer" of the disappeared at a national level. Thousands of people were detained and tortured there. A considerable number of them – at least an estimated 500 – disappeared in that place between 1983 and the early part of the following decade. Some bodies were initially buried at the base, as well as in La Hoyada, located on the outskirts of the barracks. This was the old shooting range and army training ground, which started to be used as a clandestine cemetery for many detainees. Later, fearing that the scandal caused by the Accomarca massacre in August 1985 would lead to the discovery of the bodies at the base, soldiers exhumed the bodies in secret. They were taken at night to be buried at La Hoyada. Some bodies were cremated to destroy evidence (Uceda 2003). The exhumation of La Hoyada took place between 2005 and 2009 and led to the recovery of 109 bodies, 53 of which were complete, and the rest were in the form of fragments (Parra et al. 2020). Until 2014, it had only been possible to identify and return the remains of two of these bodies.

At La Hoyada, the role the families of the disappeared played in the task of identifying bodies was essential. Indeed, before carrying out any searches or genetic tests to confirm the identity of an exhumed body, there must be a claim made of their disappearance. Therefore, one possible means of identification may be the recognition of clothing found on these anonymous bodies. After the first excavations in La Hoyada, there was a problem with bodies that were unidentified and often unidentifiable due to the degradation they had suffered. As a result, the human rights NGOs Asociacion Pro Derechos Humanos (APRODEH) and EPAF[12] organized mobile exhibitions of photomontages of exhumed clothing, which were shown in different villages in the region. The aim was to discover who the clothes belonged to by searching for their families, since prisoners from all over the department of Ayacucho were taken to the Cabitos military base. Exhumed clothes and even some items found near the body (hair accessories, jewelry, shoes, etc.) were placed onto a drawing of a non-specific silhouette of a person. These mobile exhibitions did not yield the expected results in terms of identifying the disappeared.

Nevertheless, these activities continued, and from September 2014, an exhibition of the clothing recovered from 53 of the still-unidentified bodies exhumed from La Hoyada was organized. The forensic team of the Public Prosecutor's Office and EPAF publicized the event in order to attract those who may be interested – namely, the relatives – and to try to speed up the identification process. The exhibition began in Lima, in the Office of the Ombudsman, and then moved to Ayacucho, where La Hoyada is located. Those who knew or suspected that their relatives had been taken to the Cabitos military base were invited to visit the clothing exhibition, which looked like a secondhand clothing store. In Lima, three families recognized the clothes their disappeared relatives were wearing when they were detained, among them Rosa López Cuevas, who recognized the trousers her husband, Ricardo Baldeón, was wearing when he disappeared in 1984 and who hoped that DNA tests would confirm his identity so she may recover his remains (Castillo 2014). These visual recognition devices, as an alternative to DNA tests of the bodies, give rise to a real process of anthropomorphization of the unearthed clothes. Described as "orphans," they seem to be granted the power of speech, as it is said they "talk" of the identity of those exhumed.

14.7 The uncertain dates and stretched time of bad death

The exhumations that have been carried out over recent years in Peru follow a ritualized, stereotyped sequential process that leads to the "spectacularization" of the circulation of the exhumed dead through public space. Once the remains are recovered from the morgue, a funeral procession to the city center is organized. The procession is accompanied by civil commemorations in the main square or even in city hall, in the presence of political authorities and with religious celebrations in honor of the deceased (Robin Azevedo 2021). The bodies are then taken to their respective villages where the last funeral rites are performed before being buried once more. When the bodies from the grave at Cceraocro were returned, the funeral march carried out in Ayacucho stopped in the old city center before mass was celebrated in the Company of Jesus church. The 17 coffins were sent to the village in a truck hired with funds from the state (High Level Multisectoral Commission: Comisión Multisectorial de Alto Nivel, CMAN) and the International Committee of the Red Cross. On arrival, the bodies were buried in the new cemetery, as the decision had been made by the community to abandon the old cemetery as soon as the armed conflict ended. The families could finally bury their dead in individual graves or as couples. The families who had since migrated to Lima returned in order to oversee the definitive reburial of their dead. The geography of the dead was mended in Cceraocro when the mass grave disappeared from the local landscape and when the remains it housed could be buried in the new cemetery, with the rest of the village's recently deceased.

This new cartography of the funerary economy also materialized in the unique experience of time, which was revealed during the new burial of the exhumed dead. Bensa (1997) stressed that temporality can only be "lived" through individual practices that construct time. A perceived, somewhat disorderly, temporality has crystalized in the inscription of dates on the headstones. Two dates are normally specified in the biography of the deceased: those of birth and death or, at worst, only the date of death. On the graves of those reburied in Cceraocro, there seems to be a temporal interference related to the biographical rupture and the disturbance of the posthumous rites of these inhabitants who were killed in the 1980s, but whose funerals were held almost three decades later. Thus, the grave of one of the victims, laid by her brothers – the only surviving members of the family – has a concrete plaque on top with a handwritten inscription: "Catalina Farfán, remembered by her brothers Rubén and Esmael." No date appears, which reinforces the feeling of temporal uncertainty and the state of incompleteness that characterizes these deaths from the period of violence. Many of the headstones mention only the date of death. For example, the cast iron cross bearing the names of Emilio Alacote and Cecilia Vilcatoma, which had originally been put on the mass grave and was later moved to the couple's new grave, indicates only the date of their death. Another plaque, made by their children and grandchildren for the burial in the cemetery, was also added, and which again shows only the date of their death: "died on February 3, 1984." The mentioning of only one date introduces the idea of a temporality that has remained fixed on the terrible incident of the massacre, and as Baptandier (2001) notes, violent and premature death may be seen as a "preterm death, like a preterm birth." Yet, other graves have a feature that seems to symbolize even more strongly the distortion of time accompanying these dead. In fact, the first time I went to the cemetery, it took me some time to identify and understand this spatial marker of a seemingly random temporality. In effect, some headstones mention the date of death and another date that is not the date of birth, but rather the date the remains were recovered, or more precisely, reburied. For example, the headstone of another of the victims shows two associated details:

Lucia Anyosa Limaco
Date: February 3, 1984 (date of death)
Remembered by her daughter Reyna
Date: May 31, 2012 (date of reburial)

The difficulty in deciding which dates to choose for the headstone is, without doubt, the culmination of the altered temporality that accompanies exhumation processes. In general, the "fixed time of rites" (Bensa 1997) manifests in the concern that the chronological order of the multiple phases of funeral rites be strictly followed – although not always successfully. The temporality shown on the graves does not refer to the biographical time of the deceased, but rather to that of a cycle, an interval, a waiting time, a time suspended since the moment of death (in 1984), and which is brought to an end with the (*a priori*) definitive reburial in the new cemetery (in 2012). Therefore, time gradually stretches between the moment of real death and its subsequent ritualization, when the death is fully recognized by the family and social group. Reflecting on the exhumation processes of those disappeared during the military dictatorship in Argentina, Colombo (2010) talks of "time which opens up" to evoke these exhumed bodies that belong to two different temporalities simultaneously: that of the moment of disappearance and that of their "appearance" in a present where they are still something different, in terms of their meaning. When the disappeared reappear, including the dead who are buried without funeral rites but in graves known to the family, this return is necessarily truncated. It is a way, according to the author, to "be without being," because what is extracted from the ground is only a partial presence of the disappeared. Therefore, these reappearances of human remains interrupt lineal, chronological time.

Finally, there is another phenomenon related to the interference of temporalities, similar to that of the headstones mentioned above, which is the courteous production of funeral "keepsakes." These small commemorative objects, which include the name of the deceased, some biographic details, and the dates of birth and death, are distributed among those attending the funeral service for them to keep in remembrance of the deceased, as also occurs in other life cycle rituals such as baptisms or weddings. In 2011, I accompanied the daughter of a community leader, killed by the Shining Path in the Soras massacre of 1983, to the ceremony held in Ayacucho for the restitution of the exhumed remains of the victims. When her father's coffin was left in city hall for the night vigil that had been organized there, the daughter handed out her keepsakes to the public, while explaining to me her doubts as to which dates to put: should she have put the date he was killed or the date of the funeral? She chose the date of death in the end, since the date of the funeral was still not certain. This temporal discrepancy between events long passed (1983) and the holding of the funeral (2011) clearly explains why it is difficult for the bereaved to assimilate the funeral ritual's new temporality, almost three decades after the death occurred.

14.8 Body substitutes in the absence of any trace of remains

While the exhumation of human remains leads to new rituals for their treatment, it is not always possible to recover the bodies. In fact, in some exhumations, it is not possible to determine the identity of all those buried in the grave. On occasion, the remains found cannot be identified due to their extreme degradation, because of either the acidity of the soil or simply the passing of time. This means that some families do not recover any material part of their deceased relatives, not even in fragments. So, as shown in the exhumations carried out in La Hoyada, despite human remains being found, many of these will remain unidentified and unidentifiable. The vast majority of the disappeared who were incinerated in the crematory oven built by the soldiers to dispose of the tortured and executed bodies will never be able to be returned to their loved ones. This emptiness that families – who have spent years searching for their disappeared relatives – have had to confront becomes even worse as they are seemingly condemned to perpetual uncertainty, having had their hopes raised by the exhumations. Gatti (2014) has analyzed the figure of the disappeared as a semantic void that refers to an invisible presence and which represents a catastrophe for identity and language. In the face of this inescapable void with which the families are forced to contend, how can they overcome the absence of a material basis around which to center mourning practices and process this suspended grief, which the exhumations briefly ignited hope of finally closing?

In this vein, Rojas-Pérez (2013, 2017) has analyzed some of the actions introduced by the National Association of Relatives of Kidnapped, Detained and Disappeared Persons of Peru (Asociación Nacional de Familiares de Secuestrados, Detenidos y Desaparecidos del Perú, ANFASEP), the famous group of mothers, sisters, and widows of the disappeared of Ayacucho whose children, brothers, and husbands were detained and taken to the Cabitos military base, from which they never returned. In the face of the impossibility of recovering their carbonized remains, the group sought to make the site at La Hoyada a "sanctuary for memory." Inaugurated in 2011, its purpose was to convert this place of massacre into a "sacred site." The mothers decided to bury there the exhumed remains that could not be identified and to put up a cross in whose shadow they could shelter. As Rojas-Pérez shows, La Hoyada provided a space where it "might be" that the disappeared "were possibly" buried; in other words, it opens up the possibility that the disappeared "could" be dead and, therefore, "could" be there. For the author, the use of the subjunctive mood and the possibility of a "whereness," albeit imperfect and doubtful, breaks the interminable temporality of forced disappearances. Despite the absence of bodies, it is finally possible to start a grieving process through regularly organized cultural mourning practices. In a different context, Truc (2011) and Aronson (2016) have analyzed how families of victims of the attacks of September 11, 2001, confronted the problem of disappeared bodies, crushed in the collapse of the twin towers in New York, and the controversy surrounding the rebuilding of the site at Ground Zero. Truc shows that for the families who fiercely opposed the reconstruction, the site is first and foremost a mass grave that serves as a tomb for their dead. Therefore, it should be considered "sacred ground" in the sense of having been consecrated by the dead themselves, as it contains the bodies of hundreds of people whose remains were reduced to dust and who can never be recovered. These two examples show the establishment of new ritual and symbolic arrangements through which to confront the impossibility of the remains of the disappeared being recovered.

As Thomas (1980, p. 46) has shown, the presence of a corpse is a distressing symbol of loss and of the precariousness of human life, yet it is also calming: the deceased is there and is acknowledged by their family. It may be added that this is also true in the case of exhumed remains. While, as has been shown, contact with these may be disturbing and adaptation may be a laborious process, nevertheless, it is around remains that new funerary rituals are reorganized. Thomas finds that human beings need a physical basis around which to organize grief work, even though this must be qualified and put into perspective according to the religious and cultural context. Since there is perhaps nothing more tragic than the absence of the body of the disappeared, who is doubly absent for being dead and not physically present, the need to compensate for this has given rise to the practice of *substitutes* that sustain *fictitious funerals* (Thomas 1980, p. 46, author's italics). In the case of exhumations where a body will never be found, identified, and returned to the relatives, this idea of substitutes can be seen in the so-called "symbolic funerals" that have recently been held in the Peruvian Andes. In the case of the massacre of the inhabitants of Parcco and Pomatambo (Vilcashuamán, Ayacucho) carried out by the army in 1986, and after which the bodies were burned, only 4 of the 12 victims exhumed could be identified and returned to their relatives, in October 2013. To assuage the absence of human remains, substitutes allowed the eight other families to organize "symbolic funerals."[13] A photo of the deceased, sometimes adorned with items of clothing, was placed in the bottom of the casket before closing it. According to Galinier and Jamous (1997), body substitutes allow "thinking and acting by delegation." They create a bridge and a continuity between the missing body and the world, which renews the relationship between the dead and the living. The substitute does not only serve to mark the absence of the body but also replaces it, becoming the instrument that allows the dead to be represented and indirectly acted upon. The device through which the properties of the body are transferred onto its substitute involves a process of anthropomorphization of the object or objects, such that they attain human status. It is also possible to draw a parallel here with practices of the veneration of sacred images in southern European Christianity. In the case of the substitution of miraculous images, Albert-Llorca (2013) has shown that the continuity of the cult requires that the copy substituting the original is vested with the same sacredness, through establishing a link that is both metaphorical and metonymic. In the case of the "symbolic funerals," the metaphorical and metonymic link of the photo and clothes placed in the casket is precisely what "creates" the substitute. This is what allows funerals to be carried out in absentia with a ritual arrangement that offers the bereaved the chance to express their pain. The staging with the open casket, in which the body substitutes have been placed, provides the families with a material grounding and a ritualized setting in which to cry for the death of their loved one. Finally, through these substitutes, the "missing" dead could join the collective procession of caskets that crossed the city before being taken to be buried in the cemeteries of their respective villages.

14.9 Conclusion

There is broad consensus today around the need to enact "reparations policies" as an essential part of the "dignification" of those killed during the Peruvian armed conflict and thus to give room to the grieving process of the relatives and survivors. Nevertheless, there needs to be greater questioning of the implementation of the exhumations relating to the forced disappearances and massacres of that time and the terrible human experiences underpinning them. Indeed, what the state has called "burial sites" in fact describe highly dissimilar situations. Some "sites" are known, and it is also known who is buried in them. Some of the deceased are even properly buried following a previous exhumation carried out by the family but without the corresponding legal procedures. Thus, some families even prefer not to exhume their dead. Other "sites" have yet to be located, or if they have been, their contents remain anonymous, and the relatives anxiously await exhumations in the hope of finding their disappeared relatives. Death has been established in the first type of burial site but not in the second. There is a fundamental distinction regarding uncertainty about the death of relatives. Although there is a semantic proximity that unites these burial places, in the sense that the dead found there have not always been socialized or soothed by the usual posthumous rituals, it is nevertheless important to develop a typology of "burial sites," to be exhumed according to the level of urgency, as based on the needs of those affected. However, by implementing sweeping public policies on the search for the disappeared and developing a plan for exhumations, the state places different situations on the same plane as if they were identical, when in reality, they differ from each other and are different for the bereaved. In fact, in legal terms, as already mentioned, those killed during the armed conflict who do not have death certificates and who are therefore not recognized as such by the state go in the category of "disappeared."

In the case of the Peruvian armed conflict, it may be said that the exhumed victims doubly belong to the category of bad death. On one hand, they were murdered and their bodies were subject to violence, while on the other, the dead were subjected to "ritualcide."[14] They did not receive the appropriate funeral rites, be that because they were made to disappear and thrown into clandestine graves in locations unknown to their relatives or because the relatives themselves buried them in improvised graves close to where they were killed, in the midst of the turmoil of war, and before the Shining Path militants or the army returned. In general, the exhumations mean that the living project a sense of "incompleteness" onto the dead, since these victims of bad death seem to have been amputated from themselves, as Baptandier (2001) has rightly described. This incomplete state and the ambivalence of these dead are the key to an indescribable malaise and to the struggle many families feel when the time comes for them to collect what is left of the bodies from the morgue and take possession of them. Producing an *ordinary* death in terms of rituals with these exhumed fragments is far from easy, and it is hard for the bereaved to complete the mourning period. Indeed, those broken bones, those dirty and bloodstained clothes, in sum, those broken bodies that are returned, do not have the same destiny *a priori*, nor have they been subjected to the same rituals as the regular dead.

Nevertheless, the examples mentioned here of the exhumation-identification-return-reburial sequence of the dead from the Peruvian armed conflict show an incredible human capacity to create mechanisms of collective resilience, as both a psychological process (grief) and a sociocultural one in the accompaniment of the deceased and their bereaved relatives (mourning). Anthropologists working in other regions, where societies have been faced with extreme experiences of mass killings and disappearances, have reached similar conclusions with regard to people's inventiveness in recreating links and giving new meaning to past, present, and future existence. Guillou and Vignato (2012) have described the processes put into practice in Southeast Asia to overcome collective death resulting from natural disasters and genocides. They show that in the face of the large-scale destruction of their surroundings, people who are faced with the unimaginable and the unpredictable see the collapsing of their world as definitive and without alternative. At the same time, these authors remind us that multiple attempts are made to reestablish social, symbolic, and psychological order by means of local and appropriate resilience devices. One of these attempts refers precisely to the search for the dead and concern over their destiny: the development of alternative rituals seeks to frame this situation in the best way possible. In this sense, more social science research needs to be carried out on the collective burials that follow exhumations, through ethnographic studies of the mechanisms of ritual and symbolic reformulation in relation to the return of the dead who have been marked by bad death.

Notes

1. Translator's note: Our translation. Unless otherwise stated, all translations of cited foreign language material in this article are our own.
2. The expression "human remains" refers to the fact that only rarely are whole bodies exhumed. Nevertheless, such a notion may be rejected by relatives due to the associated "objectification" of the bodies of their exhumed loved ones.
3. However, these figures on the distribution of responsibility for deaths remain a subject of debate to this day. Rendon (2019) rejects the CVR figures, estimating in fact the reverse, attributing 58.3% of deaths to the Peruvian state and 38.3% to the Shining Path.
4. According to the CVR (2013), 79% were of rural origin, 75% spoke Quechua or another indigenous language – such as the Asháninka of the Amazon – while only 16% of the overall population in Peru have a language other than Spanish as their first language. For a critical reading of the construction of the "indigenous victim," see Robin Azevedo and Delacroix (2017).

5. The arrival of forensic experts took place without prior notice to the inhabitants, including some relatives of those buried in the grave. The exhumation was the result of a petition carried out in Lima by a group of siblings who wished to recover the remains of their parents in order to bury them. It is worth noting that if a person requests the exhumation of a relative buried in a mass grave, and the state grants the request, then the grave is exhumed in its entirety, without needing to consult the other families. See Delacroix (2021) and Robin Azevedo (2021) on the different forms of revictimization of the families.
6. On this point, the oneiric appearance of the dead during the exhumations in the Andes should be noted; see, for example, the beautiful writings of Cecconi (2021) and Delacroix (2018).
7. See Robin Azevedo (2008) on the mechanisms of misfortune in the context of funeral rituals.
8. *Antemortem* reference cards contain a vast amount of information provided by the family about the person at the time of their death or disappearance. These cards list all elements that may allow posthumous identification, from the clothing, shoes, and jewelry worn on the day they disappeared to biophysical details (fillings or false teeth, physical deformities, etc.). All of these elements are used to create a personalized portrait of the victims to enable the identification of exhumed remains. See Taccoen (2013) on the techniques of identification procedures.
9. For the Merina, the "return of the dead" takes place when, a few years after death, a grave is reopened and the bones taken out, to then be reburied; this rite concludes the passing from a state of death to that of ancestor (Bloch 1971).
10. See Robin Azevedo (2006, 2008) on the treatment of the body during funeral rites in the rural Peruvian Andes.
11. Gatti uses the term *"chupadero"* (literally meaning "sucker") to evoke detention and torture centers in Argentina and Uruguay that operated through devastation, pulling people out of existence, erasing them, and then throwing them out like garbage.
12. The Peruvian Team of Forensic Anthropology (Equipo Peruano de Antropología Forense, EPAF) is an NGO specializing in the search for the disappeared and the exhumation of mass graves from the Peruvian armed conflict and took part in the excavation of the Cabitos-La Hoyada complex together with the forensic team of the Public Prosecutor's Office.
13. See "Homage to the Parcco and Pomatambo victims. Chapter 5: Placing of photos and clothing in the ossuaries," CMAN premises. https://www.youtube.com/watch?v=ZzJNyStxlrY.
14. "Ritualcide" is understood as the suddenly imposed suspension of a ritual practice; see LeVine (2010), cited in Guillou and Vignato (2012, p. 170).

References

Albert-Llorca, M. (2013). Les 'vraies' statues et leurs substituts. *Archives de Sciences Sociales des Religions* **161**: 251–269.

Anstett, E. (2020). Pourquoi exhumer? L'anthropologie du funéraire face au forensic turn. In: *(Im)matérialités de la mort* (ed. R. Azevedo V), 191–199. Paris: CNRS éditions.

Anstett, E. and Dreyfus, M. (2015). *Human Remains and Identification: Mass Violence, Genocide, and the 'Forensic Turn'*. Manchester: Manchester University Press.

Aronson, J.D. (2016). *Who Owns the Dead? The Science and Politics of Death in Ground Zero*. Cambridge, MA: Harvard University Press.

Baptandier, B. (2001). Introduction. In: *De la malemort en quelques pays d'Asie* (ed. B. Baptandier), 7–22. Paris: Karthala.

Bensa, A. (1997). Images et usages du temps. *Terrain* **29**: 5–18.

Bensa, A. and Fassin, E. (2002). Les sciences sociales face à l'événement. *Terrain* **38**: 5–20.

Bloch, M. (1971). *Placing the Dead: Tomb, Ancestral Village and Kinship Organization in Madagascar*. London/New York: Seminar Press.

Castillo, M.E. (2014). Familiares de tres desaparecidos reconocen prendas exhumadas en fosas junto al cuartel Los Cabitos. *La República*, 13 de septiembre.

Cecconi, A. (2021). 'En mi sueño lo veo como si estuviera vivo, pero cuando despierto él no está'. Sueños, violencia política y exhumaciones en Perú y en España. In: *Retorno de cuerpos, recorrido de almas. Exhumaciones y duelos colectivos en América Latina y España* (Dirs. (eds. A.-M. Losonczy and R. Azevedo V), 50–70. Bogotá, Lima: Universidad de los Andes, IFEA.

Colombo, P. (2010). Exhumaciones: (des)aparecidos o cuando la tierra se abre. In: *Claves actuales de pensamiento* (eds. M. Navarro, B. Estévez, and A. Sánchez Cuervo), 63–72. Madrid–México: Plaza y Valdés editores.

Comisión de la Verdad y Reconciliación, CVR. (2003). Informe final. Lima. http://cverdad.org.pe/ifinal/ (accessed 202).

Cordeu, E., Illia, E., and Montevechio, B. (1994). El duelo y el luto. Etnología de los idearios de la muerte. *Runa. Archivo para las ciencias del hombre* **21**(1): 31–155.

Delacroix, D. (2016). *De pierres et de larmes. Mémorialisation et discours victimaire dans le Pérou d'après-guerre*. Paris: Institut Universitaire de Varenne.

Delacroix, D. (2018). Le bal des âmes. Postérité de la mort de masse en contexte péruvien, *Terrain* [En ligne], Terrains, mis en ligne le 10 septembre 2018. http://journals.openedition.org/terrain/16819. https://doi.org/10.4000/terrain.16819. (Consultado el 12 de junio 2019).

Delacroix, D. (2021). L'Etat cannibale. Rumeurs de trafic d'os exhumés au Pérou. *Cultures et conflits* **121**: 184–207.

Duterme, C. (2016). Honouring, commemorating, compensating: state and civil society in response to victims of the armed conflict in the Ixil region (Guatemala). *Human Remains and Violence* **2**(2): 3–20. doi: 10.7227/HRV.2.2.2HUMANREMAINSandVIOLENCE.

Duterme, C. (2017). Ritualités funéraires autour des morts exhumés: de l'élaboration des pratiques aux enjeux de reconstruction collective et individuelle. 35. ethnographiques.org. https://www.ethnographiques.org/2017/Duterme

Fassin, D. (2011). *Humanitarian Reason: A Moral History of the Present*. Berkeley, CA: University of California Press.

Fassin, D. and Rechtman, R. (2009). *The Empire of Trauma. An Inquiry into the Condition of Victimhood*. New York: Princeton University Press.

Ferrándiz, F. (2013). Exhuming the defeated: Civil war mass graves in 21st-century Spain. *American Ethnologist* **40**(1): 38–54.

Ferrándiz, F. and Robben, A. (2015). *Necropolitics. Mass Graves in the Age of Human Rights*. Philadelphia, PA: Pennsylvania University Press.

Galinier, J. and Jamous, R. (1997). Penser et agir par substituts. Le corps en perspective. *Ateliers* **18**: 5–10.

Gatti, G. (2014). *Surviving Forced Disappearance in Argentina and Uruguay*. New York: Palgrave Mac Milan.

Guillou, A.Y. (2012). An alternative memory of the Khmer Rouge genocide: The dead of the mass graves and the land guardian spirits. *South East Asia Research* **20**(2): 207–226.

Guillou, A.Y. and Vignato, S. (2012). Introduction. Special issue life after collective death in South East Asia. *South East Asia Research* **20**(2): 161–174.

Hertz, R. (1960 [1907]). *Death and the Right Hand*. Glencoe, IL: The Free Press.

Koc-Menard, N. (2014). Notes from the fields: Exhuming the past after Peruvian internal conflict. *International Journal of Transitional Justice* **8**(2): 277–288.

Korman, R. (2017). Bury or display? The politics of exhumation in post-genocide Rwanda. In: *Human Remains and Identification. Mass Violence, Genocide, and the 'Forensic Turn'* (eds. E. Anstett and J.-M. Dreyfus), 203–220. Manchester: Manchester University Press.

Kwon, H. (2012). Rethinking traumas of war. *South East Asia Research* **20**(2): 227–237.

Lefranc, S. (2012). A critique of "bottom-up" peacebuilding. Do peaceful individuals make peaceful societies? In: *Peacebuilding, Memory and Reconciliation: Bridging Top-Down and Bottom-Up Approaches* (eds. B. Charbonneau and G. Parent), 34–50. NY: Routledge.

Losonczy, A.M. and Robin Azevedo, V. (dirs.) (2021). *Retorno de cuerpos, recorrido de almas. Exhumaciones y duelos colectivos en América Latina y España*. Bogotá/Lima: Universidad de los Andes/IFEA.

Ministry of Justice and Human Rights. (2020). Reporte estadístico n.° 1. Registro Nacional de Personas Desaparecidas y de Sitios de Entierro. Lima. https://www.gob.pe/institucion/minjus/informes-publicaciones/1666390-reporte-estadistico-n-01-renade (Consultado el February 2, 2021).

Office of the Ombudsman, Republic of Peru. (2013). A diez años de la verdad, justicia y reparación. Avances, retrocesos y desafíos de un proceso inconcluso. Informe N° 162. Lima. https://www.defensoria.gob.pe/wp-content/uploads/2018/05/Resumen-Ejecutivo-ID-162.pdf (accessed 202).

Panizo, L.M. (2012). Ausencia y desaparición: el caso de los desaparecidos de la última dictadura militar en Argentina. *Argos* **29**(57): 94–125.

Panizo, L.M. (2021). De la muerte desatendida a su reconocimiento social: Prácticas y sentidos en torno a la desaparición de personas en Argentina. In: *Retorno de cuerpos, recorrido de almas. Exhumaciones y duelos colectivos en América Latina y España* (eds. A.M. Losonczy and V. Robin Azevedo), 77–98. Bogotá/Lima: Universidad de los Andes/IFEA.

Panizo, M.L. and Robin Azevedo, V. (2021). Reconvertir la "mala muerte" en época del Covid-19. In: *Emociones y Pandemia: Esbozos de la Incertidumbre* (eds. Colin et al.), 55–63. Buenos Aires: Editorial Triángulo.

Parra, R.C., Palma, M.R., Calcina, O., Tejada, J., et al. (2020). Peruvian forensic experience in the search for missing persons and the identification of human remains: History, limitations, and future challenges. In: Forensic Science and Humanitarian Action: Interacting with the Dead and the Living (eds. R.C. Parra, S.C. Zapico, and D.H. Ubelaker), 635–652. Hoboken, NJ: John Wiley & Sons.

Rendon, S. (2019). Capturing correctly: a reanalysis of the indirect capture–recapture methods in the Peruvian Truth and Reconciliation Commission. *Research & Politics* **6**(1) https://doi.org/10.1177/2053168018820375.

Ricoeur, P. (2004). *Memory, History, Forgetting*. Chicago, IL: University of Chicago Press.

Robin Azevedo, V. (2006). Caminos a la otra vida. Ritos funerarios en los Andes peruanos meridionales. In: *Etnografías de Cuzco*. Cuzco: Centro de Estudios Regionales Andinos Bartolomé de Las Casas/Instituto Francés de Estudios Andinos.

Robin Azevedo, V. (2008). *Miroirs de l'Autre vie. Pratiques rituelles et discours sur les morts dans les Andes de Cuzco (Pérou).* Nanterre: Société d'ethnologie.
Robin Azevedo, V. (2021). ¿Devolver la dignidad a los desaparecidos del conflicto armado peruano? Exhumaciones, justicia transicional y políticas de la compasión. In: *Retorno de cuerpos, recorrido de almas. Exhumaciones y duelos colectivos en el mundo hispanohablante* (eds. A.-M. Losonczy and V.R. Azevedo), 27–54. Bogotá/Lima: Universidad de los Andes/IFEA.
Robin Azevedo, V. and Delacroix, D. (2017). Categorización étnica, conflicto armado interno y reparaciones simbólicas en el Perú post - Comisión de la Verdad y Reconciliación (CVR). *Nuevo Mundo Mundos Nuevos* [En línea]. HYPERLINK "http://journals.openedition.org/nuevomundo/71688"http://journals.openedition.org/nuevomundo/71688
Rojas-Pérez, I. (2013). Inhabiting unfinished past: Law, transitional justice, and mourning in Postwar Peru. *Humanity: An International Journal of Human Rights, Humanitarianism, and Development* **4**(1): 149–170.
Rojas-Pérez, I. (2017). *Mourning Remains. State Atrocity, Exhumations, and Governing the Disappeared in Peru's Postwar Andes.* Stanford, CA: Stanford University Press.
Sanford, V. (2003). *Buried Secrets. Truth and Human Rights in Guatemala.* New York: Palgrave Macmillan.
Taccoen, M. (2013). Cuerpos y violencia de masa: las informaciones que pueden proveer los profesionales de medicina legal. In: *Cadáveres impensables, cadáveres impensados. El tratamiento de los cuerpos en las violencias de masa y los genocidios* (eds. E. Anstett, J.-M. Dreyfus, and S. Garibian), 51–58. Buenos Aires: Miño y Dávila.
Thomas, L.-V. (1980). *Le cadavre. De la Biologie à l'anthropologie.* Paris: Editions complexe.
Truc, G. (2011). Ground zero entre chantier et charnier. Sur les rapports entre pulvérisation de corps humains, mémoire et lieux. *Raisons Politiques* **41**: 33–49.
Uceda, R. (2003). *Muerte en el Pentagonito.* Bogotá: Planeta.
Uribe, M.V. (2018). *Antropología de la inhumanidad.* Bogotá: Universidad de los Andes.

CHAPTER 15

Migrant death and the ethics of visual documentation in forensic anthropology

Krista E. Latham[1,2], Alyson J. O'Daniel[3] and Tanya Ramos[4]

[1]*Department of Biology and Anthropology, University of Indianapolis, USA*
[2]*Human Identification Center, University of Indianapolis, USA*
[3]*Department of Anthropology, University of Indianapolis, USA*
[4]*Department of Biology, University of Indianapolis, USA*

15.1 Introduction

Forensic anthropology is at a historically important crossroads. Like many academic disciplines across the US, calls for racial justice amid the stark realities of police brutality, income inequality, and health disparities exacerbated by the global COVID-19 pandemic have brought questions of social responsibility to the forefront of scholarly debate within the field. Important work on the effects of cognitive bias (see, for example, Dror et al. 2021; Nakhaeizadeh et al. 2014a, 2014b; Hartley 2007; Jeanguenat et al. 2017; Winburn 2018) and the role of theory in shaping forensic methods and analyses (Wylie 1992; Winburn and Clemmons 2021) make clear how culture shapes the supposedly objective spaces of forensic science. While social scientists have long examined science as a culturally constructed social milieu inseparable from conditions of social life (Latour and Woolgar 1986), more recent iterations of this critical work powerfully call into question notions of objectivity as harmful to, rather than necessary for, the provision of justice and the pursuit of knowledge and understanding (Winburn and Clemmons 2021; see also Rodriguez Almada et al. 2021).

In this vein, some forensic anthropologists have also recently begun to question the ways in which forensic anthropology values and practices fail to foster conditions necessary for a diverse and inclusive discipline (Tallman and Bird 2022). Calls for the critical assessment of disciplinary methods, practices, missions, and

Anthropology of Violent Death: Theoretical Foundations for Forensic Humanitarian Action, First Edition.
Edited by Roberto C. Parra and Douglas H. Ubelaker.

values (Winburn et al's 2021), therefore, aim to recognize the fallibility of current forensic science, to appreciate the existing diversity of forensic science practitioners, and to move the discipline accordingly toward a more socially responsible model of leadership and practice. Such a task requires, as Winburn and Clemmons (2021) demonstrate, a meaningful reckoning with the role of sociocultural conditions in shaping the state of forensic anthropology today.

In the pages that follow, we seek to advance a socially responsible forensic anthropology by considering the real and potential impacts of contemporary visual documentation practices in the field's publication platforms. We focus in particular on the inclusion of photographs involving human remains within publications concerning mass casualty events in the US. Such an analysis enables us to explicate the unspoken ethical norms and values structuring decisions to publish images of human remains and antemortem images. We then, in turn, consider how such ethical norms and values articulate with broader sociocultural contexts of inequality in America. In so doing, we move beyond theorizing the crossroads of change to take an active step toward a disciplinary reckoning.

The present analysis is based on Winburn et al. (2021) premise that an inclusive forensic science will require us to build a new, more robust code of ethics. We contend that a revised ethical code that is responsive to the values of diversity and inclusion will be rooted in a deep appreciation of little-discussed trends in disciplinary practices, those taken-for-granted aspects of the work, as well as how such taken-for-granted practices reflect and may reproduce structural inequalities. In short, we contend that our ethics are not just what we say *we should do*; they are also what we are *enabled to do*. Through the lens of three politically charged mass casualty scenarios, the September 11th terrorist attacks, Hurricane Katrina, and the US–Mexico migrant death crisis, we explicate trends in how forensic anthropologists circulate, discuss, and use photographs of human remains within contexts of publication and under contemporary conditions of racialization too often ignored as important to our work. We explore such trends as examples of how the ethics of visual representation in our field, however implicit they may be, are shaped by historically driven scientific racism, public sentiment, and the broader socio-political conditions circumscribing the events. Such a perspective offers an entry point for making explicit the connection of our work to culture and otherwise tacit understandings of the ethical that may warrant further scrutiny and change.

15.2 Disciplinary ethics and social change: contextualizing forensic anthropology practices

Anthropologists have long studied how communities, societies, and disciplines compose and experience notions, social relations, and processes of "the ethical"

(Csordas 2013; Ortner 2016, p. 59), including anthropology's disciplinary obligation to protect individuals and communities on whom we base our work (Hymes 1974; Price 2011; Scheper-Hughes 1995). From at least as early as Franz Boas' censure for speaking against scientists' use of their professional identities as a cover for government-driven spying (Fluehr-Lobban 2003) anthropologists have debated the proper role of our discipline within public political processes (Heyman 2010). Decades of debate concerning the ethical imperatives of the discipline have led to widespread acceptance that ethics are indeed a traceable social and analytical domain that are created, enacted, and reproduced at complex intersections of personal, local, and global social life (Bornstein and Redfield 2010; Fassin 2012). In other words, a code of ethics does not exist apart from social actions occurring within and shaped by sociopolitical contexts of everyday life. On the contrary, the meaning of what counts as ethical in theory and in practice is interwoven with the material, ideological, and political conditions of community and society (Cassaniti and Hickman 2014; Ticktin 2006) and to what ends practices of the ethical are breached and/or reproduced (Howell 1996). As conditions of daily life, community, and society change, so too do the meanings and practices of the ethical. Indeed, as Fluehr-Lobban (2003) illuminates, general anthropological ethics have come into the clearest view as they shift under conditions of sociopolitical crisis.

General anthropology thus teaches us that ethics are enacted in the everyday spaces of our lives, including the spaces of our daily habits of work (Mattingly 2014). Ethics are what we *do* in the field, how we speak in our shared disciplinary spaces, what we imagine as the values of our discipline, and the limits of appropriate behavior therein. A formal ethical code can therefore provide us with abstracted values, but they become meaningful only within specific referential and material contexts where that abstracted value is at stake or in question. Shared ethics, in other words, require a shared referential context. Take, for example, the code of ethics for the American Board of Forensic Anthropology (ABFA), the certifying body for Forensic Anthropologists in the US (American Board of Forensic Anthropology, Inc. 2020).

Like the code of conduct for the American Academy of Forensic Sciences (see Winburn et al. 2021), the Code of Ethics and Conduct for the ABFA reveals a set of guidelines meant to clarify and protect the discipline's scientific authority. The code prioritizes the professional and scientific behavior of the *individual as it relates to the integrity of and public trust within the position held by the discipline's diplomates*. For example, tenet b concerns the misrepresentation of professional credentials and tenet c concerns the individual obligation to avoid misrepresentation of the scientific data. Tenet d further asserts that forensic scientists must refrain from making public statements or providing testimony based on epistemological frameworks other than science. In other words, testimony that is not "scientifically based" must be avoided. Clearly, the referential context against which the

American Board of Forensic Anthropology, Inc. CODE OF ETHICS AND CONDUCT

SECTION I – THE CODE: As a means to promote the highest quality of professional and personal conduct of its members, the following constitutes the Code of Ethics and Conduct, which is endorsed and adhered to by all Diplomates of the ABFA

Diplomates of the ABFA shall:

a) refrain from exercising professional or personal conduct adverse to the best interests and purposes of the ABFA;

b) refrain from providing any material misrepresentation of education, training, experience, or area of expertise. Misrepresentation of one or more criteria for certification shall constitute a violation of this section of the code;

c) refrain from providing any material misrepresentation of data upon which an expert opinion or conclusion is based. Diplomates shall render opinions and conclusions strictly in accordance with the evidence in the case (hypothetical or real) and only to the extent justified by the evidence;

d) not make statements in his/her written reports, public addresses, or testimony that is not technically correct and scientifically based;

e) act at all times in a completely impartial manner by employing scientific methodology to reach logical, unbiased conclusions, and by reporting all findings in a clear, concise manner;

f) set a reasonable fee for services if it is appropriate to do so; however, no services shall be rendered on a contingency fee basis;

g) treat all information from an agency or client with the confidentiality required;

h) refrain from issuing public statements that appear to represent the position of the ABFA without the specific authority first obtained from the Board of Directors

ABFA code of ethics registers as meaningful is that of our claim to the cultural value of scientific authority.

Such an approach to defining the ethical perhaps places exclusive importance on the reproduction of the discipline – the assurance of its survival within a broader cultural context that prioritizes the value of scientific authority. To be fair, legitimation of the field is important, especially when practice within the US criminal justice system can impact an individual's freedom or imprisonment; the need for standards, which outline the difference between science and pseudoscience, is important to safeguard in this respect. Yet, an ethical code that, at best implies or attests that forensic anthropology and forensic anthropologists somehow operate independently of culture is based on a belief that contradicts longstanding social scientific findings. The imperative to be impartial and unbiased is presented as self-evident and achievable within the frameworks of science (see Winburn and Clemmons (2021), for an insightful critique of scientific objectivity). However, one might question the value of being unbiased within a disciplinary history, which normalized owning and displaying the racialized dead in the name of scientific and forensic "progress." The notion of science as value-free or politically neutral is widespread and, among the ranks of forensic scientists, a deeply sensitive issue. Conversations regarding the fallacy of scientific objectivity and implicit and cognitive biases in relation to forensic science are beginning, such as the thought-provoking response (Winburn et al. 2021) discussed in the introduction (see also, Winburn and Clemmons 2021), but deeper reflections on the impact of our disciplinary fallibility must be systematically explored. Perhaps instead of basing forensic anthropology ethics upon a presumption of scientific objectivity, we might do well to consider the complicated relationships our disciplinary practices have to cultural processes and historical conditions that are decidedly non-neutral and the potential for these practices to be harmful to the communities we strive to serve.

For example, understanding the use of visual documentation as a tool for institutionalizing racism in the sciences requires an understanding of the context and goals of the human biological sciences at the time of emergence. Early studies of the earth and its living inhabitants were conducted by "naturalists," who were funded by the Christian Church, and who subscribed to the *Great Chain of Being* concept. The Great Chain of Being, or *scala naturae* was based on Aristotelian notions of perfection, and posited that God had created several varieties of humans, which could be hierarchically ranked according to their closeness to God. The concept sought to explain the ethnocentric notion that certain populations had progressed to civilization, while other populations languished in a state of what they viewed as biological degeneracy (Aristotle 1910, 1912a 1912b; Harris 2001, pp. 80–99). Based on this premise, scholars held in high esteem by the field of biology even today, like Linnaeus, categorized human races based on subjective ideas of superiority and inferiority that were couched in the language of rationality and science, which then granted the findings a façade of objectivity and authority. For example, Linnaeus's *Systema Natura* (1740) offers a taxonomy of humans that includes four varieties of man based largely on geography, including *Americanus rubescens, Europaeus albus, Asiaticus fuscus,* and *Africanus niger*. In a later published edition, Linnaeus (1758) imbued these categories with moral and behavioral attributes, ultimately investing popular thought with the currency of scientific observation (Linnean Society of London 2021). The hierarchical arrangement of man's varieties formed the ideological basis for justifying continued conquest and enslavement. This linear sequence of ranking human types based on their perceived moral attributes held a prominent place in Western thought and subsequently formed the foundation for sciences of the human body yet to come, including osteology, a precursor to forensic anthropology (Blakey 2020; Nee 2005; Brace 2005).

While theories of polygenesis, that human races were different species, faded in Europe over time, the quest to scientifically "prove" the biological superiority of European populations to justify material and political conditions of inequality and slavery continued to fuel early nineteenth century anatomists and osteologists in the US (Gould 1981). Osteology, in its earliest years and like other biological sciences, was an academic enterprise that gained legitimacy through its work sorting human populations into racial groups for purposes of confirming the false notion of discrete human races that could be hierarchically ranked in ways that corresponded to biological differences (Brace 2005; Ahmed 2002). Morton (1839), for example, curated one of the world's largest collections of human skulls as part of his work in linking cranial capacity to intellectual and moral prowess. The findings of his studies reaffirmed popularized notions of non-white peoples as inferior races of humankind. Such sentiments were often conveyed through imagery establishing visual "proof" of the legitimacy of a social hierarchy based on ideologies of white superiority. For example, images created by the Dutch anatomist Petrous Camper in the eighteenth century illustrating the facial angle, or prognathism, in various human and non-human primate populations catalyzed craniometric approaches to racial classification and were subsequently used as "evidence" for polygenesis (Camper 1770). His images depicted what was considered an idealized craniofacial profile of a Greek statue (100°) through a progressive lowering of 80° for European populations, 70° for Asian and African populations, 58° for Orangutans, and finally 42° for monkeys (Camper 1770; Meijer and Camper 1997).

Another iconic image of scientific racism can be found in a text published by students of Morton aimed at advocating for polygenesis. The image displays drawings of three faces and their corresponding skulls: a European, an African, and a Chimpanzee. The image is meant to depict Black people as closer to apes because of the appearance of certain physical features (Nott et al. 1854). From the notion that humans are inheritably biologically unequal and can be categorized and ranked based on their skeletal features to the entitled belief of bringing a universal truth to others, was born the field of American biological anthropology and later, its subspecialty of forensic anthropology (Blakey 2020; Brace 2005; Menand 2001–2002; Baker 1998, pp. 14–15).

Seen in this light, racist ideology and visual documentation have historically provided a twinned foundation for the establishment of scientific authority in the biological sciences, including forensic anthropology. As Ahmed (2002, p. 49) explains, "While Western Science legitimated itself as objective, disinterested and value-free, it was interested, situated and value-laden. It sought to legitimate itself by defining its object ('race') as "the nature" that must be understood in order to be controlled." Visual documentation provided "proof" that race was an objective natural fact; one needed only to inspect the difference and otherness depicted in images produced by authorities imbued with the power of science. The notion of scientific authority was built on the untenable and socially subjective foundation of racism and, as is currently constructed in relation to myths of objectivity, is ill-suited as an unqualified referential context for a contemporary ethical code. Seen in this light, the uncritical use of a historically given and generalized referential context of scientific authority for our contemporary ethical code leaves unexamined the legacies of scientific racism in forensic anthropology and the ways in which contemporary processes of race may continue to seep through the porous social boundaries of our disciplinary practices, such as visual documentation.

In the spirit of engaging with these thorny questions of history, authority, and social responsibility in forensic science, we use the remainder of this chapter to explore contemporary visual documentation practices in major publications associated with the field of forensic anthropology. We argue that visual documentation provides a window into tacit ethical norms of the work and the disquieting ways in which these norms articulate with sociocultural and historical contexts of inequality.

15.3 Methods and scope

This analysis stems from a generalized concern with the visual display of perished migrants' remains in US popular media. Photographs of skeletal remains, bodies in various states of decomposition, and personal effects, such as identification cards and family photographs, are ubiquitous across media outlets covering stories about migrant death.[1] It is in this context that the authors began to consider their own visual display practices and the potential meanings of human remains visual display within the field's scientific and academic publication platforms.

The display of graphic images underscores the violence and devastation occurring at the US southern border. In *Regarding the Pain of Others,* Sontag (1993, p. 21) explains that "Something becomes real – to those who are elsewhere, following it as 'news' – by being photographed." The more vivid the image, the more real it becomes and, perhaps, the pain of others becomes a subject of public concern. At the same time, however, Sontag reminds us that photographs are viewed by multiple audiences who will interpret their meaning in varied and unintended ways. For example, photographs intended to invoke concern may also be viewed as aggressive and hostile. This concern for the meanings of visual displays of human remains in the contexts of migrant death and the history of the biological sciences leads us to consider the use and meanings of contemporary visual display practices within forensic anthropology publications. Understanding that the inclusion of visual sources in forensic anthropology publications, may differ from the use of visual sources in the media, we have chosen to refer to visual displays in forensic anthropology media contexts described below as "visual documentation." This linguistic choice, however, is an uneasy one because forensic scientists do sometimes choose to share photographs with public media outlets and may have varied intentions in whatever context they use visual communication.

Following Maier et al. (2020), we examine forensic science literature to assess otherwise tacit contemporary attitudes and practices in the field. We concede that ours is but an exploratory foray into practices of visual documentation; this project was necessarily narrow in scope at the time we undertook the work. That is to say that we examined but a small slice of visual documentation practices in order to gauge the appropriateness of broader studies related to this issue. For this "pilot," we chose two journals in which to analyze images related to the three mass casualty events associated with the September 11, 2001, terrorist attacks, Hurricane Katrina, and the ongoing US–Mexico border migrant death crisis. These events were chosen because they not only represent mass casualty events of public interest but also represent catalysts for improvements in the technologies associated with human identification in the field of forensic science, both criteria which increase the chances of high publication rates. The Journal of Forensic Science (JFS) and the American Journal of Physical Anthropology (AJPA) were chosen because they publish the majority of forensic science and more specifically, forensic anthropology articles focusing on the US and encompassing the time frames in question. While a newer journal *Forensic Anthropology*, which is devoted to advances and issues in the field of forensic anthropology, would be an ideal place to search for articles focusing on the identification of human remains, its first issue was published in 2018, and therefore was not an avenue for publication during the earlier two incidents. Thus, we chose to utilize the two journals with the highest volume of forensic anthropology articles related to US policy and practice that spanned the time frame of interest.

We conducted an advanced keyword search through each journal's webpage[2] that encompassed all issues published through August 25, 2021. The same keywords were used for each journal for consistency: "World Trade Center," "September 11," "9/11," "Hurricane Katrina," "Border deaths," "US–Mexico border," and "Undocumented border crossers."

The initial results provided more articles than were relevant to our research (9953 articles). This is because all articles using those terms were included, whether or not they focused on victim identification. For example, one article included in the initial keyword search of "US–Mexico border" focused on the concordance between a decedent's social race affiliation and the forensic anthropologist's classification into an ancestral category. The key word was used when referencing "US–Mexico border casework" (Winburn and Algee-Hewitt 2021). Another example of an article included in the initial keyword search for "Hurricane Katrina" explores relationships between gun suicides, past trauma, and gun access and storage (Ramchand et al. 2018). The term "Hurricane Katrina" was mentioned as a catalyst for purchasing a firearm and as past trauma. Therefore, each article was downloaded as a portable document format (PDF) and read to ensure that the dataset included only articles that focused specifically on victim identification or treatment of the dead. In addition, our search yielded duplicate articles for the same event in instances when the article included more than one of the searched keywords. Duplicates for the same event were deleted from the dataset, while duplicates that discussed more than one event were not. In total, our search yielded 56 articles corresponding to 62 results to explore for visual documentation practices (Table 15.1).

Table 15.1 Final search results.

Journal	Keyword	Results
JFS	"World Trade Center"	14
JFS	"September 11"	4
JFS	"9/11"	1
JFS	"Hurricane Katrina"	12
JFS	"Border deaths"	4
JFS	"US–Mexico border"	16
JFS	"Undocumented border crossers"	3
AJPA	"World Trade Center"	0
AJPA	"September 11"	0
AJPA	"9/11"	1
AJPA	"Hurricane Katrina"	1
AJPA	"Border deaths"	0
AJPA	"US–Mexico border"	2
AJPA	"Undocumented border crossers"	4
	Total articles	56*

*Note that several articles discuss more than one of these mass casualty events. Therefore, the total number of articles is smaller than the total number of "Results."

All 56 articles were read and reviewed by the authors to determine the following:

Question Set 1: Did the article contain visual images? What are the subjects of any included images? Did any articles contain antemortem or postmortem images of the victims? Did any articles include identifying information regarding the victims? How were included images discussed or contextualized within the text?

Once we answered these initial descriptive questions, we considered them in the aggregate, considering such questions as:

Question Set 2: Is there a difference in the frequency of visual documentation between the two journals? Is there a difference in the frequency of visual documentation use among the three mass casualty events? Is there a difference in the frequency of victim photos within included visual documentation among the three mass casualty events?

In the final stage of qualitative analysis, we considered:

Question Set 3: Through what sociocultural contexts might we make sense of any observed trends in visual documentation practices?

15.3.1 Findings

15.3.1.1 Question set 1

Did the article contain visual images? What are the subjects of any included images? Did any articles contain antemortem or postmortem images of the victims? Did any articles include identifying information regarding the victims? How were included images discussed or contextualized within the text?

15.3.1.1.1 The September 11th terrorist attacks A close review of the images in the articles associated with the September 11, 2001 terrorist attacks, reveals only five articles have visual depictions of antemortem images or human remains: a total of 8 photographs and 17 radiographs all limited to JFS (Tables 15.2 and 15.3) (Adams and Aschheim 2016; Vehit and Christensen 2019; Klavens et al. 2020; Simpson et al. 2007; Baraybar 2008). One article discusses dental records as a means of personal identification. Dental data from the World Trade Center victims were discussed and two images of dental radiographs appear in the article. However, the radiographs are not identified as belonging specifically to victims of that event (Adams and Aschheim 2016). Another focuses on sorting commingled remains in mass fatality events, such as the September 11th World Trade Center Victims, and contains an image of a radius. However, the bone is from the anatomical collection from which the sorting method was derived and does not belong to a victim (Vehit and Christensen 2019). An article focusing on DNA identifications discusses DNA typing success in a World Trade Center sample

Table 15.2 Articles with visual images.

Journal	Keyword	Results	Articles containing visual images	Number of images
JFS	"World Trade Center"	14	3	4
JFS	"September 11"	4	2	21
JFS	"9/11"	1	0	0
JFS	"Hurricane Katrina"	12	3	33
JFS	"Border deaths"	4	1	10
JFS	"US–Mexico border"	16	3	10
JFS	"Undocumented border crossers"	3	1	8
AJPA	"World Trade Center"	0	0	0
AJPA	"September 11"	0	0	0
AJPA	"9/11"	1	0	0
AJPA	"Hurricane Katrina"	1	0	0
AJPA	"Border deaths"	0	0	0
AJPA	"US–Mexico border"	2	0	0
AJPA	"Undocumented border crossers"	4	1	6
	Totals	56*	14*	92*

*Note that several articles discuss more than one of these mass casualty events. Therefore, the total number of articles is smaller than the total number of "Results."

Table 15.3 Articles with visual images

Event	Total visual images	Photographs of skeletal remains or rntemortem images	Radiographs
The September 11th terrorist attacks	25	8	17
Hurricane Katrina	33	3	30
US–Mexico migrant death crisis	34	33	1
Totals	92*	44*	48*

*Note that several articles discuss more than one of these mass casualty events. Therefore, the total number of articles is smaller than the total number of "Results."

and includes an image of a femur that has been cut for DNA analysis. The bone in this particular image was obtained from a body donation facility (Klavens et al. 2020). Two articles discuss challenging human identifications, and the World Trade Center victims are mentioned as an example. However, the focus of the articles is on international cases. One of these articles includes 15 radiographs and images of bones containing orthopedic implants, which are case studies from Australia (Simpson et al. 2007). The other contains three images of a skull representing a case study from Peru (Baraybar 2008). Additionally, two articles that met the search criteria include images of non-human remains (Christensen et al. 2012; Antinick and Foran 2019).

In summary, for the articles related to the September 11 terrorist attacks, a total of 25 antemortem images or images of human remains are included. Two of these images are radiographs that are being used to explain the process of dental identification. Two articles discuss advances in identification techniques and include images of bones from donors. These images are clean bones in a laboratory setting and are included to demonstrate the methods of a new technique. The final two articles include images of victims, but they are not World Trade Center victims. One includes antemortem and postmortem radiographs and bones with surgical implants. The other contains photographs of three skulls of victims of an army patrol in Peru from 1983. None of the reviewed World Trade Center articles published images of the actual victims of the terrorist attack.

15.3.1.1.2 Hurricane Katrina Three articles in the Hurricane Katrina Category have visual depictions of antemortem images or human remains: a total of 3 photographs and 30 radiographs all limited to JFS (Tables 15.2 and 15.3) (Danforth et al. 2009; van der Meer et al. 2010; Simpson et al. 2007). One article focuses on the use of The AribexTM NOMADTM portable hand-held dental radiation emitting device in identification efforts following Hurricane Katrina. Four dental radiographs are presented as example images produced by the machine on training mannequins (Danforth et al. 2009). Another also focuses on the importance of dental identification in the aftermath of Hurricane Katrina. This article enlists volunteer forensic scientists to compare postmortem and antemortem dental radiographs. The radiographs come from "actual forensic dental identification cases completed at the Bexar County Forensic Sciences Center, San Antonio, Texas between the years 1999 and 2008" and not victims of Hurricane Katrina (van der Meer et al. 2010). The final article was included in the previous section because it mentions the challenges of victim identification after both the World Trade Center terrorist attacks and Hurricane Katrina and contains 15 radiographs and images of bones containing orthopedic implants that are case studies from Australia (Simpson et al. 2007). In addition, one article discusses identification techniques associated with Hurricane Katrina and includes the image of an upper and lower denture belonging to a test subject and not a victim (Richmond and Pretty 2009). One additional article in this category discusses the impact of underwater decomposition on victims like those associated with Hurricane Katrina and includes images of non-human remains (Cartozzo et al. 2021).

In summary, for the articles related to victim identification in the aftermath of Hurricane Katrina, a total of 33 images of humans/human remains are included. Four of these are dental radiographs of training mannequins with real human teeth. Another includes 11 antemortem and postmortem dental radiographs representing real casework. The final article in this group was discussed previously and contains antemortem and postmortem radiographs and bones with surgical implants. None of the reviewed Hurricane Katrina articles published images of the actual victims of the hurricane or its aftermath.

15.3.1.1.3 US–Mexico migrant death crisis Six articles associated with the US–Mexico migrant death crisis have visual depictions of antemortem images or human remains: a total of 33 photographs and 1 radiograph are found in five articles in the JFS and one in the AJPA (Tables 15.2 and 15.3) (Beck et al. 2015; Hefner et al. 2015; Beatrice and Soler 2016; Beatrice et al. 2021; Fenton et al. 2008; Fulginiti 2008). One article focuses on the scavenging and scattering of remains in the Sonoran Desert and includes an image of human rib fragments located in the desert. The same article includes eight images of non-human remains used as proxies in a decomposition study (Beck et al. 2015). Another focuses on assessing Hispanic ancestry from skeletal remains and displays an image of two crania: one "SW Hispanic" and one "Guatemalan." The "SW Hispanic" cranium displays an autopsy cut and both appear to be forensic specimens (Hefner et al. 2015). Two articles, one from the JFS and another from the AJPA, focus on skeletal indicators of stress in migrant skeletal remains. The JFS article includes four figures identified as coming from a "UBC" (unidentified border crosser): two images display portions of three crania, another includes two dental images and the fourth is a radiograph of a cranium (Beatrice and Soler 2016). The AJPA article features similar images: five of crania and one of a mandible of presumed unidentified migrants (Beatrice et al. 2021[3]). Another article in this set focused on a case study using skull-photo superimposition as an identification tool. This article includes two antemortem photos of the decedent identified by name in one figure, two figures each containing images of two skulls of unidentified persons who perished while crossing the US–Mexico border, and two figures with four images of skull-photo superimposition (Fenton et al. 2008). The final article in this set includes images of the decedents bound and blindfolded, as well as images of remains with sharp force and ballistic trauma. Two images of crania with gunshot wounds are included as well (Fulginiti 2008).

In summary, in all six of the articles that utilized photographs or radiographs of human remains to discuss processes of victim identification in the context of US–Mexico border casework, images of actual border-context decedents were published.

15.3.1.2 Question set 2

Is there a difference in the frequency of visual documentation between the two journals? Is there a difference in the frequency of visual documentation use among the three mass casualty events? Is there a difference in the frequency of victim photos within, including visual documentation of the three mass casualty events?

In the JFS, we found 54 articles meeting our search criteria (Table 15.1). In 13 of those articles, we identified 92 images of human remains or antemortem images (Tables 15.2 and 15.3). A total of eight articles in the AJPA met our search criteria (Table 15.1). Only one of those articles contained antemortem images or images of human remains (Tables 15.2 and 15.3). However, that single article contained six images. There are statistically significantly more articles (54 vs. 8) and images (86 vs. 6) in the JFS as compared to the AJPA (chi-squared is $p = 0.0001$ for each). This could be due to the devotion of the JFS to forensic science content, while the AJPA publishes on all aspects of biological anthropology, of which forensic anthropology is just one specialty.

Quantitatively, the numbers do not speak to the differential treatment of decedent images as much as a qualitative evaluation does. Twenty-five images are included in articles related to the September 11, 2001, terrorist attacks, 33 to identification efforts in the aftermath of Hurricane Katrina, and 34 in articles related to the US–Mexico border migrant death crisis. Therefore, transitioning from the numbers to better understanding the subject types in terms of context and representation of victims or other images provides more meaningful information to address the posed questions. Removing the two international articles that present examples of casework outside the US and outside the context of the three mass fatality events investigated here provides an interesting opportunity to compare the subject types among the events and between the two journals. Both the September 11th terrorist attacks and Hurricane Katrina are mass casuality events that provided experiences for the forensic science community to learn and prepare in case of a similar event in the future. As a result, these new techniques and approaches were published in scientific journals as a way to distribute the information to other practitioners. While the articles discussed the challenges of identification in the aftermath of these events and incorporated discussions of the identification processes utilized in specific cases and even analyzed some of the identification data, none of these articles released images of individuals who perished during or as a result of these disastrous events. When we visit the articles focused on the identification of migrants, we see a wider variety of topics being published. For example, not only do we see articles focused on improving the identification of this decedent population, but also case studies and analyses that seek to better understand the lived experience of this group of people. Another difference in this set of readings regards the image subjects themselves. When advances were discussed in reference to the World Trade Center or Hurricane Katrina victims, proxy bones were used to illustrate the technique. In the publications discussing migrant death, all images, whether they be photographs or radiographs, represent victims of this mass fatality event. While some images are cleaned bones photographed in laboratory settings, others represent actual scene photos depicting human bones and personal effects. One includes antemortem photographs of the decedent as well as identifying information including her name and age. One includes images of bodies bound, blindfolded, decomposing, and with lethal trauma.

Our dataset, thus indicates that publications involving migrant death at the US–Mexico border display a higher frequency of visual documentation as well as *graphic* visual documentation involving human remains. By graphic, we refer to the condition of offering vivid detail that might be considered striking or upsetting to an audience. Visual documentation involving human remains did appear in publications concerning Hurricane Katrina and the September 11th terrorist attacks, but they were materially and qualitatively different from those found in the migrant death literature. In other words, the absolute number of images for each event is roughly the same. However, the victims of the September 11 terrorist attacks and Hurricane Katrina are being protected by the use of donated remains and example images to illustrate the new techniques developed for identification in those situations. In articles describing the development of new techniques aimed at migrant identification, actual case photos and/or victim images are published instead of proxies.

15.3.1.3 Analysis: question set 3

Through what sociocultural contexts might we make sense of any observed trends in visual documentation practices?

The visual documents included in the migrant death publications tended more often to be direct images of decedents or decedent remains in the context of trauma. In some cases, personal information contextualized the photographs of remains. These photographs could be perhaps charitably viewed as simply anomalous within the forensic anthropology literature explored here. We contend, however, that read against the backdrop of the field's disciplinary history and contemporary conditions of race and racism, disproportionate and graphic displays of certain categories of people are in keeping with the meanings of visual documentation as a tool for the production of otherness in forensic science.

Migration and migrant death are highly publicized, politically charged topics in American policy circles, academic debates, and popular media. Images of migrants circulate through news stories, television, radio, and in scholarly publication venues. These images circulate in relation to the reality that the US demand for migrant labor has never led to the imagination of migrants as part of the US community and thus as deserving of social resources. "The Latino threat," as Chavez (2008) aptly describes, posits that Latinos (and especially Mexicans) are too socially different and too tied to their countries of origin to ever be fully integrated into US society.

As well, the American cultural values of rugged individualism and personal responsibility (Goode and Maskovsky 2001) preclude meaningful public recognition of structural conditions producing undocumented migration, instead focusing on notions of individual choice and, in turn, criminality (Chavez 2008). In contrast, remains associated with Hurricane Katrina and the September 11th terrorist attacks are typically associated with victimhood borne of conditions beyond individual control. Undocumented migrants are discursively construed as quintessential "others" in an American imaginary populated with visual imagery that reflects their difference. Migrants, in other words, are not "us" and so the ethics of visual documentation reserved for other mass casualty events do not apply.

A generous interpretation of how otherness may operate in this context could suggest that well-intentioned scholars may unwittingly reveal their emotional response to readers when they more frequently publish graphic visuals of migrant remains. Breaking unstated norms of visual documentation may, in a sense, reflect the novelty of migrant death and identification work as part of the landscape of forensic anthropology. A less generous interpretation, however, suggests that scholars reveal their own culturally constructed assumptions about whose privacy is worth protecting, whose remains require delicate social handling, and who constitutes the audience reading their publications. In either interpretation, the effect is still the same: the remains of undocumented migrants are documented in US forensic anthropology publishing venues differently than remains associated with other mass casualty events. History, it seems, repeats itself; bodies of color are othered through visual practices, and they disproportionately carry the load of visually documenting methodological and theoretical developments in the biological sciences.

15.4 Making the case for a more socially aware practice of forensic anthropology

Clearly, forensic anthropology's publication record suggests unequal treatment of human remains along sociocultural lines. The ABFA's code of ethics does not address specific practices, such as visual documentation, the historical or contemporary sociocultural contexts of the discipline, or the realities of fallibility and bias that shape the methods, theories, and outcomes of the work. The exclusive focus on maintaining scientific authority via notions of objectivity obscures messier realities of forensic anthropology, including its reliance on practices that reproduce otherness.

However, even if our code of ethics does not overtly recognize our imbrication with the sociocultural contexts in which we work, recent developments specific to humanitarian forensic anthropology have spotlighted conceptual space in which to envision a new ethics of praxis. By ethics of praxis, we refer to forensic science procedures and norms deeply informed by a theoretical commitment to dismantling social inequalities reproduced through the work. An ethical code that references higher-order virtues, such as human rights, social justice, and/or victims' rights, may provide us with the conceptual space necessary to move the discipline forward.

For example, several decades of humanitarian work by forensic anthropologists aimed at identifying victims of human rights violations has ushered in acceptance of, if not enthusiasm for, forensic science practice in support of human rights (Latham and O'Daniel 2018). Clyde Snow's training of the *Equipo Argentino de Anthropologia Forense* (EAAF, Argentine Forensic Anthropology team) marked the beginning of a profound shift in the politics of the discipline, rendering clear that the practice of forensic anthropology is non-neutral precisely because of the contexts in which it may be useful. Thousands of people were disappeared during Argentina's Dirty War, which spanned the years of 1976–1983. The forensic anthropology team recruited and trained by Dr. Snow would go on to exhume, analyze and identify many victims of the *Junta*. As such, the first objective of the mission of the EAAF is to "apply forensic scientific methodology to the investigation and documentation of human rights violations" (Dorretti and Snow 2003, p. 293). While focusing on the professional and scientific behavior of the individual practitioner, this objective also highlights the fact that forensic investigations are not always neutral.

More recently, a similar notion and practice of humanitarian forensic science have been extended to the identification of unidentified migrants along the US–Mexico border. In the early 2000s, The Pima County Office of the Medical Examiner (PCOME) in Tucson, Arizona experienced an increase in the number of death investigations associated with unidentified foreign nationals of Latin American descent (Birkby et al. 2008). Approximately a decade later, Texas experienced a similar increase in migrant deaths, but unlike Arizona, did not have the medical examiner system in place that could centralize death investigations. As a result, the large number of deaths constituted a mass disaster situation in which local resources were overwhelmed and volunteer forensic scientists offered their services to what was considered a humanitarian crisis at the southern US border (Anderson and Spradley 2016; Soler and Beatrice 2018; Spradley and Gocha 2020). The application of forensic science in these contexts created a politically complex set of conditions in which the forensic scientists paradoxically worked *with* and *against* governmental institutions in that the mass death events were a result of hostile governments and hostile policies. This paradox has led to deeper conversations within the discipline about the political underpinnings of our work and the implications of our standards of practice within politically charged contexts, such as migrant death (Latham and O'Daniel 2018). These conversations have largely stopped short of explicitly discussing perceived or desired shifts in our collective understanding of forensic anthropological ethics, but offer a promising place to work through such questions as we have demonstrated here.

More implicitly, however, some forensic anthropologists seem to have begun a pivot toward a sense of the ethical based on perspectives that prioritize the needs of decedent families over the educational value of human remains, an emerging referential context that could be thought of as *rights of the dead and their survivors*. Training in forensic anthropology requires the utilization of human skeletal material for teaching and demonstration purposes. Much of the real skeletal material was legally obtained or donated for educational purposes (Muller et al. 2017; Dayal et al. 2009; Hunt and Albanese 2005). However, as more educators embrace the tenet that what is legal is not always ethical, universities have experienced a shift in the ways in which human remains are used in these situations (Coman et al. 2019; Caplan and DeCamp 2019). While the Native American Graves Protection and Repatriation Act (NAGPRA), initially enacted in 1990, is aimed at removing Indigenous American remains from educational settings, it has also catalyzed the search for other sources of human skeletal material. Legally purchased skeletal material from South Asia, Russia, and China may also be found in educational settings (Rodrigues 2021) and likely represent unclaimed or culturally unaffiliated individuals who did not consent in life to being used for educational purposes (Halperin 2007). For example, Nash (2018) described that, while the collection of human remains at the Denver Museum of Nature and Science was 80% Native American, the remaining 20% was a "ghoulish hodge-podge" of unidentified non-Native human remains. Additionally, laboratories that conduct forensic investigations may utilize unidentified casework for training and educational purposes. As such, many programs that train students and practitioners have switched to using high-quality casts of human skeletal remains and bodies donated specifically for educational purposes as an acknowledgment that not all purchased materials represent individuals who consented for their bodies to be used in laboratory settings as teaching material.

15.5 Closing

Forensic anthropologists have traditionally distanced ourselves from our work by dehumanizing our cases as a way to complete the tasks associated with the unemotional analysis of the dead. In so doing, we have also distanced ourselves from the more theoretical groundings of what it means to be an anthropologist. As such, we have neglected to consider how institutionalized notions of acceptable practice reproduce conditions of otherness and, in turn, racial inequality. Training and advancement in the field require sharing new techniques aimed at improving human identification in various challenging contexts. Therefore, the publication and presentation of visual materials as part of case studies and new identification techniques are accepted as an essential form of continuing education in the field of forensic anthropology. However, the data in this pilot study demonstrate the differences in how human remains are visually depicted in various contexts. The mass fatality events associated with the September 11 terrorist attacks, Hurricane Katrina, and crossing the US–Mexico border illustrate how an ethical code that does not consider the sociopolitical aspects of our work may inadvertently enable ethics of practice that are socially unjust. All three events catalyzed new techniques and approaches to identification. All three events are recognized as events that spawned forensic innovation. However, in the presentation of these new innovations in scientific publication, there is an unequal treatment of decedent antemortem and postmortem images.

The reproduction of images of dead migrants in contrast to the use of proxy images of donated or contextually devoid images associated with the other mass fatality events highlights otherwise unspoken notions of who should and should not be protected in death. Here, we question why these images are so easily shared in contrast to other decedent populations. We also propose a more socially aware practice of forensic anthropology in which practitioners consider the potential ramifications of the particular images they release of decedents that have not consented for participation in a research or training program. A revised ethical code must therefore account for the historically driven sociopolitical contexts in which the work of forensic anthropology is completed.

Acknowledgments

The authors would like to thank Roberto Parra and Dr. Douglas Ubelaker for organizing and editing this volume. The authors would also like to thank Dr. Allysha Winburn for reviewing drafts of this chapter and providing invaluable feedback and Dr. Stephen Nawrocki for assistance in the statistical analyses.

Notes

1. It is important to note that one author (KEL) is mentioned in at least one of these news stories. We feel it is important to note this to demonstrate the authors are active participants in the field who are also in the process of reflecting on how our

own practices have contributed to these conversations and behaviors.https://www.washingtonpost.com/world/2019/06/26/father-daughter-who-drowned-border-dove-into-river-desperation/https://www.washingtonpost.com/national-security/summer-migrant-deaths-southern-border/2021/06/03/a03d7bb8-c3a6-11eb-8c34-f8095f2dc445_story.htmlhttps://www.nytimes.com/2019/04/18/us/mexico-border-deaths.htmlhttps://www.usatoday.com/border-wall/story/mass-disaster-grows-u-s-mexico-border/1009752001/https://www.nytimes.com/interactive/2017/05/04/us/texas-border-migrants-dead-bodies.html?mtrref=undefinedandgwh=EACD4A70ECF957D0C4471D8198A69AFCandgwt=payandassetType=PAYWALL
2. https://onlinelibrary-wiley-com.ezproxy.uindy.edu/loi/15564029 https://onlinelibrary-wiley-com.ezproxy.uindy.edu/loi/10968644
3. It's important to note that one author (KEL) contributed data to this publication. We feel it is important to note this to demonstrate the authors are active participants in the field who are also in the process of reflecting on how our own practices have contributed to these conversations and behaviors.

References

Adams, B.J. and Aschheim, K.W. (2016). Computerized dental comparison: A critical review of dental coding and ranking algorithms used in victim identification. *Journal of Forensic Sciences* **61**(1): 76–86. doi: 10.1111/1556-4029.12909.

Ahmed, S. (2002). Racialized bodies. In: *Real Bodies: A Sociological Introduction* (eds. M. Evans and E. Lee), 46–63. London: Palgrave Publishers.

American Board of Forensic Anthropology, Inc (2020) https://www.theabfa.org/ (accessed 2022).

Anderson, B.E. and Spradley, M.K. (2016). The role of the anthropologist in the identification of migrant remains in the American Southwest. *Academic Forensic Pathology* **6**(3): 432–438. doi: 10.23907/2016.044.

Antinick, T.C. and Foran, D.R. (2019). Intra- and inter-element variability in mitochondrial and nuclear DNA from fresh and environmentally exposed skeletal remains. *Journal of Forensic Sciences* **64**(1): 88–97. doi: 10.1111/1556-4029.13843.

Aristotle (1910). *Historia Animalium* (translated by W. Ogle). Oxford: Clarendon Press.

Aristotle (1912a). *De Partibus* Animalium (translated by W. Ogle). Oxford: Clarendon Press.

Aristotle (1912b). *De Generatione Animalium*. Oxford: Clarendon Press.

Baker, L.D. (1998). *From Savage to Negro: Anthropology and the Construction of Race, 1896–1954*. Berkeley, CA: University of California Press.

Baraybar, J.P. (2008). When DNA is not available, can we still identify people? Recommendations for best practice. *Journal of Forensic Sciences* **53**(3): 533–540. doi: 10.1111/j.1556-4029.2008.00709.x.

Beatrice, J.S. and Soler, A. (2016). Skeletal indicators of stress: A component of the biocultural profile of undocumented migrants in Southern Arizona. *Journal of Forensic Sciences* **61**(5): 1164–1172. doi: 10.1111/1556-4029.13131.

Beatrice, J.S., Soler, A., Reineke, R.C., and Martínez, D.E. (2021). Skeletal evidence of structural violence among undocumented migrants from Mexico and Central America. *American Journal of Physical Anthropology* **176**(4): 584–605. doi: 10.1002/ajpa.24391.

Beck, J., Ostericher, I., Sollish, G., and De León, J. (2015). Animal scavenging and scattering and the implications for documenting the deaths of undocumented border crossers in the Sonoran Desert. *Journal of Forensic Sciences* **60**: S11–S20. doi: 10.1111/1556-4029.12597.

Birkby, W.H., Fenton, T.W., and Anderson, B.E. (2008). Identifying Southwest Hispanics using nonmetric traits and the cultural profile. *Journal of Forensic Sciences* **53**(1): 29–33. doi: 10.1111/j.1556-4029.2007.00611.x.

Blakey, M.L. (2020). Understanding racism in physical (biological) anthropology. *American Journal of Physical Anthropology* **175**(2): 316–325. doi: 10.1002/ajpa.24208.

Bornstein, E. and Redfield, P. (eds.) (2010). *Forces of Compassion: Humanitarianism between Ethics and Politics*. Santa Fe: School for Advanced Research.

Brace, C.L. (2005). *"Race" is a Four-Letter Word: The Genesis of the Concept*. Oxford: Oxford University Press.

Camper, P. (1770). *Report of the Content of Two Lecture*. Utrecht: R. Wild and J. Altheer.

Caplan, I. and DeCamp, M. (2019). Of discomfort and disagreement: Unclaimed bodies in Anatomy Laboratories at United States Medical Schools. *Anatomical Sciences Education* **12**(4): 360–369. doi: 10.1002/ase.1853.

Cartozzo, C., Singh, B., Swall, J., and Simmons, T. (2021). Postmortem submersion interval (PMSI) estimation from the microbiome of sus scrofa bone in a freshwater lake. *Journal of Forensic Sciences* **66**(4): 1334–1347. doi: 10.1111/1556-4029.14692.

Cassaniti, J.L. and Hickman, J.R. (2014). New Directions in the anthropology of morality. *Anthropological Theory* **14**(3): 251–262. doi: 10.1177/1463499614534371.

Chavez, L.R. (2008). *The Latino threat: Constructing immigrants, citizens, and the nation*. Stanford, CA: Stanford University Press.

Christensen, A.M., Smith, V.A., Ramos, V., Shegogue, C., et al. (2012). Primary and secondary skeletal blast trauma. *Journal of Forensic Sciences* **57**(1): 6–11. doi: 10.1111/j.1556-4029.2011.01938.x.

Coman, J., Kelly, A.-M., Savulescu, J., and Craig, S. (2019). Skeletons in the closet: Towards the dignified disposal of all human bones acquired for Medical Education. *British Medical Journal* **367**: l6705. doi: 10.1136/bmj.l6705.

Csordas, T.J. (2013). Morality as a cultural system? *Current Anthropology* **54**(5): 523–546. doi: 10.1086/672210.

Danforth, R.A., Herschaft, E.E., and Leonowich, J.A. (2009). Operator exposure to scatter radiation from a portable hand-held Dental Radiation Emitting Device (Aribex™ Nomad™) while making 915 intraoral dental radiographs. *Journal of Forensic Sciences* **54**(2): 415–421. doi: 10.1111/j.1556-4029.2008.00960.x.

Dayal, M.R., Kegley, A.D.T., Štrkalj, G., Bidmos, M.A., et al. (2009). The history and composition of the Raymond A. Dart collection of human skeletons at the University of the Witwatersrand, Johannesburg, South Africa. *American Journal of Physical Anthropology* **140**(2): 324–335. doi: 10.1002/ajpa.21072.

Dorretti, M. and Snow, C.C. (2003). Forensic anthropology and human rights: The Argentine experience. In: *Hard Evidence: Case Studies in Forensic Anthropology* (ed. D.W. Steadman), 290–310. Upper Saddle River, NJ: Prentice Hall.

Dror, I., Melinek, J., Arden, J.L., Kukucka, J., et al. (2021). Cognitive bias in forensic pathology decisions. *Journal of Forensic Sciences* **66**(5): 1751–1757. doi: 10.1111/1556-4029.14697.

Fassin, D. (2012). *Humanitarian Reason: A Moral History of the Present*. Berkeley, CA: University of California Press.

Fenton, T.W., Heard, A.N., and Sauer, N.J. (2008). Skull-photo superimposition and border deaths: Identification through exclusion and the failure to exclude. *Journal of Forensic Sciences* **53**(1): 34–40. doi: 10.1111/j.1556-4029.2007.00624.x.

Fluehr-Lobban, C. (2003). Ethics in anthropology 1890-2000: A review of issues and principles. In: *Ethics and the Profession of Anthropology: Dialogue for Ethically Conscious Practice* (ed. C. Fluehr-Lobban), 1–28. Walnut Creek: AltaMira Press.

Fulginiti, L.C. (2008). Fatal footsteps: Murder of undocumented border crossers in Maricopa County, Arizona. *Journal of Forensic Sciences* **53**(1): 41–45. doi: 10.1111/j.1556-4029.2007.00613.x.

Goode, J. and Maskovsky, J. (2001). Introduction. In: *New Poverty Studies: The Ethnography of Power, Politics, and Impoverished People in the United States* (eds. J. Goode and J. Maskovsky), 1–36. New York: New York University Press.

Gould, S.J. (1981). *The Mismeasure of Man*. New York: W.W. Norton and Company.

Halperin, E.C. (2007). The poor, the black, and the marginalized as the source of cadavers in United States Anatomical Education. *Clinical Anatomy* **20**(5): 489–495. doi: 10.1002/ca.20445.

Harris, M. (2001). *The Rise of Anthropological Theory: A History of Theories of Culture*. Walnut Creek: AltaMira Press.

Hartley, R.J. (2007). To massacre: a perspective on demographic competition. *Anthropological Quarterly* **80**(1): 237–251.

Hefner, J.T., Pilloud, M.A., Black, C.J., and Anderson, B.E. (2015). Morphoscopic trait expression in "Hispanic" populations. *Journal of Forensic Sciences* **60**(5): 1135–1139. doi: 10.1111/1556-4029.12826.

Heyman, J.M. (2010). Activism in anthropology: Exploring the present through Eric R. Wolf's Vietnam-era work. *Dialectical Anthropology* **34**(2): 287–293. doi: 10.1007/s10624-010-9186-6.

Howell, S. (eds.) (1996). *The Ethnography of Moralities*. London: Routledge Press.

Hunt, D.R. and Albanese, J. (2005). History and demographic composition of the Robert J. Terry Anatomical Collection. *American Journal of Physical Anthropology* **127**(4): 406–417. doi: 10.1002/ajpa.20135.

Hymes, D. (1974). Introduction: The use of anthropology, critical, political, personal. In: *Reinventing Anthropology* (ed. D. Hymes), 3–61: Vintage Books.

Jeanguenat, A.M., Budowle, B., and Dror, I.E. (2017). Strengthening forensic DNA decision making through a better understanding of the influence of cognitive bias. *Science and Justice* **57**(6): 415–420. doi: 10.1016/j.scijus.2017.07.005.

Klavens, A., Kollmann, D.D., Elkins, K.M., and Zeller, C.B. (2020). Comparison of DNA yield and STR profiles from the diaphysis, mid-diaphysis, and metaphysis regions of femur and tibia long bones. *Journal of Forensic Sciences* **66**(3): 1104–1113. doi: 10.1111/1556-4029.14657.

Latham, K.E. and O'Daniel, A. (eds.) (2018). *Sociopolitics of Migrant Death and Repatriation: Perspectives from Forensic Science. Bioarcheology and Social Theory*. Cham: Springer.

Latour, B. and Woolgar, S. (1986). *Laboratory Life: The Social Construction of Scientific Facts*, 2 e. Princeton, NJ: Princeton University Press.

Linnaeus, C. (1740). Systema naturae, Ed. 2 - The Linnean collections. http://linnean-online.org/119958/ (accessed 2022).

Linnaeus, C. (1758). Systema naturae, Ed. 10 - The Linnean collections. http://linnean-online.org/119965/ (accessed 2022).

Maier, C., Craig, A., and Adams, D.M. (2020). Language use in ancestry research and estimation. *Journal of Forensic Sciences* **66**(1): 11–24. doi: 10.1111/1556-4029.14601.

Mattingly, C. (2014). *Moral Laboratories: Family Peril and the Struggle for a Good Life*. Berkeley, CA: University of California Press.

Meijer, M.C. and Camper, P. (1997). Petrus Camper on the origin and color of blacks. *History of Anthropology Newsletter* **24**(2): 3–9.

Menand, L. (2001–2002). Morton, Agassiz, and the origins of scientific racism in the United States. *The Journal of Blacks in Higher Education* **34**: 110. doi: 10.2307/3134139.

Morton, S. (1839). *Crania Americana, or, a Comparative View of the Skulls of Various Aboriginal Nations of North and South America: To Which Is Prefixed an Essay on the Varieties of the Human Species.* Philadelphia, PA: J. Dobson.

Muller, J.L., Pearlstein, K.E., and de la Cova, C. (2017). Dissection and documented skeletal collections: Embodiments of legalized inequality. In: *The Bioarchaeology of Dissection and Autopsy in the United States. Bioarchaeology and Social Theory* (ed. K. Nystrom), 185–201. Cham: Springer. doi: 10.1007/978-3-319-26836-1_9.

Nakhaeizadeh, S., Dror, I.E., and Morgan, R.M. (2014a). Cognitive bias in forensic anthropology: Visual assessment of skeletal remains is susceptible to confirmation bias. *Science and Justice* **54**(3): 208–214. doi: 10.1016/j.scijus.2013.11.003.

Nakhaeizadeh, S., Hanson, I., and Dozzi, N. (2014b). The power of contextual effects in forensic anthropology: A study of biasability in the visual interpretations of trauma analysis on skeletal remains. *Journal of Forensic Sciences* **59**(5): 1177–1183. doi: 10.1111/1556-4029.12473.

Nash, S. (2018). The skeletons in the museum closet. SAPIENS. https://www.sapiens.org/column/curiosities/natural-history-museum-human-remains/ (accessed 2022).

Nee, S. (2005). The great chain of being. *Nature* **435**(7041): 429–429. doi: 10.1038/435429a.

Nott, J.C., Gliddon, G.R., Morton, S.G., Agassiz, L., et al. (1854). *Types of Mankind: Or, Ethnological Researches Based Upon the Ancient Monuments, Paintings, Sculptures, and Crania of Races, and Upon Their Natural, Geographical, Philological and Biblical History; Illustrated by Selections from the Inedited Papers of Samuel George Morton and by Additional Contributions from L. Agassiz, W. Usher, and H.S. Patterson.* London: Grambo and Company, Lippincott.

Ortner, S.B. (2016). Dark anthropology and its others: Theory since the eighties. *HAU: Journal of Ethnographic Theory* **6**(1): 47–73. doi: 10.14318/hau6.1.004.

Price, D. (2011). *Weaponizing Anthropology.* Petrolia, CA: AK Press.

Ramchand, R., Franklin, E., Thornton, E., Deland, S.M., et al. (2018). Violence, guns, and suicide in New Orleans: Results from a qualitative study of recent suicide decedents. *Journal of Forensic Sciences* **63**(5): 1444–1449. doi: 10.1111/1556-4029.13742.

Richmond, R. and Pretty, I.A. (2009). The use of radio-frequency identification tags for labeling dentures-scanning properties. *Journal of Forensic Sciences* **54**(3): 664–668. doi: 10.1111/j.1556-4029.2009.01010.x.

Rodrigues, M. (2021). *Haunted by My Teaching Skeleton.* https://www.sapiens.org/archaeology/where-do-teaching-skeletons-come-from/ (accessed 2022).

Rodriguez Almada, H., Passalacqua, N.V., Congram, D., and Pilloud, M. (2021). As forensic scientists and as people, we must not confuse objectivity with neutrality. *Journal of Forensic Sciences* **66**(5): 2067–2068. doi: 10.1111/1556-4029.14785.

Scheper-Hughes, N. (1995). The primacy of the ethical: Propositions for a militant anthropology. *Current Anthropology* **36**(3): 409–440. doi: 10.1086/204378.

Simpson, E.K., James, R.A., Eitzen, D.A., and Byard, R.W. (2007). Role of orthopedic implants and bone morphology in the identification of human remains. *Journal of Forensic Sciences* **52**(2): 442–448. doi: 10.1111/j.1556-4029.2006.00370.x.

Soler, A. and Beatrice, J.S. (2018). Expanding the role of forensic anthropology in a humanitarian crisis: An example from the USA-Mexico border. In: *Sociopolitics of*

Migrant Death and Repatriation: Perspectives from Forensic Science. Bioarcheology and Social Theory (eds. K.E. Latham and A. O'Daniel), 115–128: Springer.
Sontag, S. (1993). *Regarding the Pain of Others*. New York: Picador Press.
Spradley, K. and Gocha, T.P. (2020). Migrant deaths along the Texas/Mexico border: A collaborative approach to forensic identification of human remains. In: *Forensic Science and Humanitarian Action: Interacting with the Dead and the Living* (eds. R.C. Parra, S.C. Zapico, and D.H. Ubelaker), 535–548. Hoboken, NJ: John Wiley and Sons.
Tallman, S. and Bird, C. (2022). Diversity and inclusion in forensic anthropology: where we stand and prospects for the future. *Forensic Anthropology* **5**(2): 84–101.
Ticktin, M. (2006). Where ethics and politics meet. *American Ethnologist* **33**(1): 33–49. doi: 10.1525/ae.2006.33.1.33.
Van Der Meer, D.T., Brumit, P.C., Schrader, B.A., Dove, S.B., et al. (2010). Root morphology and anatomical patterns in forensic dental identification: A comparison of computer-aided identification with traditional forensic dental identification. *Journal of Forensic Sciences* **55**(6): 1499–1503. doi: 10.1111/j.1556-4029.2010.01492.x.
Vehit, U. and Christensen, A.M. (2019). Bilateral asymmetry of nutrient foramen position in forearm bones: Implications for its use in sorting commingled remains. *Journal of Forensic Sciences* **64**(1): 186–189. doi: 10.1111/1556-4029.13853.
Winburn, A. (2018). Subjective with a capital S? Issues of objectivity in forensic anthropology. In: *Forensic Anthropology: Theoretical Framework and Scientific Basis* (eds. C.C. Boyd and D.C. Boyd), 21–38. Hoboken, NJ: John Wiley and Sons.
Winburn, A.P. and Algee-Hewitt, B. (2021). Evaluating population affinity estimates in forensic anthropology: Insights from the forensic anthropology database for assessing methods accuracy (FADAMA). *Journal of Forensic Sciences* **66**(4): 1210–1219. doi: 10.1111/1556-4029.14731.
Winburn, A.P. and Clemmons, C.M.J. (2021). Objectivity is a myth that harms the practice and diversity of forensic science. *Forensic Science International: Synergy* **3**: 100196. doi: 10.1016/j.fsisyn.2021.100196.
Winburn, A.P., Clemmons, C.M.J., Delgado, T.A., Hartley, S., et al. (2021). Responding to the American Academy of Forensic Sciences Vision, mission, and values statements: Comments, revisions, and proposed actions. *Forensic Science International: Synergy* **3**: 100197. doi: 10.1016/j.fsisyn.2021.100197.
Wylie, A. (1992). On "heavily decomposing Red Herrings": Scientific method in archaeology and the ladening of evidence with theory. In: *Metaarchaeology. Reflections by Archaeologists and Philosophers* (ed. L. Embree), 269–288. Boston, MA: Kluwer Academic. doi: 10.1007/978-94-011-1826-2_12.

CHAPTER 16

Bedeviling binaries: an integrated and dialectical approach to forensic anthropology in northern Uganda

Tricia Redeker Hepner[1] and Dawnie W. Steadman[2]

[1]*MA Program in Social Justice and Human Rights, School of Social and Behavioral Sciences, Arizona State University, USA*
[2]*Department of Anthropology, University of Tennessee, USA*

16.1 Introduction

Tenacious binaries bedevil forensic anthropology's theory and practice in human rights contexts. Perhaps none more so than the persistent humanitarian/judicial distinction, in which "the forensic" mediates uncomfortably as both positivist producer of evidence before the law and potential palliative for survivors' suffering. When positioned within the larger global universes of human rights and transitional justice, moreover, forensic anthropology engages with other often apparently opposing forces: positivism/interpretivism, universalism/relativism, science/culture, and even living/dead.

In recent years, scholars and practitioners of forensic anthropology have richly debated these binaries, with some suggesting that opposition may represent new opportunities for synthesis and growth (Kim 2018; Moon 2016; Rosenblatt 2019). Stalemated dichotomous relationships may, therefore, become productive, dialectical ones through the critically engaged application of forensic science in the service of human rights. Indeed, the boundaries of forensic anthropology's theory and practice have been expanding, as evidenced in new terminologies like "forensic humanitarian action" (Cordner and Tidball-Binz 2017; Parra et al. 2020) and in other ways for which we have yet to develop adequate descriptive and analytical vocabularies.

While historically forensic scientists limit the definition of "the forensic" in order to preserve its legal potency and scientific integrity, others seek to push

Anthropology of Violent Death: Theoretical Foundations for Forensic Humanitarian Action, First Edition. Edited by Roberto C. Parra and Douglas H. Ubelaker.

boundaries and trouble taken for granted meanings and methods in order to enhance forensic science's relevance and sensitivity to political, cultural, and ethical contexts (Elgerud and Kim 2020; Ferrandiz and Robben 2015; Hepner et al. 2018; Kim 2018; Kim et al. 2020; Rosenblatt 2019; Steadman and Wagner 2020; Tuller 2018; Mundorff and Wagner 2020). Our long-term collaboration as a cultural anthropologist (Hepner) and a forensic anthropologist (Steadman) embodies these myriad tensions and aims to overcome them by actively working with and through them. Together we have co-led a team project since 2012 in the former war zone of Acholiland, Northern Uganda, where we have trained and learned from former and current graduate students working across subdisciplines and engaged deeply with Acholi survivors whose lives are inseparable from the spiritual and material traces of the dead and disappeared.[1] Through this work, we have arrived at the argument we advance in this chapter: the potential and practice of forensic anthropology remain always–already situated within, and shaped by, culture, cosmology, and highly localized and contextualized forms of evidence, some of which are ephemeral and nonscientific, but hold immense significance and legal potential nonetheless. In elaborating what core team member Jaymelee Kim has called an "integrated approach" (2018), we illustrate how the persistent binaries noted above may effectively move from dichotomous to dialectical. The implications for theory and practice are salutary and significant, as they reflect the larger effort to expand the theory and practice of forensic anthropology through clarifying the range of its contributions in different contexts.

We approach our contribution to this volume in two ways. First, we provide an overview of our ongoing work in Uganda and some of the key findings by our team to date that illustrate how situations that may appear not to be forensically relevant become so when carefully situated in terms of culture, history, politics, cosmology, and human experience. In this way, ethnographic grounding shifts what we recognize as "forensic" and its potential. Second, we show how deploying ethnographic inquiry as intrinsic, even *a priori*, to forensic intervention makes the latter more intelligible to survivors so they may determine whether its application is desirable and for what purposes. That is, the question facing scholars and practitioners today should not be whether and how a survivor-centered forensic anthropology can contribute to humanitarian goals, wherein researchers, scientists, and/or international non-governmental organizations (INGOs) primarily define what is meant by "survivor-centered," as well as the terms "forensic" and "humanitarian." Rather, we must investigate carefully what these concepts and terms mean to people in substantive and often shifting and contradictory situations, and explore with them whether and how forensic anthropology's deployment might articulate meaningfully with their worlds, their lives, their needs, and their goals. This inevitably entails being open to both long-term ethnography and the finding that forensic intervention cannot and should not occur. Such non-intervention may be, above all, the most "humanitarian" course of action.

16.2 Restless spirits and human remains in Acholiland, Uganda

War, political violence, and mass death have stalked many parts of Uganda (RLP 2014), but none perhaps as brutally and infamously as the Northern Acholi region (Figure 16.1). From 1986 to 2006, Joseph Kony and the Lord's Resistance Army (LRA) rebels wreaked bloody havoc across Northern Uganda (and later over international borders) as they battled the National Resistance Army (NRA) and Uganda People's Defense Forces (UPDF), using their own abducted people – many of them children – as soldiers. Referred to in its time by United Nations under-secretary-general for humanitarian affairs and emergency relief, Jan Egeland, as "the biggest neglected humanitarian emergency in the world," by 2004, 90% of the Acholi population had been forcibly displaced from their

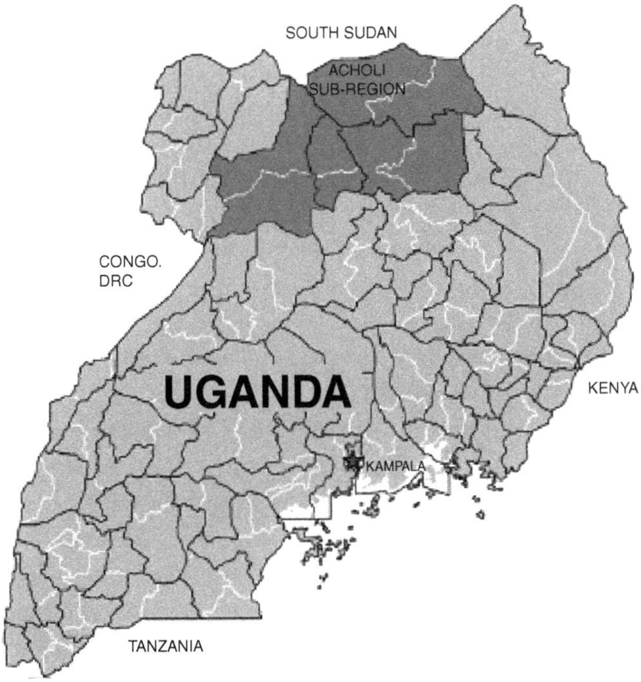

Figure 16.1 Map of Uganda with Acholi sub-region highlighted. Source: Created by Julia R. Hanebrink.

villages and homes into government established camps. Ostensibly created to protect civilians from rebel attacks and abductions, the camps themselves precipitated further suffering and death. Often caught in the crossfire among rebels and military, sometimes sites of brutalization by government soldiers due to inhabitants' suspected rebel sympathies and collaboration, the displacement camps and their overcrowded, unsanitary conditions spread communicable and sometimes fatal diseases and disrupted all elements of previously established norms, lives, and livelihoods. Clans and communities lost their wealth in land and livestock, which were seized, looted, and destroyed by rebels and military alike; women lost both children and husbands, and thus whatever claims to land or safety they may have held through virilocal marriage. Education, business, and infrastructural development were thrown in reverse. As more and more people died in the camps or in massacres committed by both factions, or were abducted from one region and killed in another, the vast and fertile agricultural lands became riddled with open, clandestine, and atrocious graves.

It is difficult to describe, let alone overstate, the extent of the damage throughout Acholiland.[2] In addition to the death and destruction noted above, the psychosocial impacts on survivors, returned rebel soldiers, and former abductees have been devastating (see Neuner et al. 2012; Victor and Porter 2017). Sexual violence against both men and women, witnessing or forcibly committing atrocities, enduring loss of resources and other means of social survival and mobility, and the extreme fragmentation of families and cultural frameworks, all continue to reverberate throughout Acholi society more than 15 years after the 2006 ceasefire.

A particularly acute and enduring form of suffering with far-reaching consequences has been the cosmological rupture between living and dead. In Acholiland, as in many parts of Africa (and elsewhere), the living and dead share intimate and ongoing relationships, with important proscriptions for mortuary rituals that often blend Acholi indigenous beliefs in spirits with Anglican, Catholic, and/or born-again Christian elements. Ideally, burials should take place on ancestral land and within the homestead itself, with the appropriate slaughtering of animals, gathering of kin and community, prayers, and proper treatment of the corpse (Seebach 2016; Figure 16.2). In cases of murder or wrongful death, reconciliation rituals among the perpetrator's and victim's clans must occur. If violent death has occurred, cleansing rituals for the surrounding landscape and those who may have come into contact with the remains must occur to help the spirit of the deceased move into the realm of ancestors. Should these elements of proper burial not occur, a range of consequences may follow for the living, as the spirit of the deceased becomes vengeful and destructive: possession, nightmares, hallucinations, mental and physical illness, infertility in the land, animals, or people, social conflict, personal misfortune, and many other

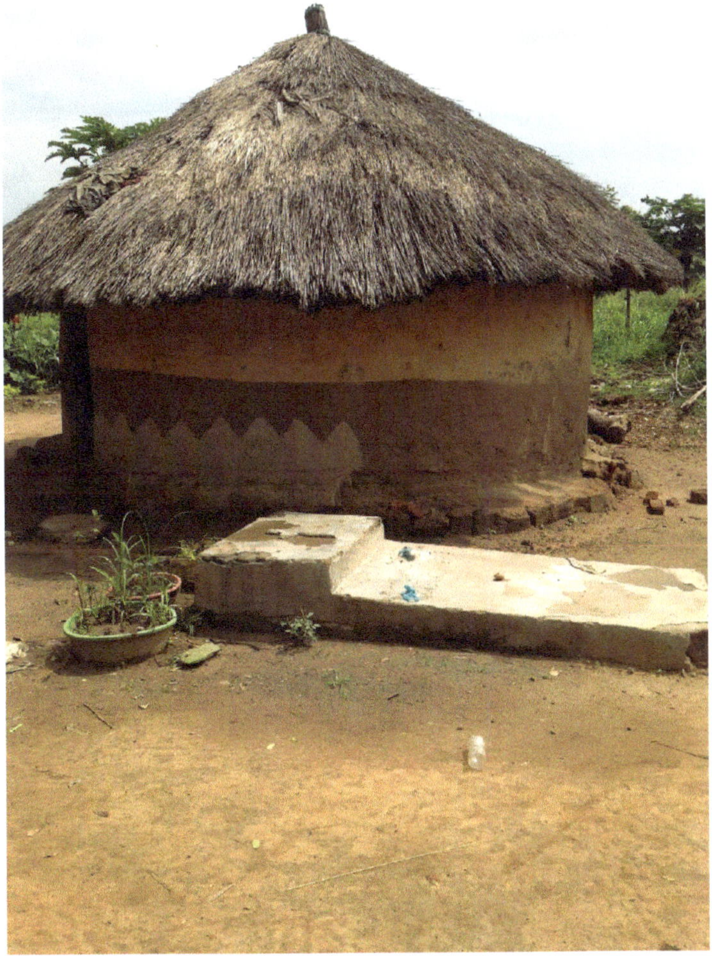

Figure 16.2 Proper burial on a homestead. Source: Tricia Redeker Hepner (Co-Author).

ramifications may occur as a result of improperly ritualized and conducted burials (Figure 16.3).

In contexts such as Acholi, where the living perceive the dead as actively exerting agency, clandestine graves, mass burials, displacement camp graves, surface scatters of those killed and left in the open, or sites where atrocities occurred but no remains are left, cause ongoing suffering, instability, and harm. The spirits of the violently killed and improperly buried dead impinge on the everyday mental and physical lives of survivors and affect their material well-being. For instance, land used for farming or building may be rendered unusable by the presence of graves, and the accidental discovery of remains while digging or building may precipitate illness and misfortune. For clans displaced onto the

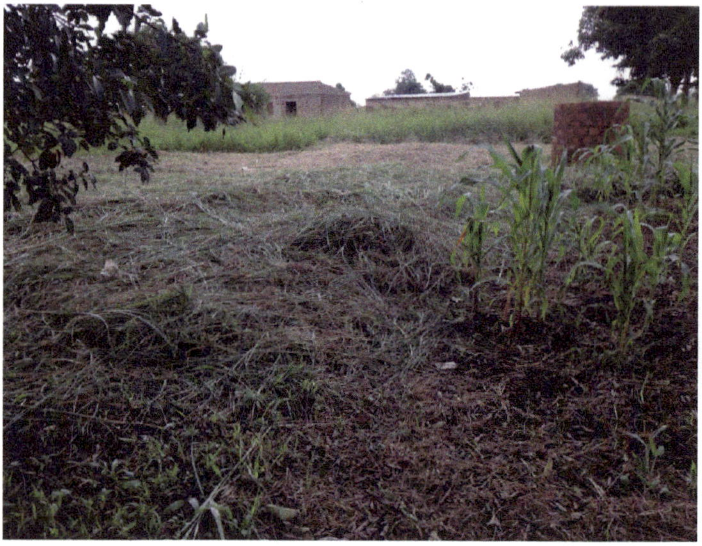

Figure 16.3 Improper burial in former IDP camp. Source: Tricia Redeker Hepner (Co-Author).

land of others, their deceased loved ones may call to them for repatriation and proper burial, but families lack the necessary resources, which include goats for sacrifice at exhumation and reburial; access to transportation for the body and those conducting the reburial; coffins, shrouds, and cement; and the ability to both pay laborers and to host kin and community. Most importantly, fulfilling exhumation and reburial depends upon survivors knowing or remembering the locations of loved ones' graves. In instances where graves have been lost or forgotten, or in cases of mass burials and surface scatters, survivors contend with the problem of identification and the recognition that burying the wrong bones can do more to exacerbate than mend the cosmological breach.

Much excellent scholarship (Baines 2007, 2010, 2017; Behrend 1999; Kembel 2015; Komakech 2018b; Meinert and Whyte 2013; Seebach 2016) has addressed the agentive dead and documented the multifarious impacts of "bones in the wrong soil" (Jahn and Wilhelm-Solomon 2015; Jahn 2016) on Acholi survivors, including the ways that graves and grave markers are entangled in land disputes (Meinert et al. 2017). The questions our team sought to explore and answer focused on how different burial and deposition contexts (surface scatters of unknown people, mass graves, and displacement camp burials of both known and unknown dead) may have different implications for survivors. We wanted to understand the full range of meanings and impacts of improper burials, from their political and legal significance to their spiritual and material effects. Amid Uganda's broader transitional justice process, with both national and local dimensions, did survivors see an important role for the dead, and if so, how? What various approaches and remedies had survivors taken to address the problem of restless spirits and human remains, and what were the outcomes? And finally, we wanted to explore what role – if any – forensic anthropology and archaeology might play in ultimately addressing the needs of both living and dead.

With the support and assistance of colleagues working with two different research and advocacy organizations, the Justice and Reconciliation Project (JRP) and the Refugee Law Project (RLP), as well as guidance from elders and cultural/religious leaders, we identified specific communities and sought approvals from the hierarchical layers of political leaders (regional district commissioners, or RDCs, and local councilpersons, or LCs), as well as clan chiefs (*rwodi*), to conduct fieldwork. Once these approvals had been secured, we worked directly with the *rwodi* and LCs to arrange a series of focus group discussions with people at the village level to get a handle on the nature and extent of improper burials and associated material or spiritual consequences. The communities we worked with represented six different villages and four different clans with known existing improper burials on their land. In addition, one of the clans had been displaced into camps located on another clan's land during the war, meaning that survivors each had unique experiences of the camp graves and intrinsically related interests in their possible exhumation, removal, and reburial. Eventually, we expanded into individual interviews with a stratified sample of villagers, many of whom included women who had married into the patriclans, and the majority of whom identified as "farmers." Over the course of six seasons, we completed 170 individual interviews and approximately two dozen focus group discussions.

Each season that our team returned, we worked to refine and adjust our research questions and methods as we continued to learn from and engage with the survivor communities and our local Acholi collaborators. As we began to understand the range of ways the improper burials affected survivors, and then began working with them to explicitly connect these impacts to their needs and aspirations for redress, we discovered that the concepts of "transitional justice" and especially "forensic science" were too abstract or unfamiliar for most interlocutors. It became clear that in order to effectively explore with people their priorities for accountability and redress, the ongoing impact and role of the dead, and possible resolutions to the myriad problems precipitated by improper burials, including the use of forensic methods, we needed to establish a baseline for communication (Tuller 2018). We did so by first exploring what participants knew, including specific cultural forms of knowledge, seeking to understand their perspectives. We then built on that with the use of pictorial images that depicted abstract concepts in concrete ways. One set of images represented various features of transitional justice, from memorialization and material compensation to amnesty and prosecution. We also provided a series of images that illustrated how forensic scientists excavate and exhume remains, how the remains are collected and stored, and then how DNA identifications might help identify who the people were in life. We were then able to deepen our discussions with participants about how these scientific methods might articulate or conflict with existing knowledge as well as cultural and religious beliefs, practices, and rituals, and to answer their many questions as we tried to establish a mutually realistic understanding of the potentials and limitations of forensic investigation with respect to their needs, interests, goals, and priorities for redress.

These discussions were especially important insofar as Northern Uganda has been the site of various government-mandated initiatives and extensive interventions by local, national, and international organizations, often without local knowledge and involvement, and these have strongly shaped people's expectations and concerns regarding any future interventions (Kim 2018). Among these interventions were several ritual cleansing ceremonies and/or reburials of remains that had emerged during development or infrastructure projects, as well as an excavation of a mass grave in 2004 overseen by "government doctors" in Lukodi, probably related to evidence gathering for prosecutions of rebels by the government and International Criminal Court (ICC). Local people reportedly received no information either prior to or following the excavation of the grave and found it deeply traumatizing in part because the villagers themselves were coerced to exhume the recently buried remains of their massacred loved ones (JRP 2011). According to the JRP, similar investigations took place in other districts around the same time as the Lukodi investigation (JRP 2011; Kim 2018:39). These externally driven interventions were opaque in purpose and meaning to Acholi survivors and caused considerable harm. For those who knew about them, the memory of the excavations shaped the way they engaged with our research, and in turn, informed our own approach and methodology (Kim 2018; Kim et al. 2020).

In 2017 and 2018, we introduced several new objectives to the research project. One of these included the use of archeological techniques to map sites that represented different depositional contexts, including displacement camp graves and mass graves (Elgerud and Kim 2020). We also included sites where atrocities had occurred but no human remains were present, because these were also associated with troubling spiritual and material conditions (Kim and Hepner 2019). The objective was to understand and visually document the ways that improper burials continued to be part of the daily reality of survivors, and we also wanted to demonstrate to them how much documentation of physical features could speak to their concerns in a meaningful way. Specifically, the site maps could provide records of graves that may be lost over time to memory or the environment; they could buttress oral testimony narratives that atrocities had occurred, thus preserving political memory; and the maps themselves could represent possible forms of evidence that might be mobilized to make legal claims for compensation, whether that be in the form of land, infrastructure, memorialization, reparations, or resources to enable exhumation, reburial, and/or ritual remedies. Over the course of the project, team members Jaymelee Kim, Lucia Elgerud, and Hugh Tuller, with the assistance of Joshua Oballim, Jr., Deo Komakech, and Jeffrey Opiyo, created maps and reports of about one dozen sites. Finally, team members Kim, Steadman, Tuller, and Hanebrink traveled to Kampala to conduct some basic training in forensic methods for Ugandan medicolegal and nongovernmental organization (NGO) staff and further assessed the scientific and judicial infrastructures relevant to any future forensic investigation.

A number of key findings have emerged from our research to date, chief among them that *traditional* forensic intervention, or the excavation of human remains and their identification for largely predetermined legal and/or humanitarian purposes, may not be possible or desirable in Acholiland. The reasons for this are manifold, ranging from lack of adequate and independent judicial and medicolegal infrastructures and the as-yet unimplemented transitional justice policy, which does not explicitly make room for forensic inquiry. It also requires consideration of how the selection of a specific region – in this case, Acholiland – might be justified and perceived in a country where violent conflicts and improper burials have been endemic (RLP 2014). In other words, why should excavation focus on Acholiland specifically, over and above other regions where atrocities have also left lasting impacts? Other considerations include the potential politicization of findings with respect to the locally contested mandates of the ICC and national criminal trials of former rebel leaders at a time when state-affiliated perpetrators remain in power. Not least of all, survivor communities themselves have not yet had a chance to dialog with our findings to date and to more fully explore their interests, or lack thereof, in possible next steps.

These complexities continue to be unpacked in our team's existing publications (Elgerud and Kim 2020; Hepner et al. 2018; Hepner 2020; Kim 2018; Kim and Hepner 2019; Kim et al. 2020; Komakech 2018a, 2018b; Tuller 2018) and will sustain our future work for some time to come. Here, however, we wish to focus on the basis of our present argument and a central finding of our work thus far: that forensic anthropology remains inherently situated within cultural webs of meaning; and that the discovery and navigation of these requires a particular kind of integrated approach among the subdisciplines of anthropology, and between anthropology and local knowledge systems and cultural contexts. Moreover, an integrated approach reveals – and may help overcome – the binaries that have bedeviled forensic anthropology's theory and practice in human rights and transitional justice contexts, helping to achieve new growth and dialectical synthesis amid a range of productive tensions.

16.3 The integrated approach

What does it mean to articulate an "integrated approach" to forensic investigation? First and foremost, the approach emerges from its embeddedness in a grounded context, or the local cultural, cosmological, and conflict-related meanings of graves and human remains. For co-PI Kim (2018), the integrated approach presupposes several features that challenge binary assumptions. First and foremost, she identifies the tensions between "forensic" and "anthropology." That is, because of their empiricist foundations and often strict scientific and judicial imperatives, forensic investigations may exist in tension with the holism of anthropology, in which the "webs of meaning" (Geertz 1973) and "vernacular" (Merry 2006) dimensions of conflict, death, and redress are prioritized. Secondly, Kim highlights the persistent "forced dichotomy of medico-legal and humanitarian forensic intervention," arguing that "an integrated approach dismisses a dichotomy, instead requiring each investigative context to critically consider the cultural context within local realities" (Kim 2018:32–33). Describing the integrated approach as "informed by context-specific information, the presence of other interventions, and grave-related concerns" (2018:29), she notes that "forensic intervention often has unintended side effects due to its dissociation from the distinct, and sometimes antagonistic, needs of the different stakeholders; it is these side effects an integrated approach mitigates" (2018:34). Such mitigation is possible because "integrated forensic anthropology acknowledges that anthropological work functions in a wide array of historical, political, legal, humanitarian, government, and nongovernment realities" (2018:34) and "requires not just knowledge of forensic anthropology, but of post-conflict reconstruction, transitional justice, and context-specific cultural practices" (2018:35).

Kim's definition of an integrated approach to forensic anthropology emerges directly from our team's sustained ethnographic fieldwork and the rich, ongoing conversations we have held with one another, with colleagues, and with members of affected communities. It is also intrinsically linked to our methods and our major findings, which have themselves embodied a dialectical and iterative relationship in which the latter continually informs the development of the former, and vice versa. For instance, one of our early emergent findings was that the right to know the fate of missing or deceased loved ones, which is a principal concern in forensic humanitarianism and forensic humanitarian action, is neither foregrounded for survivors nor separated from their other pressing concerns about unresolved graves (Kim 2018). Most of our interlocutors felt that they already knew quite well what happened to their loved ones: they witnessed the massacres and knew who occupied the mass graves in their environs; they knew if their loved ones had been abducted by rebels or otherwise disappeared that they were very likely dead, and they knew that many of their kin and community members who died in displacement camps were buried in those former camp locations. The chief problems people experienced related to these improper burials were emotional and spiritual unrest associated with the inability to conduct proper burial rituals or (re)locate the burials to the homestead on ancestral land, and the ways in which the presence of human remains and improper burials obstruct farming, building, and development.

While spiritual affliction and illnesses associated with the improperly buried and missing impacted people's psychosocial recovery, the desire to locate and recover remains largely rested on pragmatic and material concerns. The need to remove remains and the need to preserve an accurate memory of the location of graves dominated what survivors defined as "the right to know." Moreover, we also found that meaningful "justice" that encompassed both living and dead was largely defined by survivors in similarly material ways: even if forgiveness, reconciliation, and cosmological repair were important to many people, far more pressing was whether they could utilize their land or receive material compensation for losses of life and livelihood from the government (Kim and Hepner 2019). Recognizing that "an integrated forensic anthropology response to local level needs, could intervene to address the economic impacts of these graves" (Kim 2018:42), our team directed our efforts toward novel forms of documentation utilizing forensic archaeological techniques. Beyond simply supporting survivors' oral narratives of atrocities and loss, this technique produced concrete documentation of improper burials in the form of site reports (maps, photos, and measurements) that were returned to survivors and filed with LCs. Whether useful for compensation claims, buttressing a factual account of events, or helping preserve the memory and location of graves that may one day be relocated for proper burial, these site reports reflect a different meaning of "evidence" than typically defined in medicolegal and humanitarian forensic approaches, one that emerges directly from the specific context of survivors' lived experience and universe of meaning (Elgerud and Kim 2020).

Thus, far, we have focused on exploring how our fieldwork, findings, and methods challenge prevailing assumptions and approaches in forensic investigation, and how our integrated approach makes productive use of tensions that pervade forensic human rights practice. Before we move to the next section to highlight an especially significant if undertheorized binary that our research raises to the fore – to excavate/not excavate – some further key findings deserve discussion. Indeed, these are especially significant to address because they illustrate how an integrated approach allows us to leave open the possibility that *not proceeding* with the forensic investigation is a valid conclusion to reach when considering the humanitarian dimensions of forensic practice. That is, the ethnographic and documentary work we have done, and its integration of culturally specific evidence and forms of knowledge into the very question of whether to excavate or not, allows for the possibility of *non-intervention* to emerge as the recommended course of forensic humanitarian action.

A closer look at several dimensions of Acholi culture, social organization, and cosmology – specifically, kinship and family, and cultural beliefs and practices around spirits of the dead and their physical remains – helps illustrate how we might arrive at non-intervention. As we elaborate in Kim et al. (2022), Acholi clan-based patrilineal kinship structures and patrilocal/virilocal residence patterns after marriage mean that family relationships and kinship terminologies do not easily match the biological relationships traceable through DNA. In an already complex terrain in which many people were killed and buried far from their natal villages and kin groups, using DNA reference samples from living people to identify excavated human remains in their areas, even if the interred population is a closed or known one, may yield low rates of positive biological identification. However, this reality intrinsically privileges the scientific and forensic definitions of kinship and identity, which do not adequately encompass the more meaningful social designations that prevail in Acholi society and family. Rather than suggesting that Acholi norms should conform to the needs and definitions of forensic science, we would ask in what ways can we adapt forensic science to these norms and render its specific limitations intelligible and acceptable vis-à-vis the priorities of survivors? If we cannot do so, then perhaps the existing scientific approach would ultimately run counter to the humanitarian "right to know" as defined by survivors in this context.

Relatedly, Acholi beliefs and practices about the spiritual and physical residue of the deceased trouble forensic science's particular approaches to human remains and a range of attendant assumptions about the importance of physicality, presence, reconciliation, and closure. That is, one of the primary ways that Acholi survivors have struggled with the aftermath of conflict is in terms of patterns of reconciliation that require known victims and perpetrators in order to reconcile wrongs and pay compensation. In a situation in which victims and perpetrators were closely entangled in families, communities, and sometimes even individuals (with a victim also being a perpetrator), unearthing remains draws to the fore a more urgent need to acknowledge responsibility and identify who deserves compensation and who should pay it. As research on postwar Northern Uganda has elaborated (Baines 2017), this dilemma wrought by the dynamics of war itself remains unresolved. Forensic intervention, however, would very likely exacerbate the need to address these issues anew, potentially aggravating their inherent unresolvability.

Moreover, other cultural and cosmological beliefs and practices help mitigate the problem of inchoate reconciliation among living and dead, and to some extent, allow survivors to cope with the presence of improper burials and missing loved ones in the absence of known remains or locations of remains. That is, while many survivors continue to suffer from dreams, visions, hallucinations, and even illnesses and misfortune that they attribute to the spirits of unhappy, improperly buried dead, they have also turned to ceremonial practices in which the spirits of the dead may be summoned and symbolically "buried" (Kembel 2015; Seebach 2016) to help put them, and their living kin, to rest. Similarly, local ritual specialists (known as *adjwaki*) have culturally specific techniques for "determining" the identity of unknown remains. Although participants in our research readily discussed how these options are indeterminate and can be unsatisfying for proper burial of known physical remains, many people have turned to these cultural practices as a valuable and meaningful resource. To insist that a forensic intervention would achieve "better" results and closure, is therefore insensitive at best, especially because we do not actually know how successful forensic intervention would be in locating and positively identifying remains for repatriation and reburial in Northern Uganda.[3]

Finally, and more broadly, any exhumation and reburials of the deceased or similar handling of human remains (e.g. surface scatter) would likely require extensive rituals involving possible combinations of animal sacrifice, ritual cleansings using blood and cud, and the participation of indigenous ritual specialists, Anglican, Catholic, or other religious denominational leaders, clan chiefs and elders, and/or government officials. Such mobilizations are both significant and likely expensive entailments to plan, fund, and negotiate. Moreover, given the diversity and complexity of cultural and religious syncretisms in Acholi, differences among survivor communities and families obtain when it comes to the ritual aspects of exhumation and reburial. As in critiques of international and especially Western-dominated human rights and transitional justice approaches that implicitly or explicitly conceive of local culture as an "obstacle" to the more straightforward and "culture-free" objectives of positivist science, evidence, and "universal" norms and values (Merry 2003, 2006), failing to work through and with local cultural patterns and disagreements about them, could produce far greater harms and problems than non-intervention.[4]

While the above does not exhaust the range of considerations and complexities associated with improper burials, restless spirits, and human remains in Acholiland, some key findings that emerge from our integrated approach and ethnographically grounded methodology illustrate how phenomena that may appear irrelevant or even contradictory to forensic science and intervention, in fact may dramatically shape its meaning, practice, and implications, even its definitions of success or failure. In addition to pushing us to reconsider the theory and practice of forensic science itself, especially when deployed for humanitarian aims, these findings also raise a more pressing and primary question, one conditioned by an as-yet almost entirely unspoken binary: *to excavate or not to excavate?* In other words, what if the main finding of our investigation into the potential role of forensic science in postwar Uganda is that an intervention should not occur at all?

16.4 To excavate or not to excavate?

While the dichotomies discussed above have largely been interrogated with great reflection, the decision to excavate or not excavate has not risen to the same level of conscious inquiry in forensic human rights work. Of course, a mass grave must be exhumed, as the logic goes – we must know who lies within the grave and who is responsible for the deaths. To suggest otherwise would seem brutally cruel to the families missing loved ones and subvert justice as well. We wonder about the origin of this seemingly unanimous, reflexive posture related to graves of atrocity. Perhaps it can be traced to the human rights excavations in the Balkans in the 1990s, the largest-scale forensic human rights investigation to date.

The Balkans became a training ground for forensic anthropologists inspired by the Equipo Argentino de Antropología Forense (EAAF), who began excavating mass graves of desaparecidos (victims of the Junta regime who were killed and "disappeared") throughout Argentina in the 1980s. Under the tutelage of Dr. Clyde Snow, their detailed research, excavations, identifications, and testimony in war crimes trials resulted in the conviction of the three past presidents and ushered in this entirely new application of forensic anthropology and archaeology (Snow et al. 1984; Joyce and Stover 1991). With Argentina as the litmus test, archaeological exhumations of mass graves became an invaluable forensic tool that could galvanize the investigations of the atrocities in the Balkans. Thus, the International Criminal Tribunal for the former Yugoslavia (ICTY) was also motivated by the work of the EAAF as they hired dozens of anthropologists and archaeologists directly and also contracted Physicians for Human Rights, EAAF, and other organizations to help conduct excavations and document evidence of the number of graves and the approximate number and ethnicities of the victims (Cordner and Tidball-Binz 2017; Steadman and Haglund 2005; Stover and Ryan 2001).

One of the primary goals of the ICTY was to document the scale of the atrocities and demonstrate criminal activity for prosecutions, so orders were given for teams to locate and excavate, or partially excavate, as many graves as possible, conduct autopsies to assess the cause and manner of death, and determine basic demographic characteristics of the deceased (ICTY 1996; Jugo and Škulj 2015). Identifications, however, were not included in the exhumation protocols and were of lesser priority for some time until other organizations, including the International Committee of the Red Cross (ICRC) and the International Commission of Missing Persons (ICMP) were developed to meet this humanitarian need (Cordner and Tidball-Binz 2017; Hanson et al. 2016; Wagner 2015). Accordingly, how to handle the recovered bodies pre- and post-identifications was not well organized, and bodies were often stored in less than ideal circumstances (Sprogøe-Jakobsen et al. 2001). Artifacts recovered on or with the bodies, including documents, jewelry, clothing, and even ballistic evidence, served the ICTY as markers of ethnicity, but personal effects were also used for identification (Jugo 2017; Komar and Lathrop 2008). Simultaneously, the same excavation-centric approach (in contrast to victim-centered) was occurring (though on a smaller scale) under the auspices of the International Criminal Tribunal – Rwanda (ICTR) across the Rwandan landscape where nearly one million people were killed in just a three-month span during a massive genocide in 1994.

Families of the dead in both Rwanda and the former Yugoslavia had little input concerning if and how the identifications were made or the manner in which deceased family members were returned. Sarah Wagner (2008) has documented the pervasive mistrust families held of the ICTY process, which sometimes led to the dismissal of DNA evidence of identification. Perhaps the culture of expectation that every grave must be excavated and counted, and the frenetic pace in which excavations occurred, created an institutional mindset that ultimately overvalued the collective number of dead and undervalued the victims as individuals. It follows, then, that families and communities were excluded from the relevant decision-making processes. In Rwanda, memorials and public ossuaries were quickly erected as attempts to pacify the survivors, while quelling ethnic and political tensions; yet surviving family members were rarely consulted on the disposition of their recovered loved ones (Korman 2017).

Given a large number of exhumations across multiple continents in the 1990s, guidelines and protocols were established for forensic human rights investigations to standardize archaeological and anthropological approaches to mass grave exhumations and ensure proper evidence handling (Skinner et al. 2003; Haglund et al. 2001), including the "Minnesota Protocol" first written in 1991 and updated in 2016 (United Nations 1991, 2016). Emerging from these standards is a linear methodological process with limited room for "stakeholder" input (Figure 16.4). This process is viewed as objective as it is evidence-based with

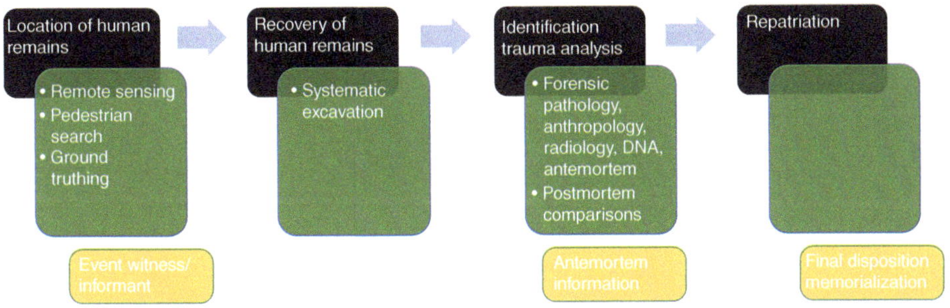

Figure 16.4 Simplified diagram of traditional tasks (black) and roles (green) of forensic scientists in humanitarian/human rights investigations. Yellow boxes are traditional areas of family/stakeholder input.

little room for "subjective" input of other stakeholders other than to help find graves or collect antemortem data or familial DNA (Ferllini 2007; Schmitt 2002; Cordner and McKelvie 2002). An integrated approach, however (see Figure 16.5), includes community input at each level, creating a mutually informed and dialectical rather than extractive relationship. An integrated approach does not necessitate that everything is negotiable; rather, it accepts the realities of contradictions and creates a path toward mutual understanding of the shared process and desired outcomes of any forensic intervention. As Rosenblatt (2015:156) states, the aspiration is to find "productive ways for forensic scientists and mourners to work together without sharing all of the same assumptions." How, then, can we evolve this process to retain the forensic integrity yet also integrate issues beyond "final disposition" input? Can engaging *a priori* and deeply with the complexities of cultural, political, and cosmological contexts actually inform and improve the forensic process? We think it can.

For example, forensic scientists may not believe that the spirits of the dead affect the living, and Acholi may not believe that the DNA "black box" can tell them where their loved one lies, yet both can be true. Importantly, an integrated approach remains evidence-based (assuming remains are found and can be analyzed) yet the context of that evidence (e.g. disturbed graves, DNA-relevant kinships) can be greatly enhanced with ethnographic data. Moreover,

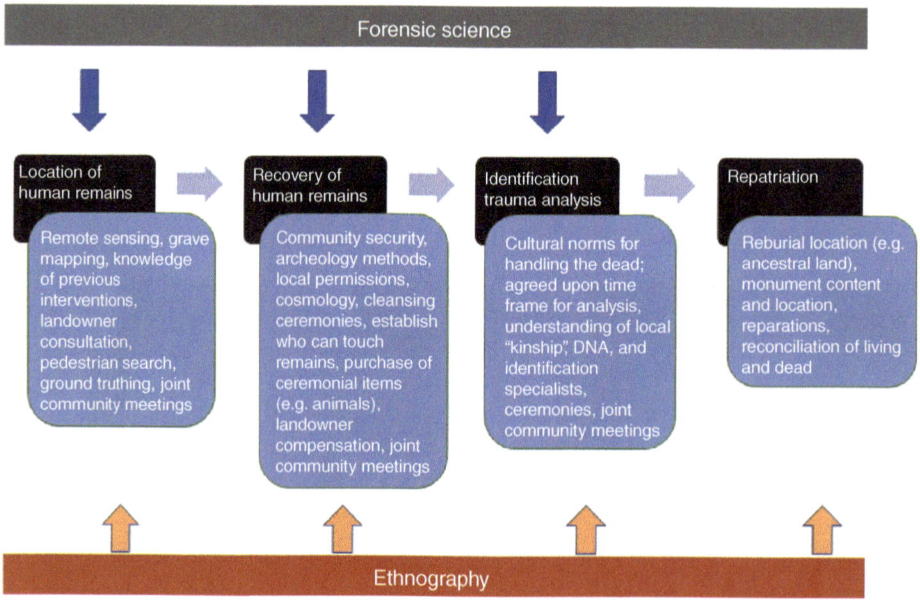

Figure 16.5 Simplified example of an integrated approach (blue boxes) deeply informed by ethnography.

situating ethnography before and during forensic intervention elevates the goal of partnership building and shared strategies (rather than the low bar of gaining "buy-in" of the forensic process by the community). Trust-building can only be produced through long-term rapport with communities. In the case of Acholi, the inclusion of rituals and ceremonies may require non-forensic resources (e.g. animals to sacrifice) and additional time and complexity, yet these neither alter the integrity of the site nor the evidence therein. Kim et al. (2021) provide specific examples whereby integration can be operationalized in seemingly disparate contexts of Northern Uganda, Cyprus, Somaliland, and Canada. Finally, the forensic footprint at the termination of an intervention can exceed the outcomes of identification and reburial and can aspire to include memorialization, improving community infrastructure (e.g. road building, water access), and contributing to local forensic capacity building (Kim et al. 2021).

While ethnography can (minimally) inform the forensic process, it is just as important that ethnographic work may reveal that the best course of humanitarian action is to not excavate. If culturally-specific and -defined parameters of integration cannot be met, such as lack of collective will, deprioritization of excavations compared to other transitional justice processes, lack of consent for familial DNA collection or unclear kinship relations, unresolvable contradictions, or lack of harmonization with spiritual beliefs, insecurity, or denial of permission by land owners, then the best course of action is to not excavate. Another mitigating factor might include tension about the time period for which remains are available for analysis (e.g. community or religious custom allows only three days of analysis before reburial, which may be untenable for forensic analysis). Some of the parameters revealed from a decade of steady ethnographic work in Acholiland may be translatable to other cultures (Kim et al. 2021), but there is no substitute for ethnography to prepare for victim-centered forensic interventions (or not). Our team agrees that if the Acholi communities/families do not wish to participate in each step of this process for any reason then the most humanitarian decision is to not disturb the graves and the spirits or take the risk of re-traumatizing the families.

To date, no excavations have begun in Acholiland. While our team has conducted nearly 200 individual or group interviews (Kim et al. 2020), many challenges require joint resolution before graves are excavated. For instance, many people wish for a non-forensic outcome to the excavations, whereby remains are simply to be moved off of private land without any strong desire to identify them, in which case there is no need for forensic involvement. Even if identification is desired, the dispersion of unknown remains across the vast landscape and displacement of victims before they were killed, means large-scale DNA databases will be required, integrating a greater number of scientific components, as well as state and private agencies. Further, some research participants feel that the grave maps are sufficient "evidence" for potential reparations from the government without excavation and/or may help define how ceremonies can be conducted that quell spiritual disturbances. Thus, our current working assessment is that excavating Acholi graves is not the right step at this time for the specific communities we have studied. However, this conclusion remains open-ended until we have the opportunity to more thoroughly share and discuss our findings with participants.[5] We recognize that as their needs and priorities and the national TJ policy continue to evolve, the decision to excavate, or not to excavate, may also change. Clearly, the binary posed by "excavate/not excavate" is itself not fixed or static; it retains a productive tension responsive to changing conditions, needs, and our ongoing engagement with survivors.

16.5 Conclusion: from binary to dialectical relationships

Rooted in her research and advocacy with Tzeltal communities in Chiapas, Mexico as they reconstructed their indigenous identity in an effort to secure autonomy under international human rights law, Speed (2006) observed how the tension between cultural relativism and universalism that long bedeviled anthropological human rights work had reached a stalemate. The dichotomous relationship posed between relativism/universalism, or culture/rights more broadly, she argued, impedes our ability to act on human rights issues and to fully grasp their meaning to people on the ground. She posed what she called "critically engaged activist research" as a method by which anthropologists unite cultural analysis with human rights action in an iterative fashion to move from binary to dialectical approaches. In this way, researchers and communities together work through messy and often contradictory phenomena, allowing persistent tensions to productively inform – and transform – both knowledge and application, processes, and outcomes.

The integrated approach we have developed through the course of our work in Northern Uganda described extensively in this chapter, relies on a similarly iterative process, undergirded by the recognition that forensic science, like human rights, cannot truly be separated from the cultural and political contexts in which it is deployed. Local conditions on the ground, from land and livelihood to kinship and cosmology, inherently shape how forensic science is apprehended by surviving communities and the multifarious implications it may have. Just as culture has often been viewed in the legal positivist tradition as an "obstacle" to realizing human rights norms and laws, which are viewed (erroneously) as "culture-free" (Merry 2003), forensic positivism may similarly view local specificities as inconvenient to a straightforward task of doing science.

Our work in Uganda demonstrates that working through dichotomies like humanitarian/judicial, science/culture, positivism/interpretivism, and even living/dead, to adopt a dialectical grasp of these relationships, produces more nuanced insights as well as greater sensitivity and humility. While this has consequently led us to the conclusion and argument that "to not excavate" may be the most humanitarian course of action in some situations, even the excavate/not excavate binary may be overcome by thinking about the many different kinds of contributions forensic anthropology can make beyond digging graves and identifying remains. From capturing intangible forms of evidence (Elgerud and Kim 2020) to stimulating deeper discussions about the meanings of justice and possible modes of redress (Hepner and Mekonnen 2022), forensic approaches can both contribute to, and catalyze, novel approaches informed by and yet exceeding a narrow scientific or medicolegal mandate. The humanitarian capacities of forensic action become more salient when imbricated with ethnographic methods, co-conceptualized in relationship to local cultural and political contexts, and receptive to forms of evidence that may be non-forensic or non-scientific. For example, mapping atrocity sites or displacement camp graves and delivering site reports to survivor communities to use for memorialization or compensation, for protection or relocation of graves from development projects, to adjudicate land disputes, and/or to retain records for future excavation and reburial of remains, illustrates how forensic science's applications become more expansive, and more responsive, in dialog with both cultural anthropology and cultural contexts.

While forensic humanitarianism and forensic humanitarian action have come a long way in better orienting forensic science toward the needs and interests of survivors, they have not yet fully integrated the power of ethnographic knowledge, methods, and contemporary theories of culture. Moreover, the prevailing definitions of "forensic intervention" continue to presuppose the imperative to excavate graves and identify remains. Our contribution to this rich and exciting conversation has focused on demonstrating that an integrated approach, one that works productively with and through the persistent binaries bedeviling forensic science in anthropological human rights contexts to arrive at a more dialectical synthesis, and which leaves open the possibility that refraining from excavation may be the most humanitarian course of action, holds considerable promise for the present and future of forensic humanitarian theory and method.

Acknowledgments

We are grateful for financial support from the following agencies and institutions: Wenner-Gren Foundation for Anthropological Fieldwork (Grant #9075), National Institutes of Health NIHMD – MHIRT Program (Grant #T37-MD001378), American Academy of Forensic Sciences-Humanitarian and Human Rights Resource Center (AAFS-HHRRC), National Institute of Justice, School for Advanced Research – NSF Team Seminars, University of Tennessee, University of Findlay, Arizona State University – School of Social and Behavioral Sciences.

Notes

1. In addition to Hepner and Steadman, the team includes Jaymelee Kim, Hugh Tuller, and Julia Hanebrink as core members. Lucia Elgerud, Deo Komakech, Wilfred Komakech, Godfrey Okot, Jeffrey Opiyo, Joshua Oballim, Jr., and others have contributed extensively.
2. A huge literature exists detailing the causes and impacts of the LRA civil war and post-conflict transitional justice, including by Ugandan research and advocacy organizations. Readers are especially directed to the Field Notes by Justice and Reconciliation Project, and the Refugee Law Project's National Memory and Peace Documentation Center. Some key works include Allen and Vlassenroot (2010), Baines (2007, 2010, 2017), Behrend (1999), Branch (2011, 2014), Dolan (2009), Finnström (2008), to name a few.
3. In instances where ritual identifications and/or symbolic burials have occurred but spiritual disturbances persisted, survivors often noted the likely "failure" of the ritual. Ritual failures can happen for a variety of reasons, including incorrect identification of the remains using spiritual divining methods. When discussing such instances, survivors were keen to understand the relative potential for failure using forensic scientific methods. This provided an opportunity to realistically discuss with them the potential and reasons for scientific failures.
4. At the same time, however, "local" cultural norms and practices are always actively being remade and leveraged for various purposes. Branch (2014) details how an inordinate emphasis on "ethnojustice" in Acholi has reinforced patriarchal power and deflected attention from the need for justice at higher levels of state accountability. In other contexts, such as societies in which conflict has generated large disaporic or exiled populations, formulating frameworks for justice and accountability require transnational approaches that blur distinctions between local, national, and international (Hepner and Mekonnen 2022). The theorization of culture as open-ended, flexible, and subject to internal power struggles is important to avoid fetishizing the "local" (Merry 2003).
5. During a recent research team seminar funded by the National Science Foundation and held at the School for Advanced Research in Santa Fe, New Mexico, team members and collaborating partners discussed a dissemination plan for participant communities and the Ugandan public that includes a visual traveling pop-up exhibit, radio interviews, and the performance of songs and skits to convey our findings and

to engage communities in discussion of next steps. Due to the COVID-19 pandemic, our ability to return to the field and to implement the dissemination plan has been delayed considerably.

References

Allen, T. and Vlassenroot, K. (eds.) (2010). *The Lord's Resistance Army: Myth and Reality*. London: Zed Books.

Baines, E.K. (2007). The haunting of alice: Local approaches to justice and reconciliation in northern Uganda. *International Journal of Transitional Justice* **1**(1): 91–114.

Baines, E.K. (2010). Spirits and social reconstruction after mass violence: Rethinking transitional justice. *African Affairs* **109**(436): 409–430.

Baines, E.K. (2017). *Buried in the Heart: Complex Victimhood and the War in Northern Uganda*. Cambridge: Cambridge University Press.

Behrend, H. (1999). Power to heal, power to kill. Spirit possession and war in northern Uganda (1986–1994). In: *Spirit Possession, Modernity, and Power in Africa* (eds. H. Behrend and U. Luig), 20–33. Madison, WI: University of Wisconsin Press.

Branch, A. (2011). *Displacing Human Rights: War and Intervention in Northern Uganda*. Cambridge: Cambridge University Press.

Branch, A. (2014). The violence of peace: Ethnojustice in northern Uganda. *Development and Change* **45**(3): 608–630.

Cordner, S.M. and McKelvie, H. (2002). Developing standards in international forensic work to identify missing persons. *Revue Internationale de la Croix-Rouge/International Review of the Red Cross* **84**: 867–884.

Cordner, S. and Tidball-Binz, M. (2017). Humanitarian forensic action: Its origins and future. *Forensic Science International* **279**: 65–71.

Dolan, C. (2009). *Social Torture: The Case of Northern Uganda, 1986-2006*. New York: Berghahn Books.

Elgerud, L.M.M.K. and Kim, J.J. (2020). Mapping the intangible: forensic human rights documentation in post-conflict Uganda. *The International Journal of Human Rights* **25**(1): 594–615.

Ferllini, R. (2007). *Forensic Archaeology and Human Right Violations*. Springfield, IL: Charles C. Thomas.

Ferrandiz, F. and Robben, A.C.G.M. (eds.) (2015). *Necropolitics: Mass Graves and Exhumations in the Age of Human Rights*. Philadelphia, PA: University of Pennsylvania Press.

Finnström, S. (2008). *Living With Bad Surroundings: War, History, and Everyday Moments in Northern Uganda*. Durham: Duke University Press.

Geertz, C. (1973). *The Interpretation of Cultures*. New York: Basic Books.

Haglund, W.D., Connor, M., and Scott, D. (2001). The archaeology of contemporary mass graves. *Historical Archaeology* **35**(1): 57–69.

Hanson, I., Holliday, M., Sullivan, K., Bomberger, K., et al. (2016). The International Commission on Missing Persons (ICMP) and the application of forensic archaeology and anthropology to identifying the missing. In: *Handbook of Forensic Anthropology and Archaeology*, 702–713: Routledge.

Hepner, T.R. (2020). On the boundaries of life and death: Notes on Eritrea and northern Uganda. *African Conflict and Peacebuilding Review* **10**(1): 127–142.

Hepner, T.R. and Mekonnen, D.R. (2022). "Justice futures": Forensic investigation and the potential for transformation in Eritrea. *Modern Africa: Politics, History and Society* **10**: 117–144.

Hepner, T.R., Wolfe Steadman, D., and Hanebrink, J.R. (2018). Sowing the dead: Massacres and the missing in northern Uganda. In: *Massacres: Bioarchaeological Interpretations of the Human Past: Local, Regional, and Global Perspectives* (eds. C.P. Anderson and D.L. Martin), 136–154. Gainesville, FL: University Press of Florida.

Jahn, I.R. (2016). Post-war development and camp-site graves: The politics of reburials in former Pabbo IDP Camp, Acholiland. *Journal of Peace and Security Studies* **2**(1): 33–44.

Jahn, I.R. and Wilhelm-Solomon, M. (2015). Bones in the wrong soil: Reburial, belonging, and disinterred cosmologies in post-conflict northern Uganda. *Critical African Studies* **7**(2): 182–201.

Joyce, C. and Stover, E. (1991). *Witnesses From the Grave: The Stories Bones Tell.* Boston, MA: Little, Brown and Company.

Jugo, A. (2017). Artefacts and personal effects from mass graves in Bosnia and Herzegovina. *Les Cahiers Sirice* **19**(2): 21–40.

Jugo, A. and Škulj, S. (2015). Ghosts of the past: The competing agendas of forensic work in identifying the missing across Bosnia and Herzegovina. *Human Remains and Violence: An Interdisciplinary Journal* **1**(1): 39. doi: 10.7227/HRV.1.1.4.

Justice and Reconciliation Project (JRP) (2011). The Lukodi Massacre: 19th May 2004. Justice and Reconciliation Project. http://justiceandreconciliation.com/wp-content/uploads/2011/04/JRP_FNXIII_Lukodi-Massacre.pdf (accessed 2021).

Kembel, A. (2015). *When the dead are not silent: The investigation of cultural perspectives concerning improper burials in northern Uganda.* Unpublished Master's thesis. Department of Anthropology, University of Tennessee.

Kim, J.J. (2018). An alternative approach to forensic anthropology: Findings from northern Uganda. *African Conflict and Peacebuilding* **8**(1): 29–53.

Kim, J. and Hepner, T.R. (2019). Of Justice and the Grave: The Role of the Dead in Post-conflict Uganda. International Criminal Law Review **19**(5): 819–843. doi: 10.1163/15718123-01905004.

Kim, J.J., Elgerud, L.M.M.K., and Tuller, H.H. (2020). Forensic archaeology and anthropology sensitization in post-conflict Uganda. *Forensic Science International* **306**: 1–9.

Kim, J.J., Baughman, J., Hanebrink, J.R., Tuller, H.H., and Emanvosky, P. (2021). Forensic biology capacity building: Challenges and opportunities in northern Uganda. Poster presentation. Humanitarian and Human Rights Resource Center.

Kim, J.J., Redeker Hepner, T., Tuller, H.H., Hanebrink, J.R., and Wolfe Steadman, D. (2022). Cultural relativity and the bounds of forensic interventions: A case study in Uganda. Poster presentation. Humanitarian and Human Rights Resource Center.

Komakech, O.D. (2018a). The mass grave scoping project: Remembering and recording memories of silenced massacres. A case in northern Uganda. *Practicing Anthropology* **40**(2): 11–13.

Komakech, W.L. (2018b). Internally displaced persons' burials in Pabbo Town Council in northern Uganda. Unpublished Master's Thesis. Department of Anthropology, University of Tennessee.

Komar, D.A. and Lathrop, S. (2008). The use of material culture to establish the ethnic identity of victims in genocide investigations: a validation study from the American Southwest. *Journal of Forensic Sciences* **53**(5): 1035–1039.

Korman, R. (2017). Bury or display?: The politics of exhumation in post-genocide Rwanda. In: *Human Remains and Identification*, 203–220: Manchester University Press.

Meinert, L. and Whyte, S.R. (2013). Creating the new times: Reburials after war in northern Uganda. In: *Taming Time, Timing Death: Social Technologies and Ritual* (eds. D.R. Christensen and R. Willerslev), 175–193. Abingdon: Ashgate Publishing Group.

Meinert, L., Willerslev, R., and Hooge Seebach, S. (2017). Cement, graves, and pillars in land disputes in northern Uganda. *African Studies Review* **60**(3): 37–67.

Merry, S.E. (2003). Human rights and the demonization of culture (and anthropology along the way). *Political and Legal Anthropology Review (PoLAR)* **26**(1): 55–76.

Merry, S.E. (2006). Transnational human rights and local activism: Mapping the middle. *American Anthropologist* **108**(1): 38–51.

Moon, C. (2016). Human rights, human remains: Forensic humanitarianism and the human rights of the dead. *International Social Science Journal* **65**(215–216): 49–63.

Mundorff, A. and Wagner, S. (2020). Immediacy and authority: Identification efforts in Bosnia and Herzegovina and the World Trade Center. In: *Silent Witness: Forensic DNA Evidence in Criminal Investigations and Humanitarian Disasters* (eds. H. Erlich, E. Stover, and T.J. White). Oxford: Oxford Scholarship Online. doi: 10.1093/oso/9780190909444.003.0013.

Neuner, F., Pfeiffer, A., Schauer-Kaiser, E., Odenwald, M., et al. (2012). Haunted by ghosts: Prevalence, predictors and outcomes of spirit possession experiences among former child soldiers and war-affected civilians in northern Uganda. *Social Science and Medicine* **75**: 548–554.

Parra, R.C., Zapico, S.C., and Ubelaker, D.H. (eds.) (2020). *Forensic Science and Humanitarian Action: Interacting with the Dead and the Living*. Hoboken, NJ: John Wiley and Sons.

Refugee Law Project (RLP) (2014). *Compendium of Conflicts in Uganda*. Kampala: Makerere University Faculty of Law.

Rosenblatt, A. (2015). *Digging for the Sisappeared: Forensic Science After Atrocity*. Stanford, CA: Stanford University Press.

Rosenblatt, A. (2019). The danger of a single story about forensic humanitarianism. *Journal of Forensic and Legal Medicine* **61**: 75–77.

Schmitt, S. (2002). Mass graves and the collection of forensic evidence: Genocide, war crimes, and crimes against humanity. In: *Advances in Forensic Taphonomy: Method, Theory, and Archaeological Perspectives* (eds. W.D. Haglund and M.H. Sorg). Boca Raton, FL: CRC Press.

Seebach, S.H. (2016). The dead are not dead: Intimate governance of transitions in Acholi. Ph.D. Dissertation. University of Aarhus.

Skinner, M., Alempijevic, D., and Djuric-Srejic, M. (2003). Guidelines for international forensic bio-archaeology monitors of mass grave exhumations. *Forensic Science International* **134**(2-3): 81–92.

Snow, C.C., Levine, L., Lukash, L., Tedeschi, L.G., et al. (1984). The investigation of the human remains of the "disappeared" in Argentina. *American Journal of Forensic Medicine and Pathology* **5**(4): 297–299.

Speed, S. (2006). At the crossroads of anthropology and human rights: Toward a critically engaged activist research. *American Anthropologist* **108**(1): 66–76.

Sprogøe-Jakobsen, S., Eriksson, A., Hougen, H.P., Knudsen, P.J., et al. (2001). Mobile autopsy teams in the investigation of war crimes in Kosovo 1999. *Journal of Forensic Science* **46**(6): 1392–1396.

Steadman, D.W. and Haglund, W.D. (2005). The scope of anthropological contributions to human rights investigations. *Journal of Forensic Science* **50**: 23–30.

Steadman, D. and Wagner, S. (2020). Taking stock: DNA testing and its complex truths. In: *Silent Witness: Forensic DNA Evidence in Criminal Investigations and Humanitarian Disasters* (eds. H. Erlich, E. Stover, and T.J. White). Oxford: Oxford Scholarship Online. doi: 10.1093/oso/9780190909444.003.0013.

Stover, E. and Ryan, M. (2001). Breaking bread with the dead. *Historical Archaeology* **35**: 7–25.

Tuller, H.H. (2018). Translating forensic science in northern Uganda. *Practicing Anthropology* **40**(2): 6–10.

United Nations (2016). The Minnesota Protocol on the Investigation of Potentially Unlawful Death. New York/Geneva: Office of the United Nations High Commissioner for Human Rights.

Victor, L. and Porter, H. (2017). Dirty things: Spiritual pollution and life after the Lord's Resistance Army. *Journal of Eastern African Studies* **11**(4): 590–608.

Wagner, S. (2008). *To Know Where He Lies: DNA Technology and the Search for Srebrenica's Missing*. Berkeley, CA: University of California Press.

Wagner, S. (2015). The quandaries of partial and commingled remains: Srebrenica's missing and Korean War casualties compared. In: *Necropolitics: Mass Graves and Exhumations in the Age of Human Rights* (eds. F. Ferrándiz and A. Robben). Philadelphia: University of Pennsylvania Press.

CHAPTER 17

Guiding principles for the dignified management of the dead in humanitarian emergencies and to prevent them from becoming missing persons

Stephen Cordner[1] and Morris Tidball-Binz[2]

[1]*Department of Forensic Medicine, Monash University, Melbourne, Australia*
[2]*UN Special Rapporteur on Extra-judicial, Summary or Arbitrary Executions, OHCHR-UNOG, Geneve, Switzerland*

17.1 Why the need for these principles?

The Guiding Principles for the dignified management of the dead in humanitarian emergencies and to prevent them from becoming missing persons were launched in 2021.[1] Since there is good existing technical guidance about the management of the dead following humanitarian emergencies, it is reasonable to ask: why do we need them? We have numerous recommendations made by international organizations over many years. These include (Conference Report 2019):

- United Nations (UN) *Manual on the Effective Prevention and Investigation of Extra-legal, Arbitrary and Summary Executions* (1991, revised in 2016)[2];
- International Committee of the Red Cross (ICRC) report *The Missing and Their Families* (2003);
- World Health Organization (WHO)/ICRC *Management of Dead Bodies after Disaster: A Field Manual for First Responders* (updated in 2016)[3];
- INTERPOL *Disaster Victim Identification (DVI) Guide* for experts in the field (updated in 2018)[4];
- Standards created by the Organization of Scientific Area Committees for Forensic Science (OSAC), part of the National Institute of Standards and Technology of the US Department of Commerce[5];

Anthropology of Violent Death: Theoretical Foundations for Forensic Humanitarian Action, First Edition. Edited by Roberto C. Parra and Douglas H. Ubelaker.

There are additional materials generated by the International Committee of Missing Persons, Justice Rapid Response, the UN Office on Drugs and Crimes, and the Disaster Mortuary Operational Response Teams, part of the US Department of Health and Human Services.

Surely we do not need more of the same. The answer is quite simple. These documents, including the WHO/ICRC Field Manual and the INTERPOL DVI Guide, do not explicitly address ***why*** it is important to manage the dead properly in these circumstances – it is assumed that all those involved, including decision makers, know this. Furthermore, despite the existence of the guidance, everyone involved in the response to humanitarian emergencies has experienced how poorly, generally speaking, the dead are managed (see Figure 17.1 for a common example). Aggravating this is the direct link between such poor management and failures to identify the dead.

All those involved in responding to humanitarian emergencies need to know that "management of the dead is a key component of the response. . . together with the search for, recovery and care of survivors, and the supply of basic services." This is part of the preamble to the Guiding Principles and is taken almost word for word from "Management of Dead Bodies after Disasters,"[6] a manual from the WHO/Pan American Health Organization (PAHO), International Committee of the Red Cross (ICRC), and the International Federation of Red Cross and Red Crescent Societies. The quote above is specifically endorsed at executive or director general level from those organizations. The main humanitarian response agencies

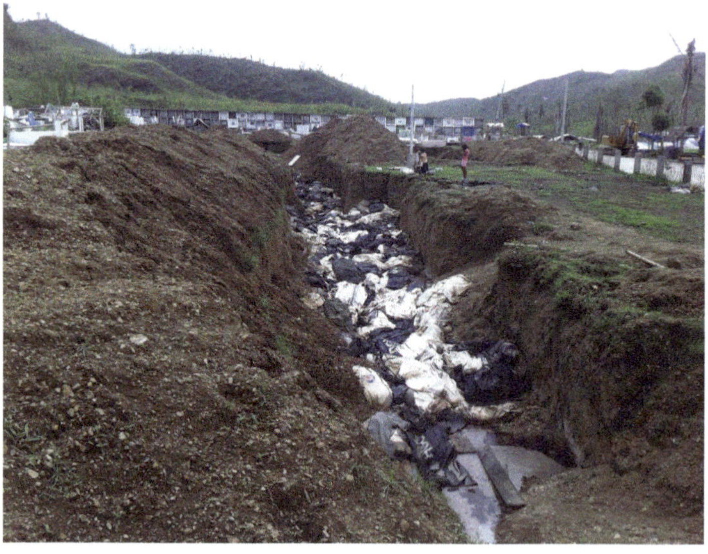

Figure 17.1 Bodies in body bags haphazardly disposed of by the authorities following a humanitarian emergency without a process in place for their identification.

worldwide explicitly state that managing the dead is one of three key components of responding to a humanitarian emergency. This priority is usually not reflected in responses on the ground by the authorities.

The substantial achievement of the principles is the direct link that is made between the dignified management of the dead and their identification. The link is made in a couple of ways. First, on a pragmatic basis. Mishandling bodies at the outset, by not giving them a unique identifying number, for example, will delay identification of that body, if not condemn that body to anonymity for ever. Such management prevents or unjustifiably delays identification and the guiding principles regards management resulting in that outcome as undignified. Second, as management of the dead extends to include interactions with their families and communities, failures there are also caught within this rubric. That is, failures to interact properly with families, including to obtain a list of the missing and antemortem information about them, aggravate the undignified management of the dead. This is not only because the failures disrespect the families but because they also complicate, unjustifiably delay, or render impossible the identification of the dead.

The direct link between dignified management of the dead and identification extends beyond the immediacy of the humanitarian disaster. It commences beforehand with planning and preparation and continues afterwards with the measures required to identify the dead as soon as feasibly possible. And the obligations identified by the Guiding Principles extend deep into the aftermath of the humanitarian emergency. Bodies that remain unidentified are not being managed in a dignified way unless steps are in place or are being taken to improve the prospects of their identification. This requirement stands in parallel to the pain and distress of the families and communities, waiting to know what happened to their missing loved one, which lasts for generations.

As important as individual identification is as an aim, there may be important variations to the priorities in different contexts. It cannot be put better than it was in the report of an early meeting that identified the need for the Principles:

> *International projects such as Below Ground: Mass Graves Exhumations and Human Rights in Historical, Transnational and Comparative Perspective hosted at the Spanish National Research Council (CSIC) examine the management or government of the dead – or necropolitics – in countries such as Spain, Argentina, Peru, Mexico, Poland, or Vietnam. In these contexts, experience has revealed strong points of tension between the forensic logic of individualization and community-oriented forms of collective body disposal. Additionally, these case studies have observed that popular representations of forensic science – the so-called "CSI effect" – have generated distorted visions of what forensic science can achieve in complex scenarios of humanitarian emergency. This has often created false expectations and produced feelings of disappointment in surviving relatives and local populations, with misguided perceptions of the forensic method.*

> *Nevertheless, according to some experts, considering forensic work in humanitarian emergencies requires attention to the tensions that emerge between law, science, and social, cultural, and religious dimensions connected to the treatment of the dead.*
> *Discussions led to the conclusion that the best way to address the deficiencies observed in the development of forensic practices in these concrete scenarios would be through the potential creation of a set of general principles. These should gather and recall, in a short and concise manner, the main norms and rules currently scattered and fragmented in the existing corpus of international humanitarian law, international human rights law, and forensic guides and manuals. This document should aim to reflect the spirit in which existing instruments and tools ought to be translated, applied, and implemented on the ground.*[7]

The Guiding Principles represent the outcome of work under the aegis of the ICRC to fill these gaps.

17.2 To whom are the guiding principles addressed?

The Guiding Principles are addressed to decision makers, managers, and practitioners involved in responding to humanitarian disasters. Effectively, this means they are addressed to all those dealing with the consequences of humanitarian emergencies resulting in fatalities. It is poor planning, organization, and decision making that has bedeviled the management of the dead in humanitarian emergencies. This has usually resulted from a lack of understanding and sensitivity to the consequences of such preparation and those decisions. Thus, the Guiding Principles are particularly relevant for high-level decision makers. But even if they make the right decisions, competent planning needs to have preceded the emergency to enable an effective response. Thus, the Guiding Principles should be compulsory reading for planners and those responsible for mitigating the effects of disasters, for example, Disaster Management Agencies.

It is the common experience of domestic forensic services that they are not consulted and are left out of disaster response planning. Planners are often focused on what they see as their priorities and often assume that someone else is responsible for planning in relation to the dead. The military authorities should be aware of these principles, since there is a considerable body of humanitarian and human rights law applicable to the military that underpins the Guiding Principles. Domestically, all levels of government, forensic services, police, fire, and other emergency services and non-governmental organization (NGO's) should have these principles brought to their attention as they are all usually involved in the response. Communities and bodies representing affected families will almost certainly become aware of the Guiding Principles in the aftermath of the humanitarian emergency, and the Guiding Principles will help them to understand what they can reasonably expect and what part they can play.

Internationally, regional organizations and NGOs as well as media outlets should be informed of these Guiding Principles.

17.3 Setting the scene

Each humanitarian emergency is unique, and the response is therefore logistically demanding as detailed requirements cannot be completely anticipated. Furthermore, local resources will inevitably be overwhelmed or as put in the Preamble to the Principles:

1. *humanitarian emergencies occur in socially, culturally, politically, and geographically diverse contexts as well as in the context of migration and result from events such as international and non-international armed conflict, other situations of violence, disasters, and epidemics*
2. *humanitarian emergencies often result in large numbers of dead persons who remain unidentified as a result of their improper or undignified management*

It is understandable that many people who have not participated in the response to disasters do not appreciate the complexities in the response. A little history might be of assistance in understanding the diversity and scale of some humanitarian disasters – their complexity (see Table 17.1).

There are a number of points emerging from this table. How dissimilar the contexts are – and taking just one difference as an example, the different nature of the humanitarian emergency has a massive impact on the response. Puerto and Tuller have set out the stark differences in response to a humanitarian emergency generated by a natural disaster to one generated by human rights violations (Salado Puerto and Tuller 2018; Table 17.2).

It does not take much imagination to see how the diversity, scale, and location – and thus the complexity – make each humanitarian emergency unique and thus the response correspondingly difficult. Puerto and Tuller further point out that the context-specific complexity and uniqueness is such that the responses to them cannot be "templated" for use in another context. In their view, the common misconceptions or missteps by experts responding to humanitarian emergencies are:

- Assuming that investigation practices are analogous to those of a mass disaster or a common domestic criminal case
- Ignoring the political, cultural, and religious aspects of the situation
- A lack of knowledge of local human variability (a technical anthropological misstep)
- Underestimating local forensic capability and overestimating their own
- Assuming that recovery and identification is always possible
- Thinking that the process should not be very arduous or long
- Managing expectations in an unrealistic manner.

Table 17.1 Humanitarian Emergencies: Diversity and Scale Equals Complexity.

Contexts	Former Yugoslavia	Tsunami (2004 Indian Ocean)	IRAQ (during Saddam regime)
Numbers of dead	140–250 000 dead[8,9] and 40 000 missing[10]	230–280 000[11,12] (including ~170 000 in Aceh)	~290 000 [13]
Geography	Numerous locations in multiple countries	Numerous locations in multiple countries	Numerous locations, one country
Time	Approx 10 yr (1990–1999)	Single event (December 26, 2004)	Approx 24 yr (1979–2003)
Circumstances	War/war crimes/crimes against humanity	Natural disaster	Crimes against humanity, murder
Civil society	Impaired	Intact – but impaired in Aceh	Destroyed
Resources	Significant (e.g. creation of ICMP[14])	Little for locals and many for internationals	Virtually none
Number identified	70% of the missing[15]	1841/2400 non-Thai deceased in Thailand.[16] Unknown total number of Thai (but 1168 id'd in the TTVI operation). Communal burials in Aceh. Unknown number in Sri Lanka.	Unknown number, but tiny

In any event, large numbers of highly experienced and knowledgeable experts with high levels of interpersonal skill will be needed in the implementation phases of properly planned responses. Of course, the availability of such people in large numbers usually does not exist, let alone at short notice, to respond to these sorts of events. This means that there will be heavy reliance on others who are inexperienced and with no special knowledge to populate the response. Many of these will be first responders.

The numbers in Table 17.1 are approximations, with considerable ranges (e.g. in Sri Lanka, the number ranges from 31[17] to >35 000[18]) (Yamada et al. 2006) and are not actual body counts or numbers based on comprehensive death certification systems. With the exception of the Great Japan Earthquake and Tsunami in 2011, where the number of deaths was based on the number of actual bodies plus confirmed reports of missing people, the authors are not aware of such precise counts following humanitarian emergencies, with the exception

Table 17.2. Response to a Humanitarian Emergency: A Natural Disaster Compared to Human Rights Violations.

Natural disaster	Human rights violations
• Full response from the affected state/country	• State often implicated and thus little support
• National and international pressure and resources to recover victims	• Investigations not initiated or supported or actively hindered
• Widespread solidarity with victims • Forensic initiatives resourced • Mechanisms implemented to care for victims and their families	• Investigations initiated years later – skeletal remains, ante mortem data, and biological reference samples more difficult to obtain
• Recovery of bodies not skeletons	• Bodies abandoned, buried in haste or destroyed
• Availability of recent ante mortem data	• Isolation of victims from their families and communities
• Immediate and long-term action by the press including disseminating information	• Limited resources • Distorted information in local or international press

of epidemics.[19] With a robust death certification system, one can at least count the number of people who have died in a particular period of interest and compare that with the average number of deaths for same period in the previous 5 years. For example, If there is a single major event, such as a pandemic, then a broad conclusion about the number of deaths in a particular period due to the pandemic can be made, relying of course on assumptions – or taking into account information – about the rates of other causes of death. There are other humanitarian emergencies where the range is much wider (e.g. the number of unlawful deaths under Saddam Hussein: the estimate in Table 17.1 from Human Rights Watch is the lowest; others extended the number to over one million). This single failure – any precision about the number of deaths – is itself disrespectful of those who died and should trigger real effort to discover more accurately the scale of the deaths in humanitarian emergencies.

At the other end of the scale, so to speak, is the figure provided by the UN Office of Disaster Risk Reduction for the deaths following Cyclone Nargis: 138 366.[20] It likely reflects the figure provided by the Myanmar authorities. This figure is provided without any evidence for how it was derived and without any indication that it is an estimate, highly likely to be substantially inaccurate – and masquerading as precision. As another example of the wide ranges in the number of deaths in humanitarian emergencies, the IFRC reports the numbers for

Cyclone Nargis as follows: 84 500 killed and 53 800 missing (which in total is very close to the UN estimate).[21]

So far, we have been considering natural disasters and human rights violations as the cause of the humanitarian emergency. The general knowledge of the number and scale of war (international armed conflicts) in the world at any one time is generally weak. Consider Table 17.3, which also shows the considerable uncertainty that exists about the number of deaths associated with them.

Consider also lower level and ongoing conflicts in:[27]

- Colombia
- Somalia
- Democratic Republic of the Congo
- Communal conflicts in Nigeria
- Insurgency in the Maghreb
- Darfur
- Islamic State insurgency in Iraq
- Mexican drug war
- Syrian civil war
- Ethnic violence in South Sudan
- Lower levels of ongoing conflict in India–Pakistan, Iran–Pakistan, Israel–Palestine, Papua–Philippines, Kurdish–Turk conflict, and many others.

Table 17.3 Active armed conflicts with >10 000 deaths in 2021 and 2022.

Country	Conflict	Date started/ deaths 2021	Cumulative deaths
Myanmar	Internal: Kachin; Karen; Rohingya; Rakhine State; protests and insurgency	1948/2000–10 997[22]	150 000–210 000
Afghanistan	Islamic State–Taliban; Panjshir	1978/36 000–42 222[23]	1.45–2.08 m
Yemen	Civil war; Al-Qaeda insurgency; Houthi–Saudi conflict; Saudi led intervention	2011/18 415[24]–310 000	377 000
Russo–Ukrainian war	Donbas; Russian Invasion	2014, 2022/8400–13 870; approx. 35 000[25]	
Tigray war	Spillover of the war; Ethiopian–Sudanese clashes	2020/8832[26]–19 200	

In addition, and finally, consider also some of the larger natural disasters from 2010 to the present:

Earthquake, Haiti, 2010: 316 000 dead and missing.
Pakistan floods, 2010: 2000 dead and missing
Great Japan Earthquake and Tsunami, 2011: 19 747 deaths
Typhoon Haiyan, Philippines, 2013: 9000–20 000 dead and missing
Ebola epidemic, West Africa, 2014: 11 308 deaths
Heat wave, India and Pakistan, 2015: 2500 deaths in each country
Earthquake, Nepal, 2015: 9000 dead and missing
Floods, India, 2019: 2000 dead
Cyclone Ida, Mozambique, 2019: >1200 dead
Mass deaths with migrations in Africa, the Middle East, Asia, Central and north America: >50 000 dead and missing.

We can proceed on the basis that most of the dead in *all* these humanitarian emergencies and the vast bulk of the dead in the majority of them, remain unidentified and are missing. With the exception of the Great Japan Earthquake (see footnote 19) and a couple of other smaller disasters,[28] the authors are not aware of publications that demonstrate effective identification of the majority of those who died in any of the above humanitarian emergencies. In the main, there was modest or ineffective state effort, and there remains little if any ongoing state effort, to find and identify those who died in these humanitarian emergencies.

The identification of 1841/2400 non-Thai deceased in Thailand following the Tsunami took extraordinary resources. To achieve this outcome, teams of forensic experts involving over 2000 people were rotated on three- to five-week missions over a 14 month period from the 31 of the 36 involved countries of Europe, North America, and the Asia Pacific region. The logistics were unprecedented, and the overall outcome was such that the INTERPOL evaluation concluded as follows: "The present thinking for a massive death toll situation is not fit for purpose in delivering our principles of forensic identification and the South East Asian Tsunami of 2004 tells us it is in urgent need of revision."[29] It was this experience that led the ICRC, PAHO, WHO, and the IFRC to collaborate on developing the manual on *The Management of Dead Bodies after Disasters* (see footnote 3).

The numbers of deaths signal the accompanying destruction and turmoil. For example, following the Tsunami, in Aceh alone, it was estimated that 500 000 people became homeless, about 800 km of coastline was destroyed, and more than 3000 hectares of land washed away or inundated with sea water.[30] At the time, there was a low-level insurrection in existence as the Acehnese were agitating for greater autonomy. In Sri Lanka, it was estimated that over 400 000 people were displaced, and direct losses were estimated at approx. US$1 billion.[31]

The above does not take into account the situation of probably hundreds of thousands of unidentified bodies passing through the world's mortuaries each year, a humanitarian emergency in its own right. Unfortunately, this remains an assertion as quantified data is simply not available.

17.4 The preamble to the Guiding Principles

Considering that:

1. *humanitarian emergencies occur in socially, culturally, politically, and geographically diverse contexts, as well as in the context of migration and result from events such as international and non-international armed conflict, other situations of violence, disasters, and epidemics*
2. *humanitarian emergencies often result in large numbers of dead persons who remain unidentified as a result of their improper or undignified management*
3. *management of the dead is a key component of the response to humanitarian emergencies, together with the search for, recovery, and care of survivors and the supply of basic services*
4. *respect due to a human being does not cease with death*
5. *for legal, religious, cultural, and other reasons, a human being's identity needs to be preserved after death*
6. *under international humanitarian law (*IHL*), families have the right to know the fate and whereabouts of relatives reported missing as a result of armed conflict, including victims of enforced disappearance. When persons go missing as a result of enforced disappearance, each victim, that is, the disappeared person and any individual who has suffered harm as the direct result of an enforced disappearance, has the right to know the truth regarding the circumstances of the enforced disappearance, the progress and results of the investigation, and the fate of the disappeared persons. In cases of gross human rights violations and serious violations of IHL, it is important that the truth about the facts surrounding such violations be made known to the victims and their relatives, and to the communities concerned, as appropriate. Forms of mourning and honoring the dead in accordance with their own religion, culture, and customs must be respected. Under international law, there are relevant obligations on the authorities, including to undertake action with regard to unidentified bodies*
7. *until identified, dead persons are likely to be missing persons whose fate and whereabouts remain unknown to their families and communities*
8. *all members of the human family possess inherent dignity and equal and inalienable rights, as recognized by the 1948 Universal Declaration of Human Rights*
9. *the authorities must respect, protect, and guarantee the dignity of the dead, including by preventing their mistreatment or despoliation, in accordance with international law, including IHL, international human rights law (*IHRL*), and international criminal law (*ICL*). International law obligations must be reflected under domestic law,*

the following principles, based on international obligations and internationally recognized standards, are relevant for all those addressing the consequences of humanitarian emergencies resulting in fatalities. Implementing these principles will help ensure the dignified management of the dead and help prevent them from becoming missing persons.

Nothing in these Guiding Principles shall be interpreted as restricting, modifying, or impairing the provisions of any international law instrument or the rules of customary international law or as derogating from the obligations of states and the rights of victims, including with regard to truth, justice, reparations, and guarantees of non-recurrence, in the aftermath of crimes under international law, including gross human rights violations or serious violations of IHL. Nothing in these Guiding Principles shall affect any rules that are more conducive to the identification and dignified management of the dead and which may be contained in domestic law or applicable international law.

The scale and contextual complexities of humanitarian emergencies as discussed are also a rehearsal of the first three statements of the Preamble. The legal and ethical responsibilities of states relating to management of the dead in these humanitarian emergencies, and the basis for those responsibilities, are set out in the remaining six preambular statements.

Preambular statement 4 of the Guiding Principles asserts that "respect due to a human being does not cease with death." There are no references provided with the Guiding Principles, but even if there were, there would be no reference for this assertion. It can be regarded as a basic humanitarian precept. By inference, states agree to this ethic when they sign up to the Geneva Conventions, which provide in some detail the protection of the dead following international armed conflict, for example.

Preambular statement 5 refers to: "for legal, religious, cultural, and other reasons, a human being's identity needs to be preserved after death." An authority for this is INTERPOL's 1996 General Assembly Resolution AGN/65/RES/13 recommending the adoption by all states of the Disaster Identification Forms "whenever appropriate and even in cases in which there is only one victim to be identified."[32] In that resolution, human beings are referred to as having a right not to lose their identities after death.

In preambular statement 6, the reader is reminded that "under international humanitarian law (IHL), families have the right to know the fate and whereabouts of relatives reported missing as a result of armed conflict, including victims of enforced disappearance."[33] Of course, the right to know the fate of such missing people includes knowing whether they are alive or dead, and if alive where they are, and if dead, how they died and where they are. The existence of this right imposes duties on the authorities. Identifying those who have died is an integral part of knowing the fate of those who are, until that point, considered missing; this is the point made in preambular 7.

In preambular 8, the reader is reminded that the Universal Declaration of Human Rights recognizes that all human beings possess inherent dignity and equal and inalienable rights. The final and ninth preambular statement reminds us that "the authorities must respect, protect and guarantee the dignity of the dead." There are obligations in this respect under IHL (Geneva Conventions)[34], IHRL,[35] and ICL[36], legal obligations that must be reflected under domestic law.

17.5 The Guiding Principles

> *I: For the purpose of these Guiding Principles, a humanitarian emergency includes its aftermath; a dead person includes all or any part of the deceased person's body, irrespective of the state of preservation; and identification is individualization by the attribution of the birth name or other appropriate name to a dead person.*
> *II: The dignity of the dead, their families, and communities should be respected at all stages and at all times: while searching for the dead; after they are found; during their recovery, analysis, and related documentation; during the storage of the remains, their return and the return of personal effects; and during the final disposition of the dead.*
> *III: Respecting the dignity of dead persons in humanitarian emergencies entails putting in place all feasible measures before, during, and in the aftermath of the events to ensure their identification as soon as possible. This enables their families, and communities as appropriate, to obtain information about their fate and whereabouts, contributes to reducing the number of persons unaccounted for, and facilitates their return for final burial or disposition.*
> *IV: Inappropriate handling of the dead and their belongings or inappropriate interactions with their families and communities, which can make identification of the dead impossible, more difficult, or unjustifiably prolonged, must be avoided, as this conduct is undignified and may be contrary to the law.*

These first principles set out the definitions and some of the scope of the dignified management of the dead in humanitarian emergencies to prevent them from becoming missing persons. Importantly, the humanitarian emergency includes its aftermath. From the point of view of the dignified management of the dead, important for its own sake but with the very practical outcome of preventing them from becoming missing persons, there is really no actual end to the humanitarian emergency. Perhaps it ends when all memory of the events has passed, but even then there are historical records. And even then, many communities revere the remains of their ancestors no matter how remote, and matters related to their management can provoke considerable upset.[37] An analogy might be Principle 7.1 in the UN Committee on Enforced Disappearances "Guiding Principles for the search for disappeared persons," where the section is headed: "The search is a continuing obligation." The principle itself states: "The search for a disappeared person should continue until his or her fate and/or whereabouts have been determined with certainty."[38]

Dignified management of the dead refers to dignified management not only of the whole body but also of any part of the body of a deceased person.

Identification, for the purposes of the Guiding Principles, is regarded as individualization by attributing the birth or other appropriate name to a dead person. There will of course be circumstances where this is neither possible nor perhaps even desirable, and the dead might be identified by reference to membership of a group or community of dead people, for example, because their remains were irretrievable and/or commingled.

The Guiding Principles apply at all stages and at all times in the process of managing the dead up to and including their final disposition – and beyond, when that management is still required to help prevent people from becoming missing persons.

Guiding Principle 3 is at the core of the document. All feasible measures must be put in place before, during, and after the humanitarian emergency to ensure the identification of the dead: this is what respecting the dignity of the dead entails. Without these measures, the dead have not been managed in a dignified way. The message for the authorities is as simple as that.

Guiding Principle 4 is the obverse of Principle 3: what makes "identification of the dead impossible, more difficult, or unjustifiably prolonged is undignified management of the dead." Thus, in Figure 17.1, it is not the visual impact (of unnumbered, unexamined, or unrecorded deceased) that renders the management of these dead undignified; it is the fact that such management renders their identification "impossible, more difficult, or unjustifiably prolonged" either in the near future or over the longer term.

> *V: The authorities must at all times respect the families, and communities as relevant, and actively encourage and enable their participation in the processes required to manage and identify the dead, including to ensure that their religious and cultural practices and beliefs regarding the handling and final disposition of dead persons are respected.*

Dignified management of the dead refers also to those who have suffered as a result of the death, including the families of the deceased.[39] In some circumstances this may extend to include a community. This is not simply the right thing to do; it is a necessary part of gaining their co-operation to maximize the dignified management of the dead, including their identification. Family, and sometimes community, will be the source of vital information (and sometimes relevant samples) to enable the identification of those who have died.

In the drafting of the guiding principles, note was taken of the view expressed in an expert meeting set out in its report as follows:

> *As a forensic community, cultural and religious aspects of managing the dead play, or should, a large part in our approach to managing the dead. But in humanitarian emergencies, one gets the sense that cultural and religious aspects are prone to misuse to justify disrespectful management to serve short term aims of dealing with the dead – often aggravated by the claim*

that the dead, if not buried immediately, will cause epidemics. . . . Or, sectarian aims are pursued through management of the dead rules which unnecessarily penalise minority groups in the community. Or management of the dead practices are pursued in the humanitarian emergency which further entrench powerlessness and disadvantage in the community at large.[40]

VI: The requirements for the dignified management and reliable identification of as many dead persons as possible will vary according to the size, context, and type of humanitarian emergency. Preparations, including a comprehensive strategy and planning, are needed to meet these requirements. Close communication and coordination are therefore necessary between all those agencies and stakeholders preparing, planning for, leading, managing, and delivering the responseas is constructive engagement with families and communities. The implementation of these plans should as far as feasible, be organized, coordinated, effective, and efficient.

VII: In particular, authorities must, irrespective of the imminence of humanitarian emergencies, adopt relevant domestic measures, including laws, policies, regulations, protocols, guidelines, and other national measures of a legal, institutional, and technical nature, including practical ones, to ensure respect for, and protection and guarantee of, the dignity of the dead. These measures must be in line with international law and should take into account these Guiding Principles and applicable best practices, including those recommended by the UN, the ICRC, the WHO, and Interpol.

VIII: All necessary information sources, such as registries and databases – including those containing data relevant to the identification of dead persons – must be gathered, managed, made available, accessed, used, and preserved with appropriate regard to data protection and in accordance with international law and internationally recognized standards.

IX: Forensic sciences and medico-legal systems play an increasingly important part in the dignified management of the dead, their reliable identification, and uncovering the cause and circumstances of their death. Thus, forensic experts and leadership from, wherever possible, the country or region in which the death occurred, should be involved in the planning for the dignified management of the dead and in the implementation of those plans in humanitarian emergencies.

X: A feature of humanitarian emergencies is that forensic experts may be in short supply or not able to access the areas in need. Thus, first responders are often relied on instead to recover, examine, document, and arrange storage of the dead in humanitarian emergencies. With appropriate training and guidance from forensic experts and if provided with the necessary resources and supervision, first responders should be relied upon to help protect the dignity of the dead and improve the chances of their identification.

Some aspects of planning were mentioned earlier in the chapter. Advance planning for the management of the dead in humanitarian emergencies is often weak, if undertaken at all. Such planning needs to encompass the main humanitarian disasters that could affect the jurisdiction and involve all necessary agencies and stakeholders. Too often, planning of the overall response omits consideration of the dead in any detail and too often makes insufficient use of advice and support from local or regional forensic experts. The outlines of an approach to planning for the management of the dead is included in the WHO/ICRC field manual management of dead bodies after disasters.[41] Implementation of the plans should be efficient and effective, as for example required under Guiding Principle 10 for the search for disappeared persons.[42] The standards set out in international law, and in the Guiding Principles, should be adopted in domestic law. All information sources that could be brought to bear to assist with identification, and thus dignified management of the dead, should be made available and utilized in accordance with applicable international law and standards.[43] The crucial importance of first responders in all stages of managing the dead following a humanitarian disaster and their need for rapid and appropriate training and guidance, including from forensic experts, must be recognized and included in planning and implementation. Proper use of first responders can contribute substantially to the dignified management of the dead, especially since local forensic experts (even with international support) will be quickly overwhelmed.

XI: The dignified management of the dead entails that they be treated without discrimination on any grounds and that they are not stigmatized. Thus, for example, acting on wrong claims that dead bodies cause epidemics should be avoided.

This principle precludes discrimination in the management of the dead on all grounds which apply to the living: race, sex, gender, age, nationality, disability, religion, culture, political affiliation, or other grounds of stigmatization, for example, wrong claims that the dead bodies cause epidemics. Dead bodies in humanitarian emergencies generally do not cause epidemics. The exception is when the deaths are due to infectious epidemics and the responsible organism is transmissible in a post-mortem setting (e.g. Ebola, Lassa fever, and cholera).[44] So, management of the dead, which involves a wrong claim that the dead will cause an epidemic, for example, as justification for rapid and mass burial without steps being taken to enable identification of the dead bodies then or later, is undignified management. This is so because the dead have been stigmatized, leading to management (e.g. hurried burial in communal graves) with the consequence that identification of the dead has been rendered impossible or delayed.

XII: Dead persons and their belongings should be searched for, recovered, examined, documented, and stored in compliance with international law and applicable best practice, using standardized procedures such as those recommended by the UN, ICRC, WHO, and Interpol. Examination, in particular, should be consistent with forensic best practice and the need for reliable identification of the deceased and should take into account cultural, religious, and community beliefs.

XIII: Families, and communities as appropriate, should be actively involved, consulted, and informed at all stages of the response to the humanitarian emergency. They are the source of essential information to identify their dead, including the names of those missing, their physical description, and biological samples that will assist in the identification process.

XIV: The active involvement of appropriately trained forensic experts in the interactions with relatives and communities should be encouraged. This is likely to help engender trust with families and communities, including to make the collection and provision of relevant information more effective.

XV: The availability of unique methods of identification, such as fingerprinting, DNA analysis, or dental examination, strengthens conclusions of identity, but such methods do not replace the need for an integrated identification process as recommended by Interpol and the ICRC, nor do they reduce the importance of any of the above principles or allow them to be bypassed.

Guiding Principle 12 is a succinct encapsulation of the standards that should be aimed for in the management of the dead in a humanitarian emergency. They are encapsulated in the technical and related guidance from the UN, WHO/ICRC, and from Interpol.[45] Effective implementation of anything less will not lead to significant numbers of identifications. The existence of this standard only emphasizes the need for competent planning followed by effective implementation. The need to take into account cultural, religious, and community beliefs leads logically to Guiding Principle 13 – to take these elements into account means that families and communities must be consulted. And the families have *essential* information without which identifications will not be made. This information can be as simple as, but excruciatingly painful, information that one or more family member is missing. This information is needed to become part of the list of those missing. Without a list of missing, there will be no identifications. With a list of missing, it becomes possible to seek further *essential* information about those individuals, mainly from families of the missing. At the same time or later, if the response is well organized, obtaining samples from family members also becomes a possibility. It is difficult to appreciate, but these simple principles, the need for a list of missing and its parallel requirement to consult with families, are not understood by many of those in decision-making positions during the response to humanitarian emergencies.

Approaching families and communities at these traumatic times is a task requiring planning, preparation, and skilled implementation. It is likely to complicate the management of the dead if it is regarded as a purely transactional matter of an administrative or law enforcement kind. Thus, Guiding Principle 14 urges the involvement of forensic experts experienced in interacting with families and communities in the preparation and implementation of this phase. Such involvement maximizes the chances of trust being developed, as those interacting with families will clearly know what they are talking about.

Guiding Principle 15 also addresses a very poorly understood complexity of the management of the dead following humanitarian emergencies. The ability of a body to be identified by a unique identifier, whether dactylography (fingerprints), dentition, or DNA, does *not* enable any short cuts to be made in the proper management of the dead following a humanitarian emergency. The bodies *must:*

- Each be given a unique body code
- Each be examined
- Each have the number and findings recorded (and these records stored so they can be tracked and accessed)
- Each be stored in such a way that they can be tracked and accessed.

As set out in the ICRC/PAHO/WHO field manual, "this process allows specific bodies with distinctive, potentially identifiable characteristics or findings, or whose DNA profile is later matched with the biological relative(s) of a missing person, to be retrieved for further examination; or return of the body to relatives; or enables placement of a memorial marker with the correct name if the body is, for example, buried and will not be moved."[46] The above management of the body allows a suitable sample for DNA profiling to be obtained from the body and properly labeled and thus properly linked to a body that is traceable. And it becomes even clearer now; if it was not clear enough before, that without a list of the missing, together with ante mortem information about them (and possibly, but not necessarily, biological samples), the above work on the bodies will be meaningless! It is immaterial which modality is to be relied upon for identification technically; all of these elements are minimum requirements and mandatory – for identification and thus the dignified management of the dead following a humanitarian emergency.

XVI: Psychosocial support for affected families and communities, as well as first responders and forensic personnel, is necessary and should be an integral part of the overall response to humanitarian emergencies, while acknowledging and respecting local resources to deal with trauma.

Support to affected families and communities, as well as workers helping to manage the dead, following a humanitarian emergency needs to be provided. Guiding Principle 16 refers to psychosocial support. There is at least one true statement that can be made about this: if bodies are managed in a dignified way, including to facilitate their earliest possible identification, the need for psychosocial support will be minimized. Families and communities will have been supported in a fundamental way by having their loved ones returned to them because their dignified management has enabled them to be identified. Workers will know that their arduous work was important and rewarded if its aims were met. If large numbers of bodies have to be managed simply for them to be buried in communal graves with no identifications and families still having to cope with all the uncertainties and consequences of their family member being missing, the psychosocial needs and demands will be substantial and on-going and can leave scars for generations.

Hofmeister and Navarro have conceived psychosocial action (which is significantly more than psychosocial support) and forensic work as complementary to each other in the aftermath of humanitarian emergencies. "For forensic investigations to be restorative – the ultimate humanitarian objective – there are certain additional conditions apart from those of scientific quality and ethics: respect, information, and coordination are among the main pillars for forensic action with a psychosocial approach, taking into account the need to treat on an individual and collective level the continuous psychological affectations caused by the disappearance of a loved one . . . . (Forensic and psychosocial sciences are working toward a common objective and) need to work in complementary and coordinated interaction for the benefit of the families and communities (Hofmeister and Navarro 2017). In the view of the authors, this idea has equal applicability to domestic settings as well as international ones.

> *XVII: If dead persons cannot be identified or returned to their families – for example, because the families cannot be identified or contacted – they should be documented, safely stored, or buried temporarily in a manner that facilitates their traceability, future identification, and return to families, or communities as appropriate. Cremation of unidentified and unclaimed bodies should therefore be avoided.*
> *XVIII: Dignified management of the dead includes guarantees of an honorable funeral and/or resting place that accords with family, cultural, and religious preferences. Resting places, including temporary burials and memorials, should be properly recorded, marked, maintained, and protected, and be accessible to the families and communities as appropriate.*
> *XIX: Final disposition of dead persons should be undertaken in a manner that respects their dignity and privacy and that of their family members and communities. Measures should be taken to protect funerary sites and monuments from desecration or disturbance and to maintain them.*
> *XX: Family members, and communities as appropriate, should be fully informed about and have full access to grave sites or places where the bodies of their dead have been laid to rest. The authorities should take all appropriate measures to return the remains and the belongings of the deceased under dignified conditions and in accordance with the wishes of the relatives. Where exhumations are needed, the procedures should be undertaken in compliance with applicable best practice and must be in line with international law. Family members, and communities as appropriate, should be given the opportunity and the necessary support from the authorities to re-bury or cremate the dead according to their own religious and cultural beliefs and practices.*

The fact that families of the deceased cannot be identified does not absolve authorities of the responsibility to manage the dead bodies so they can be traced and if necessary accessed to facilitate their possible future identification and return to their families.[47] It follows logically that unidentified and unclaimed bodies should not be cremated. For the final disposition of the dead to be dignified, family, cultural, and religious preferences need to be followed, and as mentioned above, this can happen only if there are communication channels with the families.

XXI: Where necessary, international cooperation, including forensic assistance, capacity-building, and training should be called upon by those concerned for the purpose of responding to humanitarian emergencies, to ensure the proper and dignified management, and identification of the dead, to prevent them becoming missing persons.

Following a humanitarian emergency, it is unlikely that the local or national authorities will have sufficient resources and capability to deal with all aspects of the management of the dead. This is particularly so with forensic expertise. Cooperation and assistance should be sought. Planned international arrangements lag behind the need for such cooperation and is an area that needs attention and development. Countries with considerable experience in responding to humanitarian emergencies (for example, Indonesia) may well be willing to respond to such requests (Cordner et al. 2011).

17.6 The process of producing the Guiding Principles

In 2018, the ICRC's Missing Persons Project and its Forensic Unit, together with the Right to Truth, Truth(s) through Rights (RTTR) Project (of the Swiss National Science Foundation and the Law Faculty of the University of Geneva), convened a meeting of experts to discuss the need to develop general recommendations on the dignified management of the dead in humanitarian emergencies.

Based on recommendations from that meeting,[48] and from a series of consultations held in 2019 – in Europe,[49] Africa,[50] the Middle East,[51] and Asia and the Pacific,[52] the Guiding Principles were drafted. In May 2020 there was a final round of online consultations, which included participants from the 2018 meeting. The guidelines were launched by the ICRC at the June 2021 meeting of the International Academy of Legal Medicine, held in Geneva. There would be some precedence, therefore, for the shorthand reference to the principles being called "The Geneva Principles."

17.7 Conclusions

The Guiding Principles on the dignified management of the dead in humanitarian emergencies are aimed at everyone involved, including decision makers, to prevent the dead from remaining what at that point they are: missing persons. They are missing because relatives do not know if they are dead or what has happened to them, unless and until they are identified. Their dignified management – which includes that of their families and communities – is necessary for this outcome.

The Guiding Principles do not define "dignified management" but *"connect the 'dignified' management of the dead to the particular social, familial, cultural, and religious demands that emerge in concrete situations of humanitarian emergency as well as to the need to negotiate these with existing ethical assumptions entertained in international forensic protocols and practice."*[53] This process will challenge established notions about the proper identification and burial of the dead where individualized versus collective forms of body disposal might be in tension.

What is not in dispute is the need for planning and preparation; that legal, institutional, and technical measures are required domestically; that forensic science and medicine have crucial contributions to make at all stages of the process; that with proper training and guidance, first responders can be relied upon to make indispensable contributions; that the dead must be managed without adverse distinction; the importance of best practices in search, recovery, examination, documentation, and storage of the dead; that integrating these together with active involvement of families and communities is the crucial approach; and the fact that fingerprints, dental examination, and DNA profiling are individually identifying does not replace the need for, or allow for short cuts in this integrated approach.

We now have an ethical, legal, and operational framework or outline for the dignified management of the dead in humanitarian emergencies which, if planned competently and implemented effectively will prevent the dead from becoming missing persons.

Notes

1. https://shop.icrc.org/guiding-principles-for-dignified-management-of-the-dead-in-humanitarian-emergencies-and-to-prevent-them-becoming-missing-persons-pdf-en.html
2. Office of the United Nations High Commissioner for Human Rights (2017).
3. WHO PAHO ICRC IFRCRCS (2016).
4. https://www.interpol.int/en/How-we-work/Forensics/Disaster-Victim-Identification-DVI
5. See OSAC, "OSAC Registry Approved Standards," https://www.nist.gov/organization-scientific-area-committees-forensic-science/osac-registry
6. See Footnote 4 above.
7. Conference Report (2019).
8. Transitional Justice in the former Yugoslavia (2009).
9. Modern conflicts database: Alternative Estimates for Death Tolls. Political Economy Research Institute. University of Massachusetts, Amherst. https://web.archive.org/web/20081011224313/http://www.peri.umass.edu/fileadmin/pdf/dpe/modern_conflicts/death_tolls.pdf

10. https://www.icmp.int/the-missing/
11. https://www.worldvision.org/disaster-relief-news-stories/2004-indian-ocean-earthquake-tsunami-facts
12. INTERPOL Tsunami Evaluation Working Group. The DVI Response to the South East Asian Tsunami between December 2004 and February 2006. https://www.interpol.int/es/content/download/588/file/INTERPOL%20Tsunami%20Evaluation%20Working%20Group.pdf
13. Human Rights Watch (2004).
14. International Commission on Missing Persons.
15. https://www.icmp.int/the-missing/
16. INTERPOL Tsunami Evaluation Working Group. The DVI Response to the South East Asian Tsunami between December 2004 and February 2006. P77. See Footnote 8 above.
17. Yamada et al. (2006).
18. Australian Department of Foreign Affairs. https://www.dfat.gov.au/news/news/Pages/indian-ocean-tsunami
19. Even in this disaster, numbers vary, in part explained by additional data available as time passes. Iino and Aoki (2016), refer to a death toll of 18 429 (with 15 892 bodies recovered and 2537 still missing). livescience.com/39110-japan-2011-earthquake-tsunami-facts.html updated in February 2022, refers to a death toll of 19 747 (which includes over 2500 still missing).
20. www.unisdr.org/files/8742_2008disastersinnumbersISDRCRED.pdf
21. www.ifrc.org/en/news-and-media/news-stories/asia-pacific/myanmar/myanmar-cyclone-nargis-2008-facts-and-figures/
22. Number of reported fatalities by country-year. Aggregated Data. Armed Conflict Location and Event Data Project: https://acleddata.com/curated-data-files/#aggregated
23. Number of reported fatalities by country-year. Aggregated Data. Armed Conflict Location and Event Data Project: https://acleddata.com/curated-data-files/#aggregated
24. Number of reported fatalities by country-year. Aggregated Data. Armed Conflict Location and Event Data Project: https://acleddata.com/curated-data-files/#aggregated
25. https://en.wikipedia.org/wiki/Casualties_of_the_Russo-Ukrainian_War#2022_Russian_invasion_of_Ukraine (as at April 23, 2022).
26. Number of reported fatalities by country-year. Aggregated Data. Armed Conflict Location and Event Data Project: https://acleddata.com/curated-data-files/#aggregated
27. https://en.wikipedia.org/wiki/List_of_ongoing_armed_conflicts
28. There were 442 deceased, mainly elderly holiday makers, following the Yangtze River Ferry disaster in 2015. All the dead were identified within 2 weeks. https://www.indiatoday.in/world/story/china-eastern-star-ship-capsized-yangtze-river-final-death-toll-442-257401-2015-06-13 In addition, there were 2753 dead in the Twin Towers outrage on September 11, 2001, with 1642 identified and 1111 still "missing" 17 years later. https://www.news.com.au/technology/science/in-a-new-york-lab-17-years-on-a-team-is-still-working-to-identify-911-victims/news-story/0b2b5f358d7eb6c300e48e491f45d9d1
29. INTERPOL Tsunami Evaluation Working Group. The DVI Response to the South East Asian Tsunami between December 2004 and February 2006. P150. See Footnote 9 above.
30. https://www.dfat.gov.au/news/news/Pages/indian-ocean-tsunami
31. Australian Department of Foreign Affairs. https://www.dfat.gov.au/news/news/Pages/indian-ocean-tsunami

32. 1996 ICPO-INTERPOL General Assembly, 65th Session, Resolution AGN/65/RES/13. https://www.legal-tools.org/doc/d6aa95/pdf/
33. Article 32 Additional Protocol 1, Geneva Conventions; International Convention for the Protection of All Persons from Enforced Disappearance, December 20, 2006, U.N.Doc. Res.A/Res/61/177, Art.24(2). https://treaties.un.org/doc/source/docs/A_RES_61_177-E.pdf
34. GCI Art 15 para. 1 and 16, para 4; GCII Art 18 para. 1 and 19 para 3; GCIII Art 122 para 9; GCIV Art art.16 para 2 and 139.
35. ICCPR Art 7; ECHR Art3; Arab Charter on Human Rights Art 8; American Convention on Human rights Art 5; African Charter on Humans and Peoples Rights Art 4,5.
36. See Footnote 57 in relation to the war crime of outrages upon personal dignity, in Elements of Crimes from the International Criminal Court. https://www.icc-cpi.int/sites/default/files/Publications/Elements-of-Crimes.pdf
37. https://www.smh.com.au/politics/nsw/aboriginal-elders-thankful-mungo-man-and-mungo-lady-will-finally-be-laid-to-rest-20220406-p5ab7d.html
38. https://documents-dds-ny.un.org/doc/UNDOC/GEN/G19/134/11/PDF/G1913411.pdf?OpenElement
39. See for example the UN Committee on Enforced Disappearances: Guiding principles for the search for disappeared persons, U.N. Doc. CED/C/7 sec. (2019). Principles 2.1, 2.3.
40. Conference Report (2019).
41. ICRC, PAHO/WHO, IFRCRC (2016). Annex 4: Mass Fatality Plan Checklist. P50–53.
42. U.N. Committee on Enforced Disappearances, *Guiding principles for the search for disappeared persons*, U.N. Doc. CED/C/7 sec. (2019), principle 10.
43. U.N. Committee on Enforced Disappearances, *Guiding principles for the search for disappeared persons*, U.N. Doc. CED/C/7 sec. (2019), principle 11.
44. ICRC, PAHO/WHO, IFRCRC (2016). Frequently asked questions. See questions 1, 2, 5, and 6. pp. 35–36.
45. ICRC, PAHO/WHO, IFRCRC (2016); INTERPOL (2018); Office of the United Nations High Commissioner for Human Rights (2017).
46. ICRC, PAHO/WHO, IFRCRC (2016). Annex 8. P60.
47. See also: Dealing with Mortal Remains. Section A.6 IASC Operational Guidelines on the protection of persons in situations of natural disasters. Inter-Agency Stanting Committee, January 2011. pp. 26–27. https://www.ohchr.org/sites/default/files/Documents/Issues/IDPersons/OperationalGuidelines_IDP.pdf
48. Conference Report (2019).
49. First International Symposium on Humanitarian Forensic Action (jointly organized by the International Committee of the Red Cross, the Faculty of Medicine at the University of Coimbra, The Portuguese Red Cross Society and the University's Center for Forensic Studies) Coimbra, November 28–30, 2019.
50. The annual meeting of the African Society of Forensic Medicine, Dar es Salaam, Tanzania. March 11–15, 2019.
51. 10th International Meeting of the Arab Union of Forensic and Toxicology. October 1–4, 2019.
52. Asia Pacific Medico Legal Agencies network meeting, Kuala Lumpur, Malaysia. April 22–24, 2019.
53. Conference Report (2019).

References

Conference Report (2019). The development of guiding principles for the proper management of the dead in humanitarian emergencies and help in preventing their becoming missing persons: First Experts' Meeting. *International Review of the Red Cross* **101**(912): 1213–1229. doi: 10.1017/S1816383120000223.

Cordner, S.M., Woodford, N., and Bassed, R. (2011). Forensic aspects of the 2009 Victorian Bushfires Disaster. *Forensic Science International* **205**(1): 2–7.

Hofmeister, U. and Navarro, S. (2017). A psychosocial approach in humanitarian forensic action. The Latin American perspective. *Forensic Science International* **280**: 35–43.

Human Rights Watch (2004). Iraq: State of the evidence. https://web.archive.org/web/20210520135506/https://www.hrw.org/report/2004/11/03/iraq-state-evidence#_ftn47 (last accessed 2 December, 2022).

ICTJ (2009). Transitional justice in the former Yugoslavia. https://www.ictj.org/publication/transitional-justice-former-yugoslavia (last accessed 2 December, 2022).

Iino, M. and Aoki, Y. (2016). The use of radiology in the Japanese tsunami DVI process. *Journal of Forensic Radiology and Imaging* **4**: 20–26.

INTERPOL (2018). Disaster victim identification (DVI) guide. Available at: https://www.interpol.int/en/How-we-work/Forensics/Disaster-Victim-Identification-DVI (last accessed 2 December, 2022).

Office of the United Nations High Commissioner for Human Rights (2017). *The Minnesota Protocol on the Investigation of Potentially Unlawful Deaths: The Revised United Nations Manual on the Effective Prevention and Investigation of Extra-Legal, Arbitrary and Summary Executions, UN Doc. HR/PUB/17/4.* (UN Doc. E/ST/CSDHA/.12, 1991). New York/Geneva: Office of the United Nations High Commissioner for Human Rights.

PAHO/WHO, ICRC, IFRCRC (2016). *Management of Dead Bodies after Disasters: A Field Manual for First Responders*, 2nd rev. e. PAHO, Washington, DC: https://www.icrc.org/en/doc/assets/files/other/icrc_002_0880.pdf.

Salado Puerto, M. and Tuller, H. (2018). Large scale investigations into the missing: Challenges and considerations. *Forensic Science International* **285**: 20–29.

Yamada, S., Gunatilake, R., Ruytman, T.M., Gunatilake, S., et al. (2006). The Sri Lanka tsunami experience. *Disaster Management and Response* **4**(2): 38–48 https://www.researchgate.net/publication/7198574_The_Sri_Lanka_Tsunami_Experience.

CHAPTER 18

Epilog: Anthropology of violent death and forensic humanitarian action

Douglas H. Ubelaker[1] and Roberto C. Parra[2,3,*]

[1]*Smithsonian Institution, National Museum of Natural History, Washington, DC, USA*
[2]*Technical Assistance Team. United Nations Joint Human Rights Office (UNJHRO). MONUSCO, Democratic Republic of Congo*
[3]*Unité mixte de recherche d'Anthropologie bio-culturelle, Droit, Éthique & Santé (UMR 7268 - ÁDES), Aix Marseille University, Marseille, France*
**The views expressed herein are those of the author and do not necessarily reflect the views of the United Nations.*

18.1 Humanity and its less violent reactions?

Contrary to the vision presented in *"The Better Angels of Our Nature"* by Steven Pinker (2011), who optimistically highlights that, over the centuries, humanity has progressively become less violent because we are more civilized. Richard Wrangham (2019), in *"The Goodness Paradox: The Strange Relationship Between Virtue and Violence in Human Evolution,"* shows us a different picture from the same evolutionary perspective as Pinker. In short, Wrangham argues that humans are increasingly docile and try to control our aggressive impulses (avoiding reactive aggression), but at the same time, we are so violent also that we have the ability to kill tens of thousands in just a few days (in the sense of proactive aggressiveness). The Rwandan genocide (1994), the atomic bombs in Hiroshima and Nagasaki (1945), and the murder of six million European Jews by the Nazi German regime (1933–1945), as well as a wide range of examples (Hobsbawm 2008; Valentino 2004; Fry 2013; Hinton and Irvin-Erickson 2014, among others) are just a few recent samples of our violent capacities in such civilized times.

Wrangham, states in his "Goodness Paradox" that chimpanzees and bonobos, which inhabit neighboring lands in the Congo and are genetically similar, are

Anthropology of Violent Death: Theoretical Foundations for Forensic Humanitarian Action, First Edition.
Edited by Roberto C. Parra and Douglas H. Ubelaker.

very useful examples of animals that not only share much of our DNA but also show emotions and behaviors similar to humans. While bonobos are relatively peaceful, chimpanzees have no qualms about killing members of their own society, including friends, lovers, and even children. This author argues that chimpanzees and bonobos demonstrate the violence and peace found coexisting in human behavior. Wrangham also offers answers about how bonobos and chimpanzees evolved so differently. For example, the violence of chimpanzees allowed them to compete with gorillas for natural resources, while bonobos lived in an area with abundant foliage and little competition. Because violent bonobos were not necessary for the evolution of the species, they became more domesticated as well as less violent. Following the principles of evolution, natural selection would favor a reduction of what Wrangham calls "reactive aggression," that is, "an immediate response to an imminent threat involving anger, fear, or both" (2019, p. 41).

This "domestication" would have evolved in response to the situation, not by another creature, while aggressiveness would have been a more useful attribute for chimpanzees who had to compete for resources. Some humans live competing for resources and some others do not, or at least do not compete necessarily on the same level. The sense in which humans are unique, Wrangham explains, is that we show a lower tendency to reactive aggression and a greater tendency to proactive aggression.[1] Thus, we have reached "civilized" levels of violence and destruction among ourselves.

Chapter 5 clearly illustrates how during ancestral societies, violent death was developed and intensified, including wars, capture and death of prisoners, and massacres of people. Certainly, archeology and history prove, among other topics, that human creativity is not only involved in discovering new modes of production, scientific knowledge, and technology development, but also in inventing new mechanisms of violence that can push us to subtle subjugation of other human beings, and if this does not work "civilized" to avoid conflict, we begin to justify violence at other levels. As Galtung (1996, p. viii) has pointed out in this regard, "*Conflict is much more than what meets the naked eye as 'trouble', direct violence. There is also the violence frozen into structures, and the culture that legitimizes violence.*" Certainly, culture multiplies the potential for violence through implicit and explicit meanings of symbols, which always remain there. Therefore, the only aspect that can be modified is the moment of aggression, the places where violence develops and its connotation, the technological effectiveness for kill, kill again and destroy, the social and political framework of the scenario, and the sense that seeks to legitimize it. Unlike ancient times, we now have the civilized capacity to cultivate an industry of violent death, where other humans die at the hands of other humans through genocides, massacres, and wars with thousands of deaths caused by bombs. Even humanity is constantly living under uncertainty of probable nuclear wars with total devastation as a consequence.

In "The Goodness Paradox," Wrangham covers an interesting number of facets, which conclussions are not necessarily according to our opinion. Nonetheless, his work provides us with some valuable science-based reminders about the human animal, our propensity to kill for "just causes or good causes" and a wide range of information that leads us to reflect on this gloomy and complex part of our human nature for the anxiety to kill, kill again, and destroy. The anthropology of violent death arises in this scenario.

18.2 Anthropology applied to forensic sciences and the notion of anthropology of violent death in the humanitarian context

18.2.1 The theoretical approach of forensic anthropology: beyond the classic empirical vision

The science supporting forensic anthropology enjoys a solid theoretical and methodological foundation derived from decades of research, experimentation, and casework. While this foundation is substantial and well-grounded in solid methods and theory, it is also dynamic and continually evolving. Each year, our journals present new methods and informative tests of old ones. However, forensic anthropologists have not been able to systematically recognize and evaluate the violence against the bodies and memories of the violated and their cultural meanings during fieldwork, nor have we been able to understand its roots, nor relate the micro-violences of everyday life with the structural forces of violence, broader and invisible, but symbolically powerful. Forensic anthropologists have concentrated on technifying our thoughts, but we have forgotten our social and cultural essence, we have classically declared ourselves as laboratory technicians for the evaluation of skeletons, their measurements, and their diversities, when the latter is not necessarily the fundamental objective of our role, but only one of the means to reach answers. In the contemporary world, forensic anthropology is much more complex, where there are not only "antiquated but also inadequate and inaccurate" considerations as Boyd and Boyd (2018) have clearly demonstrated in "*Forensic Anthropology: Theoretical framework and Scientific basis.*" The volume cited above is an excellent example for thinking and reflecting on the foundations of forensic anthropology:

> "We, therefore, recommend a more modern and realistic interpretation of forensic anthropological theory—one that, as we will see, is not hierarchical or static but based on three dynamic interacting *forms* of theory: foundational, interpretive, and methodological (Boyd and Boyd 2018, p. 6)."

Forensic anthropologists must move theoretically toward abstracting our thoughts from the connotation of the meanings of violence and the treatment of violated bodies by the actors of violence. The anthropology of violent death offers us an enormous field of knowledge foundational and a brilliant path for those who take on the challenge of following it. As forensic anthropology is an applied discipline of anthropology in general, the foundational theory is not only based on biological aspects but also on the social and cultural theory of our own knowledge. The biocultural approach, as argued by Zuckerman and Martin (2016), then becomes a powerful theoretical framework for forensic anthropologists to apply in any scenario where the contribution of modern forensic anthropology is required.

Global applications of forensic science introduce new problems seeking resolution. In growing numbers, forensic anthropologists become involved in international humanitarian action projects in diverse geographic areas and cultural contexts. Through all of this activity, contributions to humanitarian action have emerged as the core of a new subdiscipline of the field of forensic anthropology. This component of forensic anthropology not only contributes to the global judicial system but also to humanitarian and social issues. Involvement in global humanitarian action projects offers anthropologists an opportunity not only to apply their skills to help resolve contemporary world problems but also tremendous, enriching, cultural, and educational experiences that can be life-changing.

18.2.2 Anthropology of violent death and humanitarian action

The anthropology of violent death can be seen as a field of understanding that brings together diverse ways of understanding cultural visions and practices, which involve experiencing the suffering and misfortune of bloody events, as well as the intentional manipulation of bodies. The anthropology of violent death is closely linked to "bad death" and the implication of its meanings. As an example, Chapter 14 addresses the issue of bad death from a post-conflict Peru approach. However, the anthropology of violent death is not a novel approach, but it has always remained in parallel to the notion of the anthropology of death of Robert Hertz (1960), which is related to the "good death" and its cultural expressions. The anthropology of violent death is not only the contrasting of how people remember their dead from the normality of the cultural worldview and its processes of commemoration, but it is also the symbolic way in which the dead transmit their expressions violated and how they want the living to feel pressurized, which also include the meanings of those spaces where the dead are placed in a disrespectful way (negative deathscapes), which contain strong loads of meanings that alter the social, cultural, and even political landscape (Anstett 2018; Parra et al. 2022; Kwon 2006, 2008; Mueggler 2001). What happens when territories or landscapes are also places where mass death has occurred, where not necessarily another human killed another human? For example, during migratory crises, in situations of shipwrecks or long walks in deserts where people die due to suffocation, and their bodies are finally disappeared as a consequence of environmental aggression. These are important issues that must necessarily be included in the anthropology of violent death, where the missing bodies of these people were lost in the mist of large scenarios, such as the Mediterranean Ocean. This place, as well as others, concentrates hundreds of thousands of people there dead, which is understood paraphrasing Kovras and Robins (2016) as the *"wall separating Europe from Africa"* or as titled by Sheridan and McGuire (2020) in their edited work *"The border and its bodies: the embodiment of risk along the U.S-México line."*

This field of knowledge of anthropology has been preparing and developing for several years, but it has recently been made visible as a response to various episodes of human violence without limits, which leads to the particular violent treatment of the bodies, the disappearance of people and their impact on socio-cultural and political scenarios as explained by Elizabeth Anstett (Chapter 6) and Alfredo Gonzalez-Ruibal (Chapter 4). The anthropology of violent death as a field of reflection has its origins in the *École des Hautes Études en Sciences Sociales de Paris,* which took place from September 12–14, 2012, as part of the Annual Conference "Human Remains and Mass Violence" (www.corpsesofmassviolence.eu). Numerous publications have been developed since then, such as *"Destruction and Human Remains: Disposal and concealment in genocide and mass violence" (Anstett and Dreyfus 2014); "Human Remains and Identification: mass violence, genocide and the 'forensic turn'" (Anstett and Dreyfus 2015); "Human Remains and Mass Violence: Methodological approaches" (Dreyfus and Anstett 2015); "Governing the dead: Sovereignty and the politics of dead bodies"* (Stepputat 2014) among others. In addition, has been released a peer-reviewed publication called Human Remains and Violence: An Interdisciplinary Journal (www.manchesteruniversitypress.co.uk/journals/hrv/) that includes several approaches to academic research on dead bodies and the production of human remains in a massive way, whether in contexts of mass violence, genocide, or disasters.

Furthermore, we agree with Anstett and Dreyfus (2015) when they argue that:

> "These issues also address the emergence of the symbolic and legal status of corpses, a central point for all of the studies. They call for new anthropological studies of contemporary societies' relations with human remains in all their forms: whole or dismembered corpses, complete skeletons or single bones, tissues, organs, appendages, and finally ashes (Anstett and Dreyfus 2015, p. 6)."

The anthropology of violent death involves all of this, as well as the diverse cultural and political perspectives that lead to a diverse understanding regarding the treatment of the body, from approaches that for us may be unworthy, immoral, brutal, frightening, horrendous, and barbaric, but that for other cultural conceptions have diverse explanations from the performance of violence, as shown in Chapters 7 and 16. Situations that cannot necessarily be conceived as a strictly humanitarian need and its potential support to recover the body and dignify it from the forensic sciences, as explained in Chapter 9.

Moreover, we can mention some clearly manifest exceptions, as happens in African and mainly Asian societies, where the conception of posthumous dignity is not reduced to the materiality of that body, but rather to the tranquility and functionality of life beyond the material. Human groups that are often living in the core of armed conflict, organized crime, and violence without limits, are constantly creating and recreating cultural forms and mechanisms to cope and overcome the loss, along with the violent event, considering that after one violent event the next one to come might be with greater intensity. Normally, we think that professionals must indicate how to overcome these adversities when they themselves are demonstrating their own cultural mechanisms to respond to their frequent experiences. Catatumbo or Buenaventura in Colombia, Tegucigalpa or San Pedro Sula in Honduras, the Eastern region of Guatemala, and the Eastern region of DRC, among other places on the planet where human beings interact chronically with tragedy, extreme violence, death, and suffering are places where we must explore the ways in which those forms that lead to coexist anthropologically with violent death manifest themselves.

Parra et al. (2020) have described the case of Buenaventura on the Colombian Pacific coast, how a group of women who are known in that city as "mothers for life," managed to organize to fight against uncertainty, pain, to face the loss of a loved one, as well as to help other women who experience the same situation. In Buenaventura, one of the frequent characteristics of violence is the dismemberment of corpses. Even though sometimes these actions have been widely visible, the inhabitants of the port of Buenaventura know that when a person disappears, it is most likely that person has been dismembered, thrown into the sea, buried in specific areas, and even subjected to complex processes of liquefaction with chemical substances. *Mothers for life* know this situation, and they have developed practices adjusted to their reality that are known as the *"rituality of the absent body,"* which implies that *"There will be no bodies to bury, there will be no body to cry, there will be nobody to commemorate, but memories to dignify and pains to overcome."*

On the other hand, when the bodies are found, it does not necessarily mean that they must be recovered. Forensic works in the space of death and exhumations of dead bodies have brought innumerable political and cultural discussions as has been exposed in Chapters 7, 9, 13, 14, and 16. Unquestionably, there are moral standards of posthumous dignity that we must take into account to preserve the memory of our deceased, as discussed in Chapter 2 in "*The posthumous dignity of dead persons*" or in "*Battlefields and Killed in Action: Tombs of the Unknown Soldier and Commemoration*" presented in Chapter 10, and the important interactive reciprocity between the living and the dead as explained in Chapter 3; in addition to ethical values including among forensic scientists, to recognize the inclusion of diverse sociocultural contexts as shown in Chapter 15. As well as legal norms of protection and respect for the dead from international law (Londoño-Romanowsky and Silva-Chau 2020; Gaggioli 2018; Smolensky 2009) and Islamic norms, such as the considerations shown in Chapter 12 for humanitarian forensic action. Thus, important guides of good practices for the humanitarian work of forensic sciences in the face of death are explained in Chapters 11 and 17. However, according to Redeker-Hepner and Steadman (see Chapter 16), humanitarian work must also take into account that, "*While forensic humanitarianism and forensic humanitarian action have come a long way in better orienting forensic science toward the needs and interests of survivors, they have not yet fully integrated the power of ethnographic knowledge, methods, and contemporary theories of culture.*" Additionally, according to Antonius Robben in Chapter 8:

> "Forensic humanitarian work is conducted under the assumption that bereaved people need to conduct grief work to loosen the emotional tie to the dead and achieve closure, and that the relatives and friends of missing persons will be unable to mourn as long as they cannot bury their human remains. This chapter has argued instead that people may transform their relationships with the deceased or missing victims of political violence into enduring bonds. The ways in which people relate to the dead and the disappeared are culturally dependent. Ending the relationship is not a universal requirement for the bereaved's mental and physical health but only one of many forms of mourning" (see Chapter 8).

Anthropology plays a fundamental role in studying these differences and their potential similarities either to find points of balance that lead us to mechanisms of adequate humanitarian action as explained in all the chapters of this volume, or to look for ways that lead to solving a problem that more than humanitarian, can become a cultural and social problem for populations affected by violence. Not everything that seems to be humanitarian from our western conception is also for other ways of conceiving realities in other worlds (Fassin 2012). Forensic sciences can even disrupt and further damage what for a certain individual or communal views have been overcome. A greater discussion between the social sciences and the forensic sciences must be directed, and even a greater understanding with the legal sciences must be developed. For example, if there are no bodies to exhume/recover or bodies to analyze/examine, but geographical places to examine regarding the concentration of historical, including social anthropological information of the events of death or disappearance that happened in these particular deathscapes (Parra et al. 2022; Anstett and Dreyfus 2014). Anstett and Dreyfus (2014) have described the matter to us:

> "Legal scholars have concentrated on the charges relating to the destruction of bodies – and the legal status of the bodies themselves – with respect to both international criminal law and national legal systems. They also investigate the role played by corpses in the legal prosecution of perpetrators of mass violence, that is, as evidence of a crime; and when corpses are absent, legal issues arise regarding the status of the dead. Anthropologists, for their part, have addressed not only the question of how the destruction of bodies is integrated into the symbolic and social space of the societies in question but also that of the hierarchies present among these corpses and of the dead more generally. Anthropological studies of blood and body parts are of immense value for an understanding of the role of societies in the process of collective destruction (2014, p. 4)."

Humanitarian Reason by Didier Fassin (2012) formulates a very interesting question that contributes to the approach of the anthropology of violent death: Why do suffering and misfortune matter? If we suspend for a moment the clearly moral answer, which seems to be clearly obvious, the reasons why this question should matter and discuss its particularities confronts us with diverse thoughts and worldviews involving implications of its specific forms to manifest, in diverse cultures around the world. For Fassin, and for us too, the "humanitarian reason" is a cultural phenomenon in an anthropological sense, a phenomenon that must be interpreted and analyzed in terms of what it includes and excludes symbolically, and not so much in the legal sense of materiality. The nature of our thoughts is so complex, as explained by Changeux and Ricoeur (2000), that we constantly create and recreate mechanisms that, to a large extent, make us overcome extreme situations very much in spite of suffering and misfortune. Only those who survive can teach us to propose better mechanisms to face proactive aggressions and their consequences. Survivors have found specific ways to remember violence and reminisce their victims who died from that violence. Thus, their experiences could be a matter of further investigation. The anthropology of violent death becomes a meeting point to do so. It is not possible to adequately address humanitarian forensic action without this kind of knowledge.

Note

1. "Proactive violence is not immediately preceded by any equivalent arousal. There is no instantaneous threat to respond to. Proactive aggression is characterized by the presence of a deliberate plan and frequently by an absence of emotion at the time of the assault." (Wrangham 2019, p. 41)

References

Anstett, E. (2018). What is a mass grave? Toward an anthropology of human remains treatment in contemporary context of mass violence. In: *A Companion to the Anthropology of Death* (ed. A.C.G.M. Robben), 177–188. Chichester: John Wiley and Sons, Inc.

Anstett, É. and Dreyfus, J.-M. (eds.) (2014). *Destruction and Human Remains: Disposal and Concealment in Genocide and Mass Violence*. Oxford: Manchester University Press.

Anstett, É. and Dreyfus, J.-M. (eds.) (2015). *Human Remains and Identification: Mass Violence, Genocide, and the 'Forensic Turn'*. Oxford: Manchester University Press.

Boyd, C.C. and Boyd, D.C. (eds.) (2018). Forensic Anthropology: Theoretical Framework and Scientific Basic: John Wiley & Sons Ltd.

Changeux, J.-P. and Ricoeur, P. (2000). *What Makes Us Think. A Neuroscientist and a Philosopher Argue about Ethics, Human Nature, and the Brain*. Princeton, NJ: Princeton University Press.

Dreyfus, J.-M. and Anstett, É. (eds.) (2015). *Human Remains and Mass Violence: Methodological Approaches*. Oxford: Manchester University Press.

Fassin, D. (2012). *Humanitarian Reason. A Moral History of the Present*. Berkeley, CA: University of California Press.

Fry, D.P. (eds.) (2013). *War, Peace, and Human Nature: The Convergence of Evolutionary and Cultural Views*. Oxford: Oxford University Press.

Gaggioli, G. (2018). International humanitarian law: The legal framework for humanitarian forensic action. *Forensic Science International* **282**: 184–194.

Galtung, J. (1996). *Peace by Peaceful Meands: Peace and Conflict, Development and Civilization*. London: SAGE Publications Ltd.

Hertz, R. (1960). *A Contribution to the Study of the Collective Representation of Death and Right Hand*. London: Cohen and West.

Hinton, T.P. and Irvin-Erickson, D. (eds.) (2014). *Hidden Genocides: Power, Knowledge, Memory*. Ithaca, NY: Rutgers University Press.

Hobsbawm, E. (2008). War, peace and hegemony at the beginning of the twenty-first century. In: *War, Peace and Hegemony in a Globalized World: The Changing Balance of Power in the Twenty-First Century* (ed. C. Chari), 15–24. Oxon: Routledge.

Kovras, L. and Robins, S. (2016). Death as the border: Managing missing migrants and unidentified bodies at the EU's Mediterranean frontier. *Political Geography* **55**: 40–49.

Kwon, H. (2006). *After the Massacre: Commemoration and Consolation in Ha My and My Lai*. Berkeley, CA: University of California Press.

Kwon, H. (2008). *Ghosts of War in Vietnam*. Cambridge: Cambridge University Press.

Londoño-Romanowsky, X. and Silva-Chau, M. (2020). The protection of the missing and the dead under international law. In: *Forensic Science and Humanitarian Action: Interacting with the Dead and the Living* (eds. R.C. Parra, S.C. Zapico, and D.H. Ubelaker), 1 e, 25–34. Hoboken, NJ: John Wiley & Sons.

Mueggler, E. (2001). *The Age of Wild Ghosts: Memory, Violence, and Place in Southwest China*. Berkeley, CA: University of California Press.

Parra, R.C., Anstett, E., Perich, P., and Buikstra, J.E. (2020). Unidentified deceased persons: Social life, social death, and humanitarian action. In: *Forensic Science and Humanitarian Action: Interacting with the Dead and the Living* (eds. R.C. Parra, S.C. Zapico, and D.H. Ubelaker), 1 e, 79–99. Hoboken, NJ: John Wiley & Sons.

Parra, R.C., Vigo-Corea, D.M., Palma, M.R., Condori, L.A., et al. (2022). Anthropology as a humanitarian action in Peru: violent death and deathscapes out of place. *Human Organization, Society for Applied Anthropology* **81**(2): 180.

Pinker, S. (2011). *The Better Angels of Our Nature: Why Violence has Declined*. New York: Viking.
Sheridan, T.E. and McGuire, R.H. (eds.) (2020). *The Border and Its Bodies: The Embodiment of Risk Along the U.S.-México Line*. Tucson, AZ: University of Arizona Press.
Smolensky, K.R. (2009). Rights of the dead. *Hofstra Law Review* **37**(3): Article 4. https://scholarlycommons.law.hofstra.edu/hlr/vol37/iss3/4 (accessed 2022).
Stepputat, F. (eds.) (2014). *Governing the Dead: Sovereignty and the Politics of Dead Bodies*. Manchester: Manchester University Press.
Valentino, B.A. (2004). *Final Solutions: Mass Killing and Genocide in the Twentieth Century*. Ithaca, NY: Cornell University Press.
Wrangham, R. (2019). *The Goodness Paradox: The Strange Relationship Between Virtue and Violence in Human Evolution*: Penguin Random House, LLC, London, UK.
Zuckerman, M.K. and Martin, D.Ñ. (eds.) (2016). New Directions in Biocultural Anthropology. NYC: Wiley Blackwell.

Index

Anthropology of Violent Death: Theoretical Foundations for Forensic Humanitarian Action, First Edition.
Edited by Roberto C. Parra and Douglas H. Ubelaker.